2015 The Year Book of MEDICINE®

Editors

James A. Barker
Jennifer L. Barton
Kenneth R. DeVault
Renee Garrick
Michael R. Gold
Nancy M. Khardori
Colleen A. Lawton
Derek LeRoith

ELSEVIER
MOSBY

ELSEVIER
MOSBY

Vice President, Global Medical Reference: Mary E. Gatsch
Acquisitions Editor: Jessica McCool
Developmental Editor: Susan Showalter
Production Supervisor, Electronic Year Books: Donna M. Skelton
Electronic Article Manager: Mike Sheets
Illustrations and Permissions Coordinator: Dawn Vohsen

2015 EDITION

Composition by TNQ Books and Journals Pvt Ltd, India

Editorial Office:
Elsevier
Suite 1800
1600 John F. Kennedy Blvd
Philadelphia, PA 19103-2899

International Standard Serial Number: 0084-3873
International Standard Book Number: 978-0-323-35546-9

Editorial Board

Table of Contents

Journals Represented

Journals represented in this YEAR BOOK are listed below.

Alimentary Pharmacology & Therapeutics
American Journal of Gastroenterology
American Journal of Kidney Diseases
American Journal of Medicine
American Journal of Respiratory and Critical Care Medicine
Annals of Allergy, Asthma & Immunology
Annals of Internal Medicine
Annals of the American Thoracic Society
Annals of the Rheumatic Diseases
Annals of Vascular Surgery
Arthritis Care & Research
Arthritis & Rheumatology (Hoboken, N.J.)
Brachytherapy
British Medical Journal
CA: A Cancer Journal for Clinicians
Cancer
Chest
Circulation
Clinical Chemistry
Clinical Endocrinology
Clinical Gastroenterology and Hepatology
Clinical Infectious Diseases
Clinical Journal of the American Society of Nephrology
Clinical Pediatrics
Clinical Pharmacology & Therapeutics
Critical Care Medicine
Diabetes
Diabetes Care
Diabetes, Obesity & Metabolism
European Heart Journal
European Respiratory Journal
Gastroenterology
Gut
Intensive Care Medicine
International Journal of Radiation Oncology *Biology* Physics
Journal of Clinical Oncology
Journal of Infectious Diseases
Journal of the American Academy of Dermatology
Journal of the American College of Cardiology
Journal of the American Medical Association
Journal of the American Medical Association Ophthalmology
Journal of the American Society of Nephrology
JPEN Journal of Parenteral and Enteral Nutrition
Kidney International
Lancet
Lancet Oncology
Nature

New England Journal of Medicine
Oncology (Williston Park, N.Y.)
Otolaryngology-Head and Neck Surgery
Practical Radiation Oncology
Proceedings of the National Academy of Sciences of the United States of America
Public Library of Science One
Rheumatology International
Sleep
Thorax
Tuberculosis

Standard Abbreviations

The following terms are abbreviated in this edition: acquired immunodeficiency syndrome (AIDS), cardiopulmonary resuscitation (CPR), central nervous system (CNS), cerebrospinal fluid (CSF), computed tomography (CT), deoxyribonucleic acid (DNA), electrocardiography (ECG), health maintenance organization (HMO), human immunodeficiency virus (HIV), intensive care unit (ICU), intramuscular (IM), intravenous (IV), magnetic resonance (MR) imaging (MRI), ribonucleic acid (RNA), and ultrasound (US).

Note

The Year Book of Medicine is a literature survey service providing abstracts of articles published in the professional literature. Every effort is made to assure the accuracy of the information presented in these pages. Neither the editors nor the publisher of the Year Book of Medicine can be responsible for errors in the original materials. The editors' comments are their own opinions. Mention of specific products within this publication does not constitute endorsement.

To facilitate the use of the Year Book of Medicine as a reference tool, all illustrations and tables included in this publication are now identified as they appear in the original article. This change is meant to help the reader recognize that any illustration or table appearing in the Year Book of Medicine may be only one of many in the original article. For this reason, figure and table numbers will often appear to be out of sequence within the Year Book of Medicine.

PART ONE

RHEUMATOLOGY

JENNIFER L. BARTON, MD

1 Osteoarthritis

Use of a Validated Algorithm to Judge the Appropriateness of Total Knee Arthroplasty in the United States: A Multicenter Longitudinal Cohort Study

Riddle DL, Jiranek WA, Hayes CW (Virginia Commonwealth Univ, Richmond)
Arthritis Rheumatol 66:2134-2143, 2014

Objective.—In previous studies conducted outside the US, ~20% of total knee arthroplasty (TKA) surgeries were judged to be inappropriate. The present study was undertaken to determine the prevalence rates of TKA surgeries classified as appropriate, inconclusive, and inappropriate in a knee osteoarthritis population in the US.

Methods.—We used a modification of a validated appropriateness classification system and applied it to patients in the Osteoarthritis Initiative data set who underwent TKA. A variety of preoperative data were used in the classification, including Western Ontario and McMaster Universities Osteoarthritis Index pain and physical function scores, radiographic features, knee motion and laxity measures, and age.

Results.—Data on 205 patients who underwent TKA were examined. The prevalence rates for classification of the procedure as appropriate, inconclusive, and inappropriate were 44.0% (95% confidence interval [95% CI] 37–51%), 21.7% (95% CI 16–28%), and 34.3% (95% CI 27–41%), respectively.

Conclusion.—Approximately one-third of TKA surgeries were judged to be inappropriate. Variation in the characteristics of patients undergoing TKA was extensive. These data support the need for consensus development of criteria for patient selection among US practitioners treating patients who are potential candidates for TKA. Among the important issues, consensus development needs to address variation in patient characteristics and the relative importance of preoperative status and subsequent outcome.

► With a rise in obesity, a larger elderly population, and increased knee osteoarthritis (OA), total knee arthroplasties in the United States have skyrocketed. Knee replacements among adults who received Medicare between 1991 and 2010 increased by more than 160%. One potential reason for this steep rise is overutilization, or performing the procedure when it may not be indicated or appropriate. Riddle and colleagues set out to determine the prevalence of rates of total knee arthroplasty classified as "appropriate, inconclusive, and inappropriate" in an osteoarthritis population (the Osteoarthritis Initiative) using a validated classification system for appropriateness developed in Spain. The classification involved preoperative data such as a commonly used OA pain measure, function, radiologic features, knee motion and laxity, as well as age. Complete data were available for 175 of 205 patients who had a total knee arthroplasty at some point over a 5-year period. Of these 175 surgeries, 44% were deemed appropriate, with the majority of these patients having severe or intense symptoms and a high radiographic score. Classification was inconclusive for 38 of the 175 (21.7%), and although most of these patients had intense or severe symptoms before surgery, mobility was normal in up to two-thirds. In 60 of the 175 patients (34.3%), the total knee arthroplasty was classified as inappropriate. In this last group, symptoms were slight or moderate, or radiographic scores were not as severe. The authors point out that the percentage of patients classified as inappropriate was higher than anticipated. They highlight the need for consensus in the United States for total knee arthroplasty and that until consensus is established, significant variation in practice will continue. Involving patients in their care and informing them of the various modalities to treat OA will be critical moving forward. The goal of modern health care is to provide high-quality, patient-centered, and low-cost care that is appropriate based on evidence and consensus and that incorporates patient preference.

J. Barton, MD

Acupuncture for Chronic Knee Pain: A Randomized Clinical Trial

Hinman RS, McCrory P, Pirotta M, et al (Univ of Melbourne, Australia; et al)
JAMA 312:1313-1322, 2014

Importance.—There is debate about benefits of acupuncture for knee pain.

Objective.—To determine the efficacy of laser and needle acupuncture for chronic knee pain.

Design, Setting, and Participants.—Zelen-design clinical trial (randomization occurred before informed consent), in Victoria, Australia (February 2010-December 2012). Community volunteers (282 patients aged ≥50 years with chronic knee pain) were treated by family physician acupuncturists.

Interventions.—No acupuncture (control group, n = 71) and needle (n = 70), laser (n = 71), and sham laser (n = 70) acupuncture. Treatments were delivered for 12 weeks. Participants and acupuncturists were blinded to laser and sham laser acupuncture. Control participants were unaware of the trial.

Main Outcomes and Measures.—Primary outcomes were average knee pain (numeric rating scale, 0 [no pain] to 10 [worst pain possible]; minimal clinically important difference [MCID], 1.8 units) and physical function (Western Ontario and McMaster Universities Osteoarthritis Index, 0 [no difficulty] to 68 [extreme difficulty]; MCID, 6 units) at 12 weeks. Secondary outcomes included other pain and function measures, quality of life, global change, and 1-year follow-up. Analyses were by intention-to-treat using multiple imputation for missing outcome data.

Results.—At 12 weeks and 1 year, 26 (9%) and 50 (18%) participants were lost to follow-up, respectively. Analyses showed neither needle nor laser acupuncture significantly improved pain (mean difference; −0.4 units; 95% CI, −1.2 to 0.4, and −0.1; 95% CI, −0.9 to 0.7, respectively) or function (−1.7; 95% CI, −6.1 to 2.6, and 0.5; 95% CI, −3.4 to 4.4, respectively) compared with sham at 12 weeks. Compared with control, needle and laser acupuncture resulted in modest improvements in pain (−1.1; 95% CI, −1.8 to −0.4, and −0.8; 95% CI, −1.5 to −0.1, respectively) at 12 weeks, but not at 1 year. Needle acupuncture resulted in modest improvement in function compared with control at 12 weeks (−3.9; 95% CI, −7.7 to −0.2) but was not significantly different from sham (−1.7; 95% CI, −6.1 to 2.6) and was not maintained at 1 year. There were no differences for most secondary outcomes and no serious adverse events.

Conclusions and Relevance.—In patients older than 50 years with moderate or severe chronic knee pain, neither laser nor needle acupuncture conferred benefit over sham for pain or function. Our findings do not support acupuncture for these patients.

Trial Registration.—anzctr.org.au Identifier: ACTRN12609001001280

▶ People with arthritis often seek out nonpharmacologic approaches to managing pain. Chronic knee pain, most often from osteoarthritis, affects many people of age 50 and older. Acupuncture using needles has been shown to be effective in treating osteoarthritis pain; however, laser acupuncture (noninvasive use of low-intensity laser therapy) compared to needle acupuncture for knee osteoarthritis has not been studied. Hinman et al conducted a Zelen-design randomized clinical trial (participants consented to acupuncture after randomization) of adults aged > 50 years with knee pain > 30 days' duration in Australia. Participants were randomized to receive one of the following: laser acupuncture, sham acupuncture, needle acupuncture, or control (no acupuncture). Eight family physicians registered as acupuncturists delivered 20-minute treatments once or twice weekly for 12 weeks with 8 to 12 total sessions allowed. Primary outcomes were self-reported pain and function. Seventy patients were included in each of the 4 arms (71 in control and laser). At 12 weeks and 1 year, 9% and 18% were lost to follow-up, respectively. The authors report that neither needle nor laser acupuncture significantly improved pain or function compared with sham at 12 weeks. Compared with control, needle and laser acupuncture resulted in modest reduction in pain, but this did not hold up at the 1-year mark. Needle acupuncture showed some improvement in function compared with control at 12 weeks, but again this was not maintained at 1 year. There were no serious adverse events. This well-designed, negative study highlights that neither needle nor laser acupuncture is beneficial for adults over age 50 with moderate or severe knee pain.

J. Barton, MD

Effect of Weight Maintenance on Symptoms of Knee Osteoarthritis in Obese Patients: A Twelve-Month Randomized Controlled Trial

Christensen R, Henriksen M, Leeds AR, et al (Bispebjerg and Frederiksberg Hosp, The Capital Region of Copenhagen, Denmark; Univ of Copenhagen, Denmark; et al)

Arthritis Care Res (Hoboken) 67:640-650, 2015

Objective.—To compare results of obese patients with knee osteoarthritis (OA) who, after an intensive weight loss regimen, received 1 year of either dietary support (D), a knee-exercise program (E), or "no attention" (C; control group).

Methods.—We conducted a randomized, 2-phase, parallel-group trial. A total of 192 obese participants with knee OA were enrolled; the mean age was 62.5 years and 81% were women with a mean entry weight of 103.2 kg. In phase 1, all participants were randomly assigned to 1 of 3 groups and began a dietary regimen of 400–810 and 1,250 kcal/day for 16 weeks (2 8-week phases) to achieve a major weight loss. Phase 2 consisted of 52 weeks' maintenance in either group D, E, or C. Outcomes were changes from randomization in pain on a 100-mm visual analog scale, weight, and response according to the Outcome Measures in Rheumatology-Osteoarthritis Research Society International criteria.

Results.—Mean weight loss for phase 1 was 12.8 kg. After 1 year on maintenance therapy, the D group sustained a lower weight (11.0 kg, 95% confidence interval [95% CI] 9.0, 12.8 kg) than those in the E (6.2, 95% CI 4.4, 8.1 kg) and C (8.2, 95% CI 6.4, 10.1 kg) groups ($P = 0.002$ by analysis of covariance [ANCOVA]). Adherence was low in the E group. All groups had statistically significant pain reduction (D: 6.1; E: 5.6; and C: 5.5 mm) with no difference between groups ($P = 0.98$ by ANCOVA). In each group 32 (50%), 26 (41%), and 33 (52%) participants responded to treatment in the D, E, and C groups, respectively, with no statistically significant difference in the number of responders ($P = 0.41$).

Conclusion.—A significant weight reduction with a 1-year maintenance program improves knee OA symptoms irrespective of maintenance program (Fig 2).

▶ Obesity and osteoarthritis (OA) increase the risk of one in the presence of the other. Both go hand in hand. Interventions aimed at weight loss among patients with OA have been successful in improving function, with reductions as low as 5.1% of total body weight. What is unknown definitively is whether weight loss can affect the progression of OA. Christensen and colleagues in Denmark conducted a pragmatic randomized controlled trial with blinded outcome assessors to compare symptomatic outcomes of 3 different arms: 1) 1 year of continuous dietary support from a dietician (and use of "formula products" such as a shake or bar), 2) 1 year of specialized knee exercise program, or 3) a "no-attention" control group. Of note, all 3 groups first underwent a 16-week weight-loss program that enrolled obese knee OA patients. The initial 16-week program

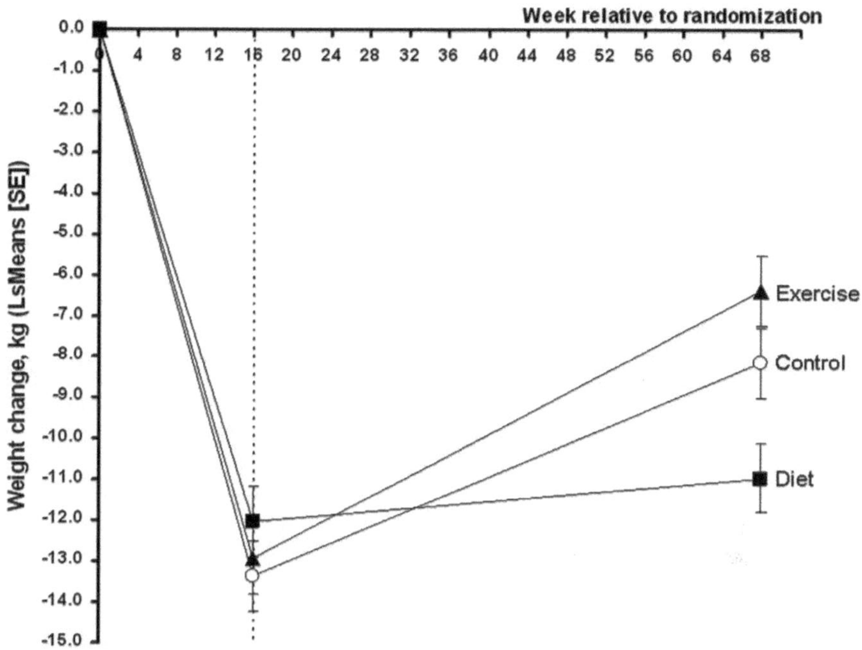

FIGURE 2.—Changes in body weight over time were explored using a repeated-measures analysis of covariance (via PROC MIXED): a factor for group, a factor for time, and a factor for the interaction between them. The outcome at baseline was applied as covariate. Values are least squares (LS) means and error bars indicate SE of the LS means. (Reprinted from Christensen R, Henriksen M, Leeds AR, et al. Effect of weight maintenance on symptoms of knee osteoarthritis in obese patients: a twelve-month randomized controlled trial. *Arthritis Care Res (Hoboken)*. 2015;67:640-650, with permission from American College of Rheumatology.)

resulted in significant weight loss and for those patients in the 1 year of continuous dietary support, they had the greatest amount of weight loss over 68 weeks (−11 kg, 95% confidence interval [CI] −12.8 to −9.1 kg; Fig 2). Weight change in the exercise group was −6.2 kg (95% CI −8.1 to −4.4 kg) and in the control group, −8.2 kg (95% CI −10.1 to −6.4 kg). In terms of participants who lost 10% or more of their body weight, the greatest percentage was in the dietary group (55%) compared with 27% in the exercise group and 31% in the control. It should be noted that attendance in the weekly dietary group was high (32 of a possible 52 sessions attended, 61.5%) where the compliance with the exercise program was much lower (13.5%, or 7 sessions attended on average out of 52 possible). This highlights that there was poor fidelity to this intervention arm, making it difficult to conclude it was ineffective. Change in symptoms did not differ among the 3 groups at the 68-week mark, and there was reduction in pain. This study highlights the effectiveness of an ongoing dietary intervention among obese individuals with OA to lose and maintain weight loss, compared with an exercise intervention (although it was not well-adhered to). Challenges to translation to general practice include the expense of a "formula product" and sustaining weekly visits with a dietician. Although changes in body mass index and body composition occurred in the diet group, symptom outcomes of OA did not differ. The search for nonpharmacologic and nonsurgical interventions for OA patients continues, and the long-term effects of weight loss require further study.

J. Barton, MD

Circulating C reactive protein in osteoarthritis: a systematic review and meta-analysis

Jin X, Beguerie JR, Zhang W, et al (Univ of Tasmania, Hobart, Australia; Austral Univ Hosp, Buenos Aires, Argentina; Univ of Nottingham, UK; et al)

Ann Rheum Dis 74:703-710, 2015

Background.—There is emerging evidence that the development and progression of osteoarthritis (OA) is associated with inflammation. C reactive protein (CRP), a systemic marker for inflammation, may be elevated in OA patients but the evidence is conflicting.

Objective.—To systematically review the literature for the relationship between serum CRP levels measured by a high sensitivity method (high sensitive CRP (hs-CRP)) and OA, as well as the correlation between circulating CRP levels and OA phenotypes.

Methods.—MEDLINE, EMBASE and CINAHL databases were systematically searched from January 1992 to December 2012. Studies were included when they met the inclusion criteria and data from studies were extracted. Two independent reviewers assessed study quality using a modified Newcastle-Ottawa Quality Assessment Scale. Meta-analyses were performed to pool available data from included studies.

Results.—32 studies met the inclusion criteria. Serum hs-CRP levels in OA were modestly but statistically significantly higher than controls (mean difference = 1.19 mg/L, 95% CI 0.64 to 1.73, $p < 0.001$) with significant heterogeneity between studies. Levels were significantly associated with pain ($r = 0.14$, 95% CI 0.09 to 0.20, $p < 0.001$) and decreased physical function ($r = 0.25$, 95% CI 0.13 to 0.39, $p < 0.001$). No significant associations were found between hs-CRP levels and radiographic OA.

Conclusions.—Low-grade systemic inflammation may play a greater role in symptoms rather than radiographic changes in OA.

▶ Osteoarthritis (OA) has long been thought of as a noninflammatory arthropathy. However, recent studies have highlighted the potential role for local inflammation and inflammatory cytokines such as tumor necrosis factor alpha, interleukin-6, and others produced by synovium and chondrocytes in the pathogenesis. A common marker for inflammation is C-reactive protein (CRP) which is often elevated in active inflammatory arthritis such as rheumatoid arthritis. Studies of CRP levels in osteoarthritis have found mixed results, with some reporting an association with increased levels of CRP and OA and others no association (especially when adjusting for body mass index [BMI]). Jin and colleagues undertook a systematic review and meta-analysis to determine whether CRP levels are elevated in OA patients compared with controls and to determine whether levels of CRP correlated with the prevalence or progression of joint symptoms in OA (joint pain, stiffness, or poor function). A total of 32 studies identified between 1992 and 2012 met their inclusion criteria. Serum CRP levels in OA were modestly elevated compared with healthy controls (mean difference of 1.19 mg/L; $P < .001$). A significant heterogeneity between studies led the authors to conduct subgroup and sensitivity analyses. CRP levels were higher in hip OA compared with knee; controlling for BMI did not change the increase in CRP in OA, but CRP was not associated with progression of OA. In analyses that examined association of CRP with pain or loss of physical function, there was a statistically significant correlation. The findings of this systematic review and meta-analysis indicate that low-grade inflammation may play a role in the symptoms of OA but not in the radiographic progression.

J. Barton, MD

2 Osteoporosis and Other Metabolic Diseases of Bone

Romosozumab in Postmenopausal Women with Low Bone Mineral Density

McClung MR, Grauer A, Boonen S, et al (Oregon Osteoporosis Ctr, Portland; Amgen, Thousand Oaks, CA; Leuven Univ, Belgium; et al)

N Engl J Med 370:412-420, 2014

Background.—Sclerostin is an osteocyte-derived inhibitor of osteoblast activity. The monoclonal antibody romosozumab binds to sclerostin and increases bone formation.

Methods.—In a phase 2, multicenter, international, randomized, placebo-controlled, parallel-group, eight-group study, we evaluated the efficacy and safety of romosozumab over a 12-month period in 419 postmenopausal women, 55 to 85 years of age, who had low bone mineral density (a T score of −2.0 or less at the lumbar spine, total hip, or femoral neck and −3.5 or more at each of the three sites). Participants were randomly assigned to receive subcutaneous romosozumab monthly (at a dose of 70 mg, 140 mg, or 210 mg) or every 3 months (140 mg or 210 mg), subcutaneous placebo, or an open-label active comparator — oral alendronate (70 mg weekly) or subcutaneous teriparatide (20 μg daily). The primary end point was the percentage change from baseline in bone mineral density at the lumbar spine at 12 months. Secondary end points included percentage changes in bone mineral density at other sites and in markers of bone turnover.

Results.—All dose levels of romosozumab were associated with significant increases in bone mineral density at the lumbar spine, including an increase of 11.3% with the 210-mg monthly dose, as compared with a decrease of 0.1% with placebo and increases of 4.1% with alendronate and 7.1% with teriparatide. Romosozumab was also associated with large increases in bone mineral density at the total hip and femoral neck, as well as transitory increases in bone-formation markers and sustained decreases in a bone-resorption marker. Except for mild, generally nonrecurring injection-site reactions with romosozumab, adverse events were similar among groups.

Conclusions.—In postmenopausal women with low bone mass, romosozumab was associated with increased bone mineral density and bone formation and with decreased bone resorption. (Funded by Amgen and UCB Pharma; ClinicalTrials.gov number, NCT00896532.)

▶ Patients with rheumatic diseases are often at risk of fracture because of use corticosteroids and systemic inflammation. Antiresorptive therapy such as the bisphosphonates to treat osteoporosis has been found to increase bone density and decrease risk of fracture; however, mechanistically it does not lead to new bone formation. The discovery of sclerostin, an osteocyte-secreted glycoprotein that regulates bone formation by impeding osteoblast proliferation and function, has led to a new target for therapy. The humanized monoclonal antibody romosozumab is an antisclerostin antibody, which was found in phase 1 trials to stimulate bone formation, decrease bone resorption, and increase bone density. McClung et al went on to conduct a phase 2, multicenter, randomized, placebo-controlled trial in 28 centers across the Americas and Europe. A total of 419 women between the ages of 55 and 85 years were randomly assigned to 1 of 8 arms (1 placebo, 1 alendronate, 1 teriparatide, and 5 romosozumab arms, which differed by time and dose; Fig 1 in the original article). The primary end-point of the study was change in bone mineral density (BMD) at the lumbar spine at 12 months. Extensive exclusion criteria were listed. At 12 months, the pooled romosozumab group compared with the pooled placebo group had a significant increase in BMD ($P < .001$) with the largest increase in the largest monthly dose of active drug, with a mean increase in BMD of 11.3% at the lumbar spine, 4.1% at total hip, and 3.7% at femoral neck (Fig 2 in the original article). There were no significant differences in safety. This study highlights a novel target for increasing bone density in women with osteoporosis; however, one should note the extensive exclusion criteria when reviewing future larger studies. The trial was supported by Amgen and UCB Pharma.

J. Barton, MD

3 Rheumatoid Arthritis

Socioeconomic Disparities in the Health of African Americans With Rheumatoid Arthritis From the Southeastern United States

Baldassari AR, Cleveland RJ, Jonas BL, et al (Univ of North Carolina at Chapel Hill; et al)

Arthritis Care Res 66:1808-1817, 2014

Objective.—To examine cross-sectional baseline data from the Consortium for the Longitudinal Evaluation of African Americans with Early Rheumatoid Arthritis registry for the association between socioeconomic status (SES) with clinical and self-report health outcomes.

Methods.—We analyzed data on 937 African Americans who provided comprehensive sociodemographic data in addition to self-reported health outcomes. SES measures included educational attainment, homeownership, household income, and occupation. Outcomes included measures of disease activity, joint damage, autoantibody status, and self-reported measures. Multivariable linear, logistic, and zero-inflated Poisson regression models were used to estimate associations of each SES measure with rheumatoid arthritis (RA) outcomes, controlling for sex, age, disease duration, comorbid conditions, body mass index, smoking, methotrexate/leflunomide use, and biologic agent use.

Results.—The mean age was 54 years, 86% were women, and the mean RA disease duration was 7.8 years. Approximately 24% had less than a high school degree, 56% had a nonprofessional occupation, 75% had a household income <$30,000, and 55% were nonhomeowners. In multivariable regression models, significantly increased associations of disease activity measures and self-reported health outcomes were observed with low household income (<$30,000/year) and nonhomeownership. Education less than high school was primarily associated with self-reported health outcomes. Among participants with disease duration <2 years, associations of SES were confined to self-reported measures.

Conclusion.—Our results indicate significant socioeconomic disparities in self-reported physical and mental health, clinical disease activity measures, and autoantibody status among African Americans with RA not explained by differences in demographics, medication use, and health behaviors.

▶ Despite tremendous advances in the treatment and approach to rheumatoid arthritis (RA), disparities in outcomes by race/ethnicity, education, and language exist. Large cohorts of diverse patients with RA are uncommon, and clinical trials of therapies for RA generally include majority populations. Baldassari and colleagues present the results of their cross-sectional analysis of more than 900 African American adults with RA in the Consortium for Longitudinal Evaluation of African Americans with Early Rheumatoid Arthritis, which was established in 2001 in the Southeastern United States. Of 937 individuals, 86% were women, 75% had an annual income of less than $30,000, 24% did not have a high school diploma, and most were not homeowners (56%). Mean disease duration was 7 years. In terms of variation in disease activity, there were clear associations between socioeconomic status (SES) and RA disease activity, with non homeowners having higher C-reactive protein levels, more tender joints, and higher Disease Activity Score—C-reactive protein compared with homeowners. Low-income participants had 34% more swollen joints. Occupation was also significantly associated with tender joints. In terms of self-reported health outcomes, SES disparities were seen, with yearly household income of less than $30,000 being associated with increases in pain and fatigue and higher Health Assessment Questionnaire scores and higher numbers of mentally and physically unhealthy days. There was no significant relationship between SES and erosive changes on radiographs. This first study of health disparities in African Americans with RA highlights the importance of financial indicators such as income and home ownership in the course of this chronic debilitating disease and that many of these disparities are preventable.

J. Barton, MD

Being overweight or obese and risk of developing rheumatoid arthritis among women: a prospective cohort study

Lu B, Hiraki LT, Sparks JA, et al (Brigham & Women's Hosp, Boston, MA; et al)
Ann Rheum Dis 73:1914-1922, 2014

Objectives.—To examine the relationship between being overweight or obese and developing rheumatoid arthritis (RA) in two large prospective cohorts, the Nurses' Health Study (NHS) and Nurses' Health Study II (NHSII).

Methods.—We followed 109 896 women enrolled in NHS and 108 727 in NHSII who provided lifestyle, environmental exposure and anthropometric information through biennial questionnaires. We assessed the association between time-varying and cumulative Body Mass Index (BMI) in WHO categories of normal, overweight and obese (18.5–<25, 25.0–<30, ≥30.0 kg/m^2) and incident RA meeting the 1987 American College of Rheumatology (ACR) criteria. We estimated HRs for overall RA and serologic subtypes with Cox regression models adjusted for potential confounders. We repeated analyses restricted to RA diagnosed at age 55 years or younger.

Results.—During 2 765 195 person-years of follow-up (1976–2008) in NHS and 1 934 518 person-years (1989–2009) in NHSII, we validated

1181 incident cases of RA (826 in NHS, 355 in NHSII). There was a trend toward increased risk of all RA among overweight and obese women (HR (95% CI) 1.37 (0.95 to 1.98) and 1.37 (0.91, 2.09), p for trend = 0.068). Among RA cases diagnosed at age 55 years or younger, this association appeared stronger (HR 1.45 (1.03 to 2.03) for overweight and 1.65 (1.34 to 2.05) for obese women (p trend <0.001)). Ten cumulative years of being obese, conferred a 37% increased risk of RA at younger ages (HR 1.37 (1.11 to 1.69)).

Conclusions.—Risks of seropositive and seronegative RA were elevated among overweight and obese women, particularly among women diagnosed with RA at earlier ages.

▶ Rates of overweight and obese Americans are rising rapidly. Increased morbidity and mortality have been associated with obesity: increased risk of diabetes, hypertension, hyperlipidemia, and cardiovascular disease. One proposed contribution of obesity to these conditions is systemic inflammation—adipose tissue produces proinflammatory adipokines such as C-reactive protein, tumor necrosis factor-alpha and interleukin-6. The etiology of rheumatoid arthritis (RA) is not 100% understood. A number of conflicting studies have examined whether there is an association between body mass index (BMI) and RA, some finding positive associations and others none. Bu et al present a rigorous examination of BMI over time and its association with incident RA in prospective cohort study of more than 200 000 women in the Nurses Health Study and Nurses Health Study II. The age-adjusted incidence rates for RA in this cohort (30 in 100 000 person years) were lower than that reported in the Olmstead County, Minneapolis study; however, were consistent with European reports and those of a Massachusetts study. The authors found that being obese increased the risk of RA in women between 40% and 70%, depending on age and serologic status. The group at highest risk of developing RA was those who were overweight or obese at age 18. Being overweight or obese throughout one's life was associated with the development of RA at age 55 or younger. The relationship between BMI and incident RA was attenuated for those diagnosed after age 55, which may reflect differences in pathophysiology of RA diagnosed at an older age or challenges with BMI capturing fat mass for women at that age. Regardless, this well-done study highlights a need to counsel young women that being overweight or obese is associated with higher risk of developing RA and that maintaining a normal weight may be important to overall health.

J. Barton, MD

Medication Risk Communication During Rheumatology Office Visits

Blalock SJ, DeVellis BM, DeVellis RF, et al (Univ of North Carolina, Chapel Hill; et al)

Arthritis Care Res 67:161-168, 2015

Objective.—We used a multidimensional framework to describe the types of information about medication risks that rheumatologists provide to rheumatoid arthritis (RA) patients during routine office visits.

Methods.—We analyzed 1,094 audiotaped rheumatology office visits involving 450 RA patients. Each patient had up to 3 visits audiotaped. In conjunction with each office visit, patients also completed a self-administered questionnaire and interview and the rheumatologists provided ratings of patient health status.

Results.—The number of medication risks discussed per visit ranged from 0–18, with a mean ± SD of 3.23 ± 2.93. The rheumatologist initiated ~80% of the medication risk discussions. Approximately one-fourth of the discussions (25.6%) were limited to an assessment of whether or not the patient was experiencing a medication side effect. More risks were discussed during visits when changes to the patient's regimen were discussed than when no changes were discussed ($X \equiv 3.93, SD = 3.10$ *and* $X \equiv 2.20, SD = 2.34,$ *respectively*; $P < 0.0001$). When medications were being proposed for addition to the patient's regimen, the most frequently discussed risk dimensions were the importance of monitoring (30%), probability (29.8%), things the patient should do to minimize risk (25.5%), and risk severity (21.8%).

Conclusion.—Most discussions of medication risks that we observed were quite limited and often restricted to an assessment of whether the patient was experiencing side effects from their current medications. The amount of information that is optimal and how to tailor information to the preferences and abilities of individual patients remain important areas for future research.

▶ The treatment and strategies used to effectively treat rheumatoid arthritis (RA) have made a tremendous impact on outcomes, with the potential for remission for many. Medications can lead to remission for some but carry risk of serious side effects or toxicity. Patients need to have a clear understanding of risks and benefits, which should also be informed to participants in their care and engage in shared decision making around treatments. How well do rheumatologists communicate risk to patients with RA? Blalock and colleagues undertook an analysis of more than 1000 audio-taped rheumatology visits of 450 RA patients located in Wisconsin and North Carolina. Using the transcripts of the visits, the investigators used a 5-step approach to analyzing medication risk discussions. The number of medication risks per visit ranged from 0 to 18 with a mean of 3.23. Rheumatologists initiated the conversation about risk 80% of the time and just more than a quarter of the discussions were limited to whether a patient was experiencing a side effect. When introducing a new medication, the most frequent risk dimension discussed was importance of monitoring (30%), probability (29.8%), things the patient should do to minimize risk (25.5%), and risk severity (21.8%). Surprisingly, the rheumatologist described potential severity/impact of risk in 8.1% of the risk discussions and when providing information about risk probability in 10.3% of discussions, the clinician almost always used qualitative terms (91.3%) as opposed to frequencies (eg, 1 in 100). This study highlights a critical gap in patient-clinician communication in rheumatology. To have true shared decision making, patients must first be informed. Patients want information from their doctors. This study highlights a need for education of rheumatologists around risk communication and better tools that synthesize the existing evidence on risk, such as decision support tools, and translate it to patients.

J. Barton, MD

4 Sjogren's Syndrome

Identification of lymphoma predictors in patients with primary Sjögren's syndrome: a systematic literature review and meta-analysis

Nishishinya MB, Pereda CA, Muñoz-Fernández S, et al (Instituto Traumatológico Quirón, Barcelona, Spain)

Rheumatol Int 35:17-26, 2015

To identify risk and predictors of lymphoma or lymphoproliferative -disease in patients with primary Sjögren syndrome. Articles were identified through a comprehensive search strategy in Medline, Embase and Cochrane CENTRAL. Studies had to investigate primary Sjögren syndrome patients, 18 years of age or older, with the goal of examining potential clinical, immunological and hematological risk factors for lymphoma or lymphoproliferative disease. The quality of the studies was graded using the Oxford Levels of Evidence Scale. Whenever possible, the authors created evidence tables and performed meta-analysis. Of 900 studies identified, 18 were selected for inclusion. These studies provided data from over 15,000 patients (90 % female) for analysis. Lymphadenopathy, parotid enlargement, palpable purpura, low C4 serum levels and cryoglobulins were the most consistent non-Hodgkin's lymphoma/lymphoproliferative disease predictors. Additionally, some of the studies identified splenomegaly, low C3 serum levels, lymphopenia and neutropenia as significant prognostic factors. The detection of germinal center-like lesions in primary Sjögren Syndrome diagnostic salivary biopsies was also proposed as highly predictive of non-Hodgkin's lymphoma. In contrast, anemia, anti-Ro, anti-La, antinuclear antibodies, rheumatoid factor, male gender and hypergammaglobulinemia were not associated with lymphoma or lymphoproliferative disease. Patients with primary Sjögren syndrome have an increased risk of lymphoma or lymphoproliferative disease compared to the general population. Ascertaining relevant and reliable predictors in this patient population would greatly facilitate the identification of patients at elevated risk for closer monitoring in the context of limited resources.

► Patients with primary Sjogren's syndrome (pSS) have an increased risk of lymphoma, mostly non-Hodgkin's lymphoma. Almost 1 of 5 pSS patients will die from lymphoma. This association has been documented for the last 40 years. Nishishinya and colleagues report the results of their systematic review and meta-analysis conducted to identify significant clinical or immunologic predictors associated with this increased risk in patients with pSS. A review of relevant literature from 1961 to January 2014 identified more than 900 articles, of which,

18 met all inclusion criteria. These studies collectively included more than 15 000 patients, of whom 90% were women with an average age of 39 to 67. Significant clinical factors associated with increased risk of lymphoma identified in at least 2 studies were parotid enlargement (6 studies), lymphadenopathy (4 studies), and palpable purpura (3 studies). Hematologic or serologic factors associated with increased lymphoma risk noted in at least 2 studies included low c3, low c4, cryoglobulins, and lymphopenia. Although this study highlights many important predictors of increased risk of malignancy, specifically lymphoma, among patients with pSS, it should be noted that the studies included in the review did not use a consistent classification criteria. Only 4 of the 18 used the American-European Consensus Group criteria, which consider a salivary gland biopsy essential to classification. A study from 2011 reported that the presence of germinal center lesions on labial salivary gland biopsies at the time of diagnosis was predictive of non-Hodgkin's lymphoma. Additionally, the review is limited by not having data on DMARD therapy and how that may influence the development of non-Hodgkin's lymphoma or lymphoproliferative disease. This review, however, does highlight clinical and serologic factors for which to remain vigilant in clinical practice when caring for patients with pSS.

J. Barton, MD

Efficacy and safety of belimumab in primary Sjögren's syndrome: results of the BELISS open-label phase II study

Mariette X, Seror R, Quartuccio L, et al (Hôpitaux Universitaires Paris-Sud, Le Kremlin Bicêtre, France; Udine Univ, Italy; et al)
Ann Rheum Dis 74:526-531, 2015

Background.—Increased expression of B cell activating factor (BAFF or B lymphocyte stimulator) may explain the B cell activation characteristic of primary Sjögren's syndrome (pSS).

Objectives.—To evaluate the efficacy and safety of belimumab, targeting BAFF, in patients with pSS.

Methods.—Patients were included in this bi-centric prospective 1-year open-label trial if they fulfilled American European Consensus group criteria, were anti-Sjögren's syndrome A-positive and had current systemic complications or salivary gland enlargement, or early disease (<5 years), or biomarkers of B cell activation. They received belimumab, 10 mg/kg, at weeks 0, 2 and 4 and then every 4 weeks to week 24. The primary endpoint, assessed at week 28, was improvement in two of five items: reduction in ≥30% in dryness score on a visual analogue scale (VAS), ≥30% in fatigue VAS score, ≥30% in VAS pain score, ≥30% in systemic activity VAS assessed by the physician and/or >25% improvement in any B cell activation biomarker values.

Results.—Among 30 patients included, the primary endpoint was achieved in 18 (60%). The mean (SD) European League Against Rheumatism (EULAR) Sjögren's Syndrome Disease Activity Index decreased from 8.8 (7.4) to 6.3 (6.6) ($p = 0.0015$) and EULAR Sjögren's Syndrome Patient

Reported Index from 6.4 (1.1) to 5.6 (2.0) ($p = 0.0174$). The mean dryness, fatigue and pain VAS varied from 7.8 (1.8) to 6.2 (2.9) ($p = 0.0021$), 6.9 (1.8) to 6.0 (2.2) ($p = 0.0606$) and 4.6 (2.6) to 4.7 (2.4) ($p = 0.89$), respectively. Salivary flow and Schirmer's test did not change.

Conclusions.—These encouraging results justify future randomised controlled trials of belimumab in a selected target population of pSS patients most likely to benefit from treatment (Fig 2).

▶ B lymphocytes serve a critical role in the pathogenesis of primary Sjogren's syndrome (pSS). Current evidence-based treatments for pSS largely treat symptoms of dry eyes and mouth. B-cell activating factor (BAFF) has been found to play roles in B-cell maturation, plasma cell survival, antibody response promotion, and immunoglobulin class switching. A relatively new biologic therapy directed at BAFF is belimumab, a monoclonal anti-BAFF antibody. It has been found to be efficacious in treating certain manifestations of systemic lupus erythematosus such as arthritis and serositis. Investigators in France and Italy sought to study the efficacy and safety of belimumab among persons with pSS. Mariette and colleagues report on the results of a 1-year, open-label study at 2 sites of

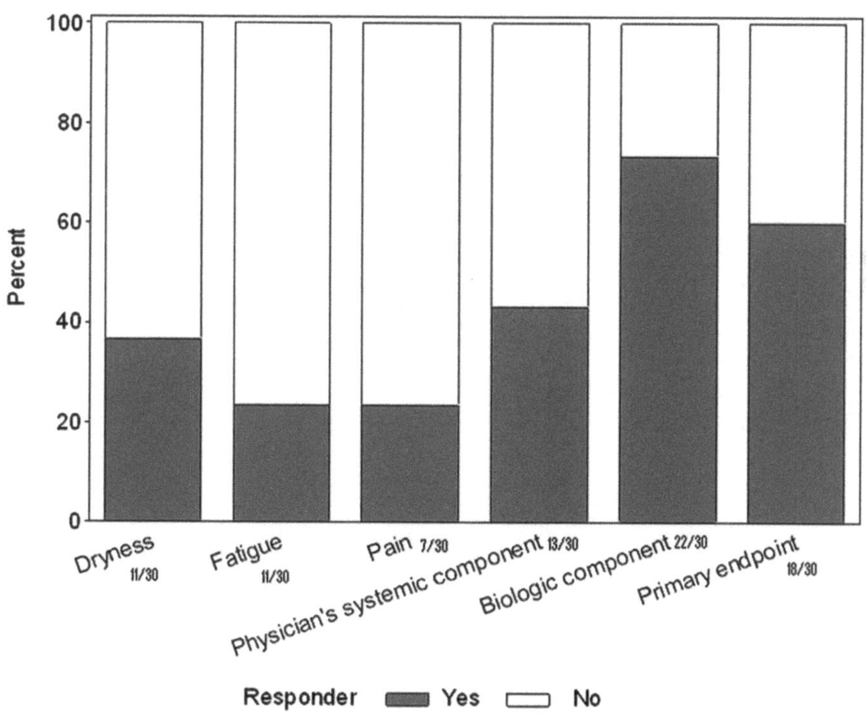

FIGURE 2.—Response to treatment for primary outcome (achieving two of five items at 28 weeks) and each component (dryness, fatigue and/or pain score; systemic activity assessed by the physician; B cell activation biomarkers). (Reproduced from Mariette X, Seror R, Quartuccio L, et al. Efficacy and safety of belimumab in primary Sjögren's syndrome: results of the BELISS open-label phase II study. *Ann Rheum Dis*. 2015;74:526-531, with permission from the BMJ Publishing Group Ltd.)

belimumab, 10 mg/kg, at 0, 2, and 4 weeks and every 4 weeks thereafter for 24 weeks. The primary outcome was assessed at week 28 and consisted of improvement by 30% or more of 2 of 5 items, which included patient-reported measures of dryness, fatigue, pain, or physician-rated systemic disease activity or a greater than 25% change in B-cell activation markers. Thirty patients were enrolled, all of whom were women with an average disease duration of 5.7 years. Two of the 30 discontinued treatment before the end of the study (one with lymphoma and cryoglobulinemic vasculitis worsened, another with meningitis). At 28 weeks, 60% of participants reached the primary endpoint. Of note, the change in individual scores of fatigue and pain did not reach statistical significance; however, visual analog scale for dryness did (Fig 2). The physician's systemic and biological components of the primary endpoint had the most response. There was no change in the Schirmer's test or saliva flow over the study period. One severe adverse event was noted during the study period (pneumococcal meningitis), and breast cancer developed in 1 patient (3 months after study end). This study should be interpreted with caution given its open-label design and small sample size; however, it does suggest potential treatment efficacy and impact on B-cell activation and possibly warrants a larger, randomized, controlled trial for this condition lacking options for therapy.

J. Barton, MD

5 Systemic Lupus Erythematosus

Treatment of Lupus Nephritis With Abatacept: The Abatacept and Cyclophosphamide Combination Efficacy and Safety Study

The ACCESS Trial Group (New York Univ; Rho Inc., Chapel Hill, NC; et al)

Arthritis Rheumatol 66:3096-3104, 2014

Objective.—To assess the efficacy and safety of a 24-week course of abatacept in the treatment of active lupus nephritis and to assess the potential of abatacept to induce "clinical tolerance," defined as sustained clinical quiescence of lupus nephritis after discontinuation of immunosuppressive therapy.

Methods.—Patients with active lupus nephritis (n = 134) were enrolled in a randomized, double-blind phase II add-on trial in which they received either abatacept or placebo in conjunction with the Euro- Lupus Nephritis Trial regimen of low-dose cyclophosphamide (CYC) followed by azathioprine (AZA). The primary efficacy outcome was the frequency of complete response at week 24. Thereafter, patients who met either complete or partial response criteria continued blinded treatment through week 52. During this phase of the study, subjects in the abatacept treatment group in whom a complete response was achieved at week 24 discontinued immunosuppressive therapy other than prednisone (10 mg/day).

Results.—There were no statistically significant differences between groups with respect to the primary outcome or any of the secondary outcomes, including measures of safety. A complete response was achieved in 33% of the subjects in the treatment group and in 31% of the subjects in the control group at week 24. Fifty percent of the subjects in the treatment group who met complete response criteria and therefore discontinued immunosuppressive therapy at week 24 maintained their complete response status through week 52.

Conclusion.—The addition of abatacept to a regimen of CYC followed by AZA did not improve the outcome of lupus nephritis at either 24 or 52 weeks. No worrisome safety signals were encountered.

▶ Effective, safe treatments for active class III or IV lupus nephritis are limited. A recent double-blind randomized, phase II add-on trial was conducted in which patients meeting American College of Rheumatology criteria for systemic lupus erythematosus, age 16 or greater, and had biopsy-proven class III or IV lupus nephritis received either abatacept or placebo in conjunction with cyclophosphamide (Euro Lupus Nephritis Trial regimen of 500 mg intravenously every 2 weeks for 6 cycles) followed by maintenance with azathioprine. The primary end point of this trial was the frequency of complete response by week 24, which was achieved by 33% of the treatment group and 31% in the control group with no significant difference between the 2. Although this study did not show any benefit of adding abatacept to cyclophosphamide in patients with lupus nephritis, there may have been several reasons for this: (1) dose of abatacept was too low, (2) dose of cyclophosphamide was too low, (3) a combination of abatacept with mycophenolate may have shown benefit, or (4) the use of corticosteroids may have interfered with the efficacy of abatacept (mouse studies that showed a synergistic effect of abatacept and cyclophosphamide did not use steroids). At present, this study showed no benefit of adding abatacept to a current regimen of cyclophosphamide (CYC) for nephritis, but it did show that the Euro Lupus CYC protocol had efficacy in a racially diverse lupus population, which had not been studied in earlier studies of largely white, European patients. The search for treatments for lupus nephritis continues.

J. Barton, MD

Increased Congenital Heart Defects in Children Born to Women With Systemic Lupus Erythematosus: Results From the Offspring of Systemic Lupus Erythematosus Mothers Registry Study

Vinet É, Pineau CA, Scott S, et al (McGill Univ Health Centre, Montreal, Canada; et al)

Circulation 131:149-156, 2014

Background.—In a large population-based study, we aimed to determine whether children born to women with systemic lupus erythematosus (SLE) have an increased risk of congenital heart defects (CHDs) in comparison with children born to women without SLE.

Methods and Results.—The Offspring of SLE Mothers Registry (OSLER) includes all women who had ≥1 hospitalization for delivery after SLE diagnosis, identified through Quebec's healthcare databases (1989—2009), and a randomly selected control group of women, matched ≥4:1 for age and year of delivery. We identified children born live to SLE mothers and their matched controls, and ascertained CHD based on ≥1 hospitalization or physician visit with relevant diagnostic codes, within the first 12 months of life. We performed multivariable logistic regression analyses, using the generalized estimating equation method, to adjust for relevant covariates. Five hundred nine women with SLE had 719 children, whereas 5824 matched controls had 8493 children. In comparison with controls, children born to women with SLE experienced more CHD (5.2% [95% confidence interval (CI), 3.7—7.1] versus 1.9% [95% CI, 1.6—2.2], difference 3.3% [95% CI, 1.9—5.2]). In multivariable analyses, children born to women with SLE had a substantially increased risk of CHD (odds ratio, 2.62; 95% CI, 1.77—3.88) in comparison with controls. In addition, in comparison with controls, offspring of SLE mothers had a substantially increased risk of having a CHD repair procedure (odds ratio, 5.82; 95% CI, 1.77–19.09).

Conclusions.—In comparison with children from the general population, children born to women with SLE have an increased risk of CHD, and an increased risk of having a CHD repair procedure, as well (Table 3).

► Systemic lupus erythematosus (SLE) most commonly affects women of childbearing age with a prevalence of about 1.5 per 1000 women age 18 to 44. Women with SLE often are concerned about the impact of the illness on pregnancy and risks to their offspring. Decision making around therapy can be complex given the teratogenicity of several medications used to treat SLE (eg, mycophenolate mofetil or methotrexate). The association between anti-Ro/SSA antibodies and congenital heart block has been studied but little data exist on whether babies of mothers with SLE are at increased risk of congenital heart disease compared with mothers without SLE, and, if so, what particular forms of congenital heart disease are most common. Vinet and colleagues examined these questions in a large population-based study of 719 children born to mothers with SLE in the

TABLE 3.—Multivariable Analyses of the Risk of All Types of Congenital Heart Defects and Subtypes in the Overall Sample of Children (n = 9212) from Quebec's Administrative Databases, Canada, 1989 to 2009

Covariates	Any CHD OR (95% CI)	ASD OR (95% CI)	VSD OR (95% CI)	Valve Anomalies OR (95% CI)
Maternal SLE				
No	Reference	Reference	Reference	Reference
Yes	2.62 (1.77–3.88)	3.32 (1.97–5.57)	2.50 (1.31–4.75)	2.95 (1.23–7.07)
Sex				
Male	Reference	Reference	Reference	Reference
Female	1.06 (0.79–1.42)	1.00 (0.66–1.53)	1.30 (0.80–2.11)	0.71 (0.35–1.44)
Education				
≤ High school	Reference	Reference	Reference	Reference
≥ College	0.94 (0.68–1.30)	0.87 (0.55–1.38)	1.16 (0.68–1.98)	1.01 (0.47–2.20)
Ethnicity				
White	Reference	Reference	Reference	Reference
Other	1.28 (0.90–1.81)	1.35 (0.84–2.19)	1.47 (0.85–2.55)	1.30 (0.57–2.94)
Pregestational diabetes mellitus				
No	Reference	Reference	Reference	Reference
Yes	2.05 (0.99–4.23)	2.54 (1.03–6.27)	3.56 (1.24–10.17)	2.14 (0.46–10.02)
Gestational diabetes mellitus				
No	Reference	Reference	Reference	Reference
Yes	1.17 (0.54–2.54)	1.01 (0.31–3.26)	3.05 (1.28–7.25)	2.07 (0.48–8.96)
Hypertension				
No	Reference	Reference	Reference	Reference
Yes	1.59 (0.70–3.64)	2.04 (0.76–5.53)	0.56 (0.07–4.24)	0.91 (0.11–7.66)
Asthma				
No	Reference	Reference	Reference	Reference
Yes	2.76 (1.63–4.71)	2.00 (0.89–4.53)	1.24 (0.38–4.02)	4.25 (1.57–11.53)

ASD indicates atrial septal defect; CHD, congenital heart defect; CI, confidence interval; OR, odds ratio; SLE, systemic lupus erythematosus; and VSD, ventricular septal defects.

Reprinted from Vinet É, Pineau CA, Scott S, et al. Increased congenital heart defects in children born to women with systemic lupus erythematosus: results from the offspring of systemic lupus erythematosus mothers registry study. *Circulation.* 2014;131:149-156, Copyright 2014, with permission from American Heart Association, Inc.

Offspring of SLE Mothers Registry compared with 8493 control children. Mothers with SLE were more likely to be a nonwhite racial/ethnic minority but otherwise had similar demographics in terms of mean age and marital status. Not surprisingly, mothers with SLE had more obstetric complications such as preterm births and preeclampsia compared with control mothers. Children born to SLE mothers had more congenital heart disease (5.1%, 95% confidence interval [CI], 3.7-7.1) compared with control children (1.9%, 95% CI, 1.6-2.2). In multivariate analysis, children born to mothers with SLE had increased risk of congenital heart disease (odds ratio, 2.62, 95% CI, 1.77-3.88, Table 3), specifically, increased risk of atrial and ventricular septal defects and valve anomalies. This large, population-based study of children of mothers with SLE is a significant contribution to the literature and hopefully will spur more research into what role drug exposure in utero, maternal antibodies, and cytokines play in the development of these congenital anomalies.

J. Barton, MD

6 Drug Toxicity

The Risk of Toxic Retinopathy in Patients on Long-term Hydroxychloroquine Therapy

Melles RB, Marmor MF (Redwood City Med Ctr, CA; Stanford Univ, Palo Alto, CA)

JAMA Ophthalmol 132:1453-1460, 2014

Importance.—Hydroxychloroquine sulfate is widely used for the long-term treatment of autoimmune conditions but can cause irreversible toxic retinopathy. Prior estimations of risk were low but were based largely on short-term users or severe retinal toxicity (bull's eye maculopathy). The risk may be much higher because retinopathy can be detected earlier when using more sensitive screening techniques.

Objectives.—To reassess the prevalence of and risk factors for hydroxychloroquine retinal toxicity and to determine dosage levels that facilitate safe use of the drug.

Design, Setting, and Participants.—Retrospective case-control study in an integrated health organization of approximately 3.4 million members among 2361 patients who had used hydroxychloroquine continuously for at least 5 years according to pharmacy records and who were evaluated with visual field testing or spectral-domain optical coherence tomography.

Exposure.—Hydroxychloroquine use for at least 5 years.

Main Outcomes and Measures.—Retinal toxicity as determined by characteristic visual field loss or retinal thinning and photoreceptor damage, as well as statistical measures of risk factors and prevalence.

Results.—Real body weight predicted risk better than ideal body weight and was used for all calculations. The overall prevalence of hydroxychloroquine retinopathy was 7.5% but varied with daily consumption (odds ratio, 5.67; 95% CI, 4.14-7.79 for >5.0 mg/kg) and with duration of use (odds ratio, 3.22; 95% CI, 2.20-4.70 for >10 years). For daily consumption of 4.0 to 5.0 mg/kg, the prevalence of retinal toxicity remained less than 2% within the first 10 years of use but rose to almost 20% after 20 years of use. Other major risk factors include kidney disease (odds ratio, 2.08; 95% CI, 1.44-3.01) and concurrent tamoxifen citrate therapy (odds ratio, 4.59; 95% CI, 2.05-10.27).

Conclusions and Relevance.—These data suggest that hydroxychloroquine retinopathy is more common than previously recognized, especially at high dosages and long duration of use. While no completely safe dosage is identified from this study, daily consumption of 5.0 mg/kg of real body weight or less is associated with a low risk for up to 10 years. Knowledge of these data and risk factors should help physicians prescribe hydroxychloroquine in a manner that will minimize the likelihood of vision loss.

▶ Hydroxychloroquine plays an important therapeutic role in systemic lupus erythematosus and rheumatoid arthritis (RA). In addition to treating these conditions, hydroxychloroquine may be effective in lowering risk of diabetes. In general, hydroxychloroquine is well tolerated and has few adverse effects; however, long-term use has been associated with irreversible retinal toxicity, which could lead to blindness. Recommendations for a daily dose based on 6.5 mg/kg of ideal body weight have come out of studies that found very little retinal toxicity below that dose. Melles and Marmor performed a retrospective case-control study of a large health organization (Kaiser Permanente) to assess the prevalence of and risk factors for retinal toxicity and ascertain the safest dosage levels. Of 3.4 million members, they identified 2361 patients who had used hydroxychloroquine at least 5 years and had visual field testing or spectral-domain optical coherence tomography. Whereas in prior studies retinal toxicity had been reported at 0.5% to 2%, this study had a prevalence of 7.5%. This prevalence varied by daily dosage (odds ratio [OR], 5.67; 95% confidence interval [CI], 4.14-7.79 for > 5 mg/kg) and with length of use (OR, 3.22; 95% CI, 2.20-4.70 for > 10 years of use). Retinal toxicity prevalence decreased to less than 2% for dosing of 4 to 5 mg/kg but was almost 20% for 20 years. Increasing daily dose and increased duration of use both resulted in increased cumulative risk (Fig 3 in the original article). Kidney disease and concomitant tamoxifen use were both risk factors of retinal toxicity. The efficacy of hydroxychloroquine in lupus and RA has been established in the literature and clearly reduces mortality and end organ damage. These findings suggest that the prevalence of retinal toxicity from hydroxychloroquine is nearly 3 times higher than previously thought. Detection methods for retinal toxicity have improved. Rheumatologists must carefully weigh the efficacy of hydroxychloroquine with safety when dosing and be vigilant about screening and prevention of toxicity. Studies are needed to closely examine efficacy in light of this potentially safer dosing by real body weight at 5 mg/kg. Future studies on pharmacogenetics may allow us to identify those patients at greater risk of retinal toxicity with hydroxychloroquine.

J. Barton, MD

Phenotype Standardization for Statin-Induced Myotoxicity

Alfirevic A, Neely D, Armitage J, et al (Univ of Liverpool, UK; Royal Victoria Infirmary, Newcastle upon Tyne, UK; Clinical Trial Service Unit, Oxford, UK; et al)

Clin Pharmacol Ther 96:470-476, 2014

Statins are widely used lipid-lowering drugs that are effective in reducing cardiovascular disease risk. Although they are generally well tolerated, they can cause muscle toxicity, which can lead to severe rhabdomyolysis. Research in this area has been hampered to some extent by the lack of standardized nomenclature and phenotypic definitions. We have used numerical and descriptive classifications and developed an algorithm to define statin-related myotoxicity phenotypes, including myalgia, myopathy, rhabdomyolysis, and necrotizing autoimmune myopathy (Fig 1 and Table 1).

► A rheumatologist commonly faces a patient with muscle aches or pain. We see many patients with multiple chronic conditions, including hypertension, diabetes, and hyperlipidemia. One condition to consider in a patient with myalgias who is on a statin is whether it is medication related. Statin-induced myotoxicity spans a spectrum of phenotypes that are important for any clinician to be aware of. The Phenotype Standardization Project was started several years ago to facilitate collaboration to better define adverse drug reactions across multiple studies and datasets. In December 2013, a group of international experts convened a workshop on statin-induced myotoxicity to develop consensus definitions of phenotypes. This effort was funded by the European Union Seventh Framework Program. Alfirevic et al then report on their phenotype criteria, which is outlined in the helpful Table 1 and spans 7 classifications of statin-related myopathy (SRM) from 0 (creatinine kinase <4× upper limit of normal and no muscle symptoms) to SRM 6 (autoimmune-mediated

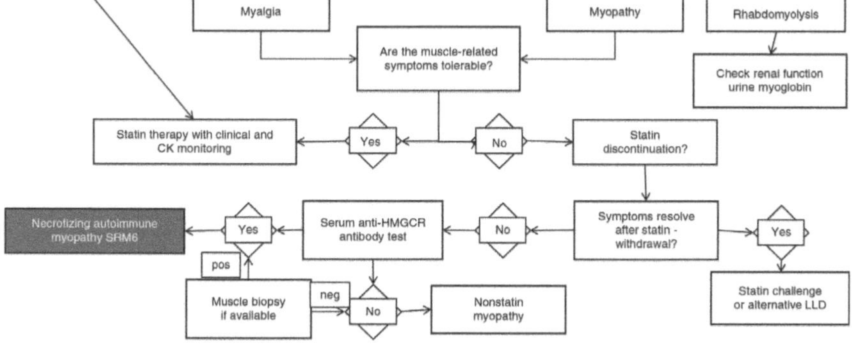

FIGURE 1.—Algorithm for defining the type of statin-related myotoxicity. New nomenclature was introduced to reflect the phenotype classification and severity (SRM 0 to SRM 6) of statin-related toxicity. CK, creatine kinase; HMGCR, 3-hydroxy-3-methylglutaryl-coenzyme A reductase; LLD, lipid-lowering drug; SRM, statin-related myotoxicity; ULN, upper limit of normal. (Reprinted from Alfirevic A, Neely D, Armitage J, et al. Phenotype standardization for statin-induced myotoxicity. *Clin Pharmacol Ther.* 2014;96:470-476.)

TABLE 1.—Statin-Related Myotoxicity Phenotype Classification

SRM Classification	Phenotype	Incidence	Definition	Reference
SRM 0	CK elevation <4× ULN	1.5–26%	No muscle symptoms	Refs. 1,20,34,35,67
SRM 1	Myalgia, tolerable	190/100,000 Patient-years; 0.3–33%	Muscle symptoms without CK elevation	Refs. 1,19,21,50,68
SRM 2	Myalgia, intolerable	0.2–2/1,000	Muscle symptoms, CK <4× ULN, complete resolution on dechallenge	Ref. 20
SRM 3	Myopathy	5/100,000 Patient-years	CK elevation >4× ULN <10× ULN ± muscle symptoms, complete resolution on dechallenge	Ref. 1
SRM 4	Severe myopathy	0.11%	CK elevation >10× ULN <50× ULN, muscle symptoms, complete resolution on dechallenge	Refs. 20,69
SRM 5	Rhabdomyolysis	0.1–8.4/100,000 Patient-years	CK elevation >10× ULN with evidence of renal impairment + muscle symptoms or CK >50× ULN	Refs. 4,6,25,44,45
SRM 6	Autoimmune-mediated necrotizing myositis	~2/million per year	HMGCR antibodies, HMGCR expression in muscle biopsy, incomplete resolution on dechallenge	Refs. 51,70

Editor's Note: Please refer to original journal article for full references.

Numeric classification was developed by an expert group; descriptive nomenclature was adapted from the recommendation of the American College of Cardiology/American Heart Association/National Heart, Lung, and Blood Institute Clinical Advisory Board.[3,7]

CK, creatine kinase; HMGCR, 3-hydroxy-3-methylglutaryl-coenzyme A reductase; SRM, statin-related myotoxicity; ULN, upper limit of normal.

Reprinted from Alfirevic A, Neely D, Armitage J, et al. Phenotype standardization for statin-induced myotoxicity. *Clin Pharmacol Ther.* 2014;96:470-476.

necrotizing myositis) with the presence of 3-hydroxy-3-methylglutaryl-coenzyme A reductase antibodies. Included in the report is an algorithm for how to approach the definition of a statin-related myopathy and steps in the evaluation (Fig 1). Through the literature search, the authors identified risk factors for statin-induced myopathy that include advanced age (> 80), female gender, low body mass index, physical exercise, and history of statin myopathy, as well as drug factors (higher dose of statin, interacting drugs such as CYP3A4 and CYP2C9 enzyme inhibitors), and diet factors (grapefruit juice). More than 25 million people worldwide are taking statins, and it is imperative that research on the prediction and prevention of serious adverse effects from these drugs continues and reaches clinicians.

J. Barton, MD

7 Seronegative Spondyloarthropathies

Risk of major cardiovascular events in patients with psoriatic arthritis, psoriasis and rheumatoid arthritis: a population-based cohort study

Ogdie A, Yu Y, Haynes K, et al (Univ of Pennsylvania, Philadelphia; Brigham and Women's Hosp, Boston, MA; et al)

Ann Rheum Dis 74:326-332, 2015

Objectives.—We aimed to quantify the risk of major adverse cardiovascular events (MACE) among patients with psoriatic arthritis (PsA), rheumatoid arthritis (RA) and psoriasis without known PsA compared with the general population after adjusting for traditional cardiovascular risk factors.

Methods.—A population-based longitudinal cohort study from 1994 to 2010 was performed in The Health Improvement Network (THIN), a primary care medical record database in the UK. Patients aged 18–89 years of age with PsA, RA or psoriasis were included. Up to 10 unexposed controls matched on practice and index date were selected for each patient with PsA. Outcomes included cardiovascular death, myocardial infarction, cerebrovascular accidents and the composite outcome (MACE). Cox proportional hazards models were used to calculate the HRs for each outcome adjusted for traditional risk factors. A priori, we hypothesised an interaction between disease status and disease-modifying antirheumatic drug (DMARD) use.

Results.—Patients with PsA (N = 8706), RA (N = 41 752), psoriasis (N = 138 424) and unexposed controls (N = 81 573) were identified. After adjustment for traditional risk factors, the risk of MACE was higher in patients with PsA not prescribed a DMARD (HR 1.24, 95% CI 1.03 to 1.49), patients with RA (No DMARD: HR 1.39, 95% CI 1.28 to 1.50, DMARD: HR 1.58, 95% CI 1.46 to 1.70), patients with psoriasis not prescribed a DMARD (HR 1.08, 95% CI 1.02 to 1.15) and patients with severe psoriasis (DMARD users: HR 1.42, 95% CI 1.17 to 1.73).

Conclusions.—Cardiovascular risk should be addressed with all patients affected by psoriasis, PsA or RA.

▶ Increased risk of incident cardiovascular events in patients with inflammatory arthritis such as rheumatoid arthritis (RA) is well established. Psoriatic arthritis (PsA) has been linked to higher prevalence of cardiovascular comorbidities such as stroke (cerebrovascular accident [CVA]) or myocardial infarction (MI), but the majority of studies to date have been cross-sectional. Ogdie and colleagues sought to answer the question of whether there were increased incidence of cardiovascular events (MI, CVA, cardiovascular death) among adults with PsA compared with adults with RA, psoriasis, and unexposed controls. They undertook a population-based longitudinal cohort study using data from 1994 to 2010 captured in a primary care medical record database in the United Kingdom. Baseline characteristics among the 3 major groups differed in that the RA population had a higher mean age and were more often women. About half of the patients with RA and PsA were prescribed a disease-modifying antirheumatic drug (DMARD) compared with 3% with psoriasis. Because of a significant interaction between DMARD use and the conditions, results were stratified by no DMARD and DMARD. The fully adjusted hazard ratio for adults with PsA not on a DMARD revealed statistically significant increased risk of incident MI (hazard ratio [HR] 1.24, 95% confidence interval [CI] 1.03-1.49) and stroke (HR 1.33, 1.03-1.71), but not cardiovascular death. The study also revealed increased risk of major adverse cardiovascular events for patients with RA not on a DMARD as well as on a DMARD, patients with psoriasis not prescribed a DMARD, and patients with severe psoriasis (DMARD users: HR 1.42, 95% CI 1.17-1.73). In conclusion, this study highlights the fact that cardiovascular risk should be addressed in all patients who are affected by any of these 3 conditions. Health care systems can be designed to systematize screening for these patients to identify modifiable risk factors for cardiovascular disease and provide needed education and treatment for patients.

J. Barton, MD

Erosions and Sclerosis on Radiographs Precede the Subsequent Development of Syndesmophytes at the Same Site: A Twelve-Year Prospective Followup of Patients With Ankylosing Spondylitis

Ramiro S, van Tubergen A, van der Heijde D, et al (Amsterdam Rheumatology Ctr and Univ of Amsterdam, The Netherlands; Maastricht Univ Med Centre and Univ of Maastricht, The Netherlands; Leiden Univ Med Centre, The Netherlands; et al)

Arthritis Rheumatol 66:2773-2779, 2014

Objective.—To analyze whether erosions, sclerosis, and squaring assessed on radiographs precede the development of syndesmophytes in patients with ankylosing spondylitis (AS).

Methods.—Patients with AS from the Outcome in Ankylosing Spondylitis International Study (OASIS) cohort were followed up for 12 years, with radiographs obtained every 2 years. Two readers (reader 1 and reader 2) scored radiographs according to the modified Stoke Ankylosing Spondylitis Spine Score (mSASSS) and recorded abnormalities per vertebral corner. Progression from erosions, sclerosis, or squaring to (bridging) syndesmophytes was investigated using multilevel longitudinal (autoregressive and time-lagged) regression analysis. Interactions with reader and spinal region were investigated.

Results.—The analysis included 211 patients (71% male, 85% HLA—B27 positive) with a mean ± SD age of 43 ± 13 years and a symptom duration of 21 ± 12 years. A total of 921 radiographs were included, with 20,509 (reader 1) and 20,568 (reader 2) vertebral corners evaluable. Erosions were found in 1% and 2.5%, sclerosis in 0.3% and 1.7%, squaring in 6.5% and 5.1%, and syndesmophytes in 25% and 27%, by reader 1 and reader 2, respectively. The odds ratio for a new syndesmophyte to occur within 2 years at the same vertebral corner if erosions, sclerosis, or squaring were present was 2.0 (95% confidence interval [95% CI] 1.7—2.3) for the cervical and lumbar spine together, 3.1 (95% CI 2.5—3.9) for the cervical spine, and 1.3 (95% CI 1.0—1.6) for the lumbar spine. When vertebral corners with erosions, sclerosis, and squaring were analyzed separately, this effect was statistically significant for erosions and for sclerosis, but not for squaring.

Conclusion.—Erosions and sclerosis occur infrequently in patients with AS, but when they do occur, they precede the development of a new syndesmophyte, and are therefore important to assess.

▶ Syndesmophyte formation in ankylosing spondylitis (AS) leads to further radiographic progression of the disease and is associated with poorer function, decreased mobility, and reduction in quality of life. The pathophysiology of syndesmophyte formation is not fully understood. Ramiro et al present the results of a longitudinal cohort study, the Outcome in Ankylosing Spondylitis International Study (OASIS), which followed up with patients who had AS up to 12 years. This evaluation of radiographs, captured every 2 years, analyzed whether erosions, sclerosis, and squaring on radiographs precede the development of syndesmophytes. They found that among 211 patients (71% males, 85% human leukocyte antigen B27 positive) and 921 radiographs with more than 20 000 vertebral corners to review, only 1% to 2.5% had erosions, 0.3% to 1.7% had sclerosis, 5.1% to 6.5% had squaring, and 25% to 27% had syndesmophytes. The odds ratio for a new syndesmophyte to occur within 2 years of the same vertebral corner if erosions, sclerosis, or squaring were present was 2.0 (95% confidence interval, 1.7—2.3) for both the cervical and lumbar spine together. This study provides insight into the pathogenesis of syndesmophytes in AS, and although erosions, sclerosis, and squaring occur infrequently, they do, in fact, precede syndesmophyte formation. It continues to be important to assess these changes radiographically in patients with AS.

J. Barton, MD

8 Myopathies

Inflammatory Muscle Diseases
Dalakas MC (Thomas Jefferson Univ, Philadelphia, PA; et al)
N Engl J Med 372:1734-1747, 2015

Inflammatory myopathies are the largest group of potentially treatable myopathies in children and adults. They constitute a heterogeneous group of disorders that are best classified, on the basis of distinct clinicopathologic features, in four subtypes: dermatomyositis, polymyositis, necrotizing autoimmune myositis, and inclusion-body myositis (throughout this review, I use this term to refer specifically to sporadic inclusion-body myositis). A fifth subtype, termed overlap myositis, is also beginning to be recognized. The identification of the correct subtype and the distinction of these conditions from other diseases that have characteristics that mimic these conditions is fundamental, because each subtype has a different prognosis and response to therapies. This review reflects the current knowledge of these conditions, highlights how best to avoid erroneous diagnoses, describes the main clinicopathologic and immunologic features, and provides practical guidelines regarding therapies.

► Advances in the identification of autoantibodies in the area of inflammatory muscle disease serve as additional pieces of data when diagnosing patients, both children and adults, with muscle weakness. Marinos A. Dalakos, MD, presents a comprehensive review of the inflammatory myopathies with a helpful glossary of newer autoantibodies associated with various forms of myopathy such as the anti-3-hydroxy-3-methylglutaryl-coenzyme A reductase or HMGCR antibody, which is an autoantibody directed at the pharmacologic target of statins—HMGCR—which is specific for necrotizing autoimmune myositis. Table 1 in the original article provides a framework to differentiate dermatomyositis, polymyositis, necrotizing autoimmune myositis, and inclusion body myositis by 5 main areas (pattern of weakness, creatine kinase level, electromyogram, muscle biopsy, and autoantibodies) as well as imaging (magnetic resonance). Various figures throughout the review colorfully illustrate pathogenesis for dermatomyositis, polymyositis, and proposed mechanisms for inclusion body myositis. Treatment approaches and drugs in development for the inflammatory myopathies are discussed, and Dr Dalakos acknowledges the improvement in 10-year survival rate for these patients of more than 90%. This article is a comprehensive narrative review of the inflammatory myopathies that emphasizes the central role of muscle biopsy for diagnosis and importance of physical therapy for all patients. More rigorous studies of newer therapies for these conditions are needed.

J. Barton, MD

9 Vasculitis

Rituximab versus Azathioprine for Maintenance in ANCA-Associated Vasculitis

Guillevin L, for the French Vasculitis Study Group (Université Paris Descartes, France)

N Engl J Med 371:1771-1780, 2014

Background.—The combination of cyclophosphamide and glucocorticoids leads to remission in most patients with antineutrophil cytoplasm antibody (ANCA)-associated vasculitides. However, even when patients receive maintenance treatment with azathioprine or methotrexate, the relapse rate remains high. Rituximab may help to maintain remission.

Methods.—Patients with newly diagnosed or relapsing granulomatosis with polyangiitis, microscopic polyangiitis, or renal-limited ANCA-associated vasculitis in complete remission after a cyclophosphamide–glucocorticoid regimen were randomly assigned to receive either 500 mg of rituximab on days 0 and 14 and at months 6, 12, and 18 after study entry or daily azathioprine until month 22. The primary end point at month 28 was the rate of major relapse (the reappearance of disease activity or worsening, with a Birmingham Vasculitis Activity Score >0, and involvement of one or more major organs, disease-related life-threatening events, or both).

Results.—The 115 enrolled patients (87 with granulomatosis with polyangiitis, 23 with microscopic polyangiitis, and 5 with renal-limited ANCA-associated vasculitis) received azathioprine (58 patients) or rituximab (57 patients). At month 28, major relapse had occurred in 17 patients in the azathioprine group (29%) and in 3 patients in the rituximab group (5%) (hazard ratio for relapse, 6.61; 95% confidence interval, 1.56 to 27.96; $P = 0.002$). The frequencies of severe adverse events were similar in the two groups. Twenty-five patients in each group ($P = 0.92$) had severe adverse events; there were 44 events in the azathioprine group and 45 in the rituximab group. Eight patients in the azathioprine group and 11 in the rituximab group had severe infections, and cancer developed in 2 patients in the azathioprine group and 1 in the rituximab group. Two patients in the azathioprine group died (1 from sepsis and 1 from pancreatic cancer).

Conclusions.—More patients with ANCA-associated vasculitides had sustained remission at month 28 with rituximab than with azathioprine.

(Funded by the French Ministry of Health; MAINRITSAN ClinicalTrials. gov number, NCT00748644; EudraCT number, 2008-002846-51.)

▶ Relapse rates for individuals with antineutrophil cytoplasm antibody (ANCA)-associated vasculitis remain high despite progress inducing remission with glucocorticoids and cyclophosphamide (CYC). Two trials found that the use of rituximab was not inferior to CYC in inducing remission by 6 months and had similar rates of adverse events. Maintaining remission in ANCA-associated vasculitis continues to be a challenge. The MAINRITSAN (Maintenance of Remission using Rituximab in Systemic ANCA-associated Vasculitis) trial sought to examine whether a rituximab-based regimen would be more effective than, and at least as safe as, azathioprine. Study investigators randomly assigned patients with newly diagnosed or relapsing granulomatosis with polyangiitis (GPA), microscopic polyangiitis, or renal-limited ANCA-associated vasculitis who had all achieved complete remission after CYC-glucocorticoid induction regimen to 1 of 2 arms for maintenance therapy: (1) experimental arm—rituximab 500 mg on days 0 and 14, then at months 6, 12, and 18 after the first infusion or (2) control arm—azathioprine 2 mg/kg/d for 12 months, then 1.5 mg/kg for 6 months, and 1 mg/kg for 4 months. Prednisone was tapered and kept at a low dose (5 mg/d) for at least 18 months after randomization. Primary outcome was the percentage of patients with major relapse (reappearance or worsening of disease with a Birmingham Vasculitis Activity Score >0 and involvement of at least one major organ, a life-threatening manifestation, or both) at month 28. One hundred fifteen patients were randomly assigned. At month 28, major relapse had occurred in 17 of the azathioprine group (29%) compared with 3 in the rituximab group (5%). Fig 2 in the original article shows the probability of remaining relapse free according to treatment group over time using Kaplan-Meier curves. Serious adverse events were similar in both groups. Two deaths occurred in the study, both in the azathioprine group, both with GPA; one died from sepsis after being treated for a relapse with methylprednisolone pulses and CYC and another died from metastatic cancer. This study shows that the use of rituximab as maintenance for ANCA-associated vasculitis is superior to azathioprine.

J. Barton, MD

Rituximab for the treatment of relapses in antineutrophil cytoplasmic antibody-associated vasculitis

Miloslavsky EM, Rituximab in ANCA-Associated Vasculitis-Immune Tolerance Network Research Group (Massachusetts General Hosp, Boston)
Arthritis Rheumatol 66:3151-3159, 2014

Objective.—Disease relapses are frequent in antineutrophil cytoplasmic antibody-associated vasculitis (AAV). This study was undertaken to evaluate outcomes in patients with AAV who are re-treated with rituximab (RTX) and prednisone for severe disease relapses.

Methods.—The Rituximab in AAV trial was a randomized, double-blind, placebo-controlled trial comparing the rates of remission induction among patients treated with RTX (n = 99) and patients treated with cyclophosphamide (CYC) followed by azathioprine (AZA) (n = 98). Prednisone was tapered to discontinuation after 5.5 months. After remission was achieved, patients who experienced a severe disease relapse between months 6 and 18 were eligible to receive RTX and prednisone on an open-label basis according to a prespecified protocol. Investigators remained blinded with regard to the original treatment assignment.

Results.—Twenty-six patients received RTX for disease relapse after remission had initially been achieved with their originally assigned treatment. Fifteen of these patients were initially randomized to receive RTX and 11 to receive CYC/AZA. Thirteen (87%) of the patients originally assigned to receive RTX and 10 (91%) originally assigned to receive CYC/AZA achieved remission again with open-label RTX (an overall percentage of 88%). In half of the patients treated with open-label RTX, prednisone could be discontinued entirely. Patients in this cohort experienced fewer adverse events compared to the overall study population (4.7 adverse events per patient-year versus 11.8 adverse events per patient-year).

Conclusion.—Re-treatment of AAV relapses with RTX and glucocorticoids appears to be a safe and effective strategy, regardless of previous treatment.

► Up to 55% of patients with antineutrophil cytoplasmic antibody (ANCA)-associated vasculitis (AAV) will have a relapse after being inducted into remission within the first 3 years. The risk of relapse over time persists. Although headway has been made in terms of alternatives to cyclophosphamide (CYC) for induction, the search for effective therapy to treat relapse continues. The Rituximab in AAV (RAVE) trial (randomized, double-blind, placebo-controlled) found that induction with rituximab and glucocorticoids was not inferior to that of CYC plus glucocorticoids. Although rituximab (n = 99) was noninferior to CYC (n = 98) to induce remission, could it also be used to treat relapse in those patients who later experienced a flare? Miloslavsky and colleagues present the results from prospective data, which followed patients from the RAVE trial who had achieved remission in the original trial and went on to have a severe relapse between months 6 and 18. These patients were eligible to receive rituximab and prednisone on an open-label basis. Investigators in this open-label phase remained blinded to the original treatment assignment. Patients who did have relapse during this 6- to 18-month period received rituximab 375 mg/m^2 weekly for 4 weeks in conjunction with glucocorticoids. In this open-label phase, 26 patients received rituximab for a relapse between months 6 and 18 (second course of ritixumab for 15 patients and first course for 11); 81% were PR3 ANCA positive and 92% had GPA. Thirteen of the 15 who initially received rituximab achieved remission (87%), and 10 of those originally assigned to CYC achieved remission with rituximab (88%). In half, prednisone was discontinued completely, and overall there were fewer adverse events compared with the larger RAVE trial participants (4.7 adverse events per patient year compared with 11.8).

This small, open-label phase of the RAVE trial found efficacy in treating relapse of AAV with rituximab. Larger studies to fully evaluate safety over time are needed.

J. Barton, MD

10 Miscellaneous Rheumatic Diseases and Therapies

Apremilast for Behçet's Syndrome—A Phase 2, Placebo-Controlled Study

Hatemi G, Melikoglu M, Tunc R, et al (Istanbul Univ Cerrahpasa Med School, Turkey; Selçuk Univ, Konya, Turkey; et al)

N Engl J Med 372:1510-1518, 2015

Background.—Oral ulcers, the hallmark of Behçet's syndrome, can be resistant to conventional treatment; therefore, alternative agents are needed. Apremilast is an oral phosphodiesterase-4 inhibitor that modulates several inflammatory pathways.

Methods.—We conducted a phase 2, multicenter, placebo-controlled study in which 111 patients with Behçet's syndrome who had two or more oral ulcers were randomly assigned to receive 30 mg of apremilast twice daily or placebo for 12 weeks. This regimen was followed by a 12-week extension phase in which the placebo group was switched to apremilast and a 28-day post-treatment observational follow-up phase. The patients and clinicians were unaware of the study assignments throughout the trial. The primary end point was the number of oral ulcers at week 12. Secondary outcomes included pain from these ulcers (measured on a 100-mm visual-analogue scale, with higher scores indicating worse pain), the number of genital ulcers, overall disease activity, and quality of life.

Results.—The mean ($\pm$SD) number of oral ulcers per patient at week 12 was significantly lower in the apremilast group than in the placebo group (0.5 ± 1.0 vs. 2.1 ± 2.6) ($P < 0.001$). The mean decline in pain from oral ulcers from baseline to week 12 was greater with apremilast than with placebo (-44.7 ± 24.3 mm vs. -16.0 ± 32.5 mm) ($P < 0.001$). Nausea, vomiting, and diarrhea were more common in the apremilast group (with 22, 9, and 12 incidents, respectively, among 55 patients) than in the placebo group (with 10, 1, and 2 incidents, respectively, among 56 patients), findings that were similar to those in previous studies of apremilast. There were two serious adverse events in patients receiving apremilast.

Conclusions.—Apremilast was effective in treating oral ulcers, which are the cardinal manifestation of Behçet's syndrome. This preliminary study was neither large enough nor long enough to assess long-term efficacy, the effect on other manifestations of Behçet's syndrome, or the risk of uncommon serious adverse events.

▶ Oral and genital ulcers are hallmark features of Behçet syndrome and are part of the International Criteria for Behçet's Disease. Current first-line therapies for mucocutaneous manifestations of Behçet syndrome include colchicine and topical agents, and, if lesions are resistant, azathioprine, thalidomide, or tumor necrosis factor (TNF) inhibitors. The search for a safe and effective treatment for oral ulcers continues. In a study funded by Celgene, a group of international investigators conducted a phase 2, multicenter, placebo-controlled trial of an oral phosphodiesterase-4 inhibitor, apremilast, in adults with Behçet syndrome who had at least 2 oral ulcers. Apremilast is a small molecule taken orally that specifically inhibits phosphodiesterase-4, increasing intracellular cyclic adenosine monophosphate, which leads to increased levels of anti-inflammatory cytokines (interleukin [IL]-10) and decreased levels of pro-inflammatory cytokines such as TNF alpha, IL-23, and interferon gamma. It has been effective among patients with psoriasis and psoriatic arthritis in clinical trials. In this study, patients were randomly assigned to receive apremilast 30 mg by mouth twice daily ($n = 55$) or placebo for 12 weeks ($n = 56$); at the end of 12 weeks, all participants received active treatment for another 12 weeks. All subjects were then followed for a 4-week follow-up phase. The primary outcome was number of oral ulcers at 12 weeks. Secondary outcomes included change in pain from oral and genital ulcers and change in disease activity. More than 90% of participants were enrolled in Turkey, nearly 70% female with an average age of 34. The authors reported statistically significant reduction in oral ulcers in the apremilast group after 12 weeks (Fig 1 in the original article), as well as significant improvement in secondary outcomes of quality of life and pain. Gastrointestinal side effects were more common in the apremilast group. Although showing positive results as another therapy for oral ulcers in Behçet syndrome, this study is limited in that nearly all patients were from Turkey, and the study length was too short and too small to assess long-term efficacy, effect on other Behçet manifestations, or the risk of uncommon serious adverse events.

J. Barton, MD

The diagnostic utility of serum IgG4 concentrations in IgG4-related disease

Carruthers MN, Khosroshahi A, Augustin T, et al (Massachusetts General Hosp, Boston; Emory Univ School of Medicine, Atlanta, GA; North Shore Hosp, Salem, MA; et al)

Ann Rheum Dis 74:14-18, 2015

Objectives.—We evaluated the sensitivity, specificity and positive and negative predictive values of elevated serum IgG4 concentrations for the diagnosis of IgG4-RD.

Methods.—Between 2001 and 2011, 190 unique patients had elevated serum IgG4 measurements. We reviewed electronic medical records to determine the indication for IgG4 measurement and underlying clinical diagnosis. Additionally, we reviewed the records of 190 other randomly selected patients from a pool of 3360 with normal results, to evaluate test characteristics of the IgG4 measurement.

Results.—Among 380 patients analysed, 72 had either probable or definite IgG4-RD. Sixty-five of the 72 IgG4-RD patients had elevated serum IgG4 concentrations (mean: 405 mg/dL; range 140–2000 mg/dL), for a sensitivity of 90%. Among the 308 subjects without IgG4-RD, 125 had elevated IgG4 (mean: 234 mg/dL; range 135–1180 mg/dL) and 183 had normal IgG4 concentrations, for a specificity of 60%. The negative predictive value of a serum IgG4 assay was 96%, but the positive predictive value only 34%. Analysis of the serum IgG4/total IgG ratio did not improve these test characteristics. Doubling the cutoff for IgG4 improved specificity (91%) but decreased sensitivity to 35%.

Discussion.—Multiple non-IgG4-RD conditions are associated with elevated serum IgG4, leading to poor specificity and low positive predictive value for this test. A substantial subset of patients with biopsy-proven IgG4-RD do not have elevated serum IgG4. Neither doubling the cutoff for serum IgG4 nor examining the serum IgG4/IgG ratio improves the overall test characteristics for the diagnosis of IgG4-RD.

► IgG4-related disease (IgG4-RD) is a relatively new systemic disease identified just 10 years ago. This fibroinflammatory disorder can involve multiple organs such as the pancreas, retroperitoneum, salivary glands, lungs, and kidneys, among others, and is often associated with elevated serum IgG4 levels. However, it is important to note that IgG4-RD has been diagnosed in the presence of normal IgG4 levels, and diagnosis relies heavily on histopathology of involved tissue, which is characterized by lymphoplasmacytic infiltrates, storiform fibrosis, and obliterative phlebitis. IgG4 levels in the serum have been used to guide diagnosis, response to therapy, and determination of future treatment, but there are limited data on the actual test characteristics of serum IgG4. Carruthers et al establish the sensitivity, specificity, and positive and negative predictive value of patients with high IgG4 levels at 1 US hospital. They compared diagnoses of 190 patients with elevated serum IgG4 levels to 190 patients with normal levels. Of the 190 patients with high IgG4, 27 had definite IgG4-RD (had at least 2 of 3 histological findings listed above on biopsy and specific immunostaining showing >10 IgG4 + plasma cells per high-powered field and IgG4/IgG ratio >40%), and 38 had probable (no tissue biopsy but typical IgG4-RD organ involvement and typical radiographic findings). Common diagnoses among patients without IgG4-RD but elevated serum IgG4 levels included chronic sinusitis (n = 46), recurrent pneumonia (n = 29), and immunodeficiency (n = 10). Mean levels of IgG4 among those with IgG4-RD (370 mg/dL) were higher than those without (115 mg/dL), $P < .0001$. Mean IgG4 levels were highest for those with definitive IgG4-RD (proven by biopsy), 670 mg/dL. The authors calculated a sensitivity of 90% (65 of 72), specificity of 60% (183 of 309), positive predictive value of 34%, and negative predictive value of 96%. This study highlights the important need for clinical awareness that not all biopsy-proven IgG4-RD has an abnormal serum IgG4 and that a normal

IgG4 serum level argues against a diagnosis of IgG4-RD but that a positive (or abnormally high) level can be associated with other diagnoses, including hematologic malignancies. The gold standard remains a histologic diagnosis until additional diagnostic markers in peripheral blood are discovered.

J. Barton, MD

11 Gout and Other Crystal Diseases

Risk of Incident Diabetes in Patients With Gout: A Cohort Study

Kim SC, Liu J, Solomon DH (Brigham and Women's Hosp, Boston, MA)
Arthritis Rheumatol 67:273-280, 2015

Objective.—Patients with hyperuricemia or gout often have metabolic syndrome. Few prospective studies have examined the risk of incident diabetes mellitus (DM) in patients with gout, and there are no data to indicate whether the risk of DM in gout differs by sex. Therefore, this cohort study was undertaken to examine the overall and sex-specific incidence rates of DM in patients with gout.

Methods.—Using data from a US commercial insurance plan (2003–2012), the overall and sex-specific incidence rates of DM in patients with gout (ages >40 years) were compared to those in patients with osteoarthritis (OA). Incident DM was defined as a diagnosis of DM and at least one dispensing of an antidiabetic drug. The sex-specific effect of gout on DM risk was also examined.

Results.—The primary study cohorts consisted of 54,075 patients with gout and 162,225 patients with OA, matched for age, sex, and index date. In both cohorts, the mean age of the patients was 56.2 years, and 84.8% were men. Over a mean followup of 1.9 years, the incidence rate of DM was 1.91 per 100 person-years in patients with gout and 1.12 per 100 person-years in patients with OA. Multivariable Cox models adjusted for age, comorbidities, medications, and health care utilization factors revealed that gout was associated with an increased risk of DM (hazard ratio 1.45, 95% confidence interval [95% CI] 1.37–1.54) in both sexes. The impact of gout on the risk of incident DM was greater in women (hazard ratio 1.78, 95% CI 1.51–2.09) than in men (hazard ratio 1.41, 95% CI 1.33–1.50), with a significant interaction between gout and sex in relation to the risk of incident DM ($P = 0.0009$).

Conclusion.—Gout was associated with an increased risk of developing DM compared to that in patients with OA after adjustment for potential confounders. In addition, the risk of incident DM associated with gout was higher among women than among men.

► Gout affects more than 4% of the US population and is now the most common form of inflammatory arthritis. Cross-sectional studies have reported an association between gout and hyperuricemia with metabolic syndrome (abdominal obesity, hypertension, dyslipidemia, hyperinsulinemia), which now affects nearly 35% of US adults and 50% of those 60 and older. A genetic link between gout and diabetes has been proposed as well as reports of higher rates of cardiovascular disease among women with gout compared with men. Kim et al conducted a large cohort study using claims data from a US health plan to ascertain whether the presence of gout is associated with increased risk of incident diabetes and whether there were sex differences. In comparing a cohort of more than 54 000 adults older than 40 with at least 1 diagnosis code for gout and 1 prescription for a gout-related medication to more than 162 000 age and sex-matched controls with osteoarthritis (OA), the authors found an increased incident rate of diabetes over a 2-year follow-up period of 1.91 per 100 person years for those with gout compared to 1.12 per 100 person years for those with OA. When stratified by sex, women with gout had a higher incident rate than men with gout, 2.21 (95% confidence interval [CI] 1.98-2.48). In fully adjusted Cox models, gout was associated with increased risk of incident diabetes in both sexes (hazard ratio [HR] 1.45, 95% CI 1.37-1.54), and that risk was greater in women (HR 1.78, 95% CI 1.51-2.09) with gout compared with their male counterparts. Even with the limitation of claims data, this study highlights a clear increased risk of incident diabetes among adults with gout and points to the need for future studies to explore whether urate-lowering therapy can help lower that risk, especially among women.

J. Barton, MD

Increased risk of vascular disease associated with gout: a retrospective, matched cohort study in the UK Clinical Practice Research Datalink

Clarson LE, Hider SL, Belcher J, et al (Keele Univ, Staffordshire, UK; et al)
Ann Rheum Dis 74:642-647, 2015

Objectives.—To determine whether gout increases risk of incident coronary heart disease (CHD), cerebrovascular (CVD) and peripheral vascular disease (PVD) in a large cohort of primary care patients with gout, since there have been no such large studies in primary care.

Methods.—A retrospective cohort study was performed using data from the Clinical Practice Research Datalink (CPRD). Risk of incident CHD, CVD and PVD was compared in 8386 patients with an incident diagnosis of gout, and 39 766 age, sex and registered general practice–matched controls, all aged over 50 years and with no prior vascular history, in the 10 years following incidence of gout, or matched index date (baseline). Multivariable Cox Regression was used to estimate HRs and covariates included sex and baseline measures of age, Body Mass Index, smoking, alcohol consumption, Charlson comorbidity index, history of hypertension, hyperlipidaemia, chronic kidney disease, statin use and aspirin use.

Results.—Multivariable analysis showed men were at increased risk of any vascular event (HRs (95% CIs)) HR 1.06 (1.01 to 1.12), any CHD HR 1.08 (1.01 to 1.15) and PVD HR 1.18 (1.01 to 1.38), while women were at increased risk of any vascular event, HR 1.25 (1.15 to 1.35), any CHD HR 1.25 (1.12 to 1.39), and PVD 1.89 (1.50 to 2.38) but not any CVD.

Conclusions.—In this cohort of over 50s with gout, female patients with gout were at greatest risk of incident vascular events, even after adjustment for vascular risk factors, despite a higher prevalence of both gout and vascular disease in men. Further research is required to establish the reason for this sex difference.

▶ Gout is the most common inflammatory arthritis and affects up to 4% of adults in the United States. Hyperuricemia has been linked to increased incidence of coronary heart disease and stroke and increased mortality caused by these conditions. The evidence regarding the relationship between gout and coronary artery disease is mixed, however. Clarson and colleagues in the United Kingdom report on the results of a retrospective cohort of more than 8000 adults older than 50 to examine whether there was increased risk of coronary heart disease, cerebrovascular disease, or peripheral vascular disease among those with gout. They were able to track data from patients with no prior vascular history over a ten-year period after their initial gout diagnosis. They found that men were at increased risk of any of the 3 vascular events with the hazard ratios (HR) ranging from 1.06 (95% confidence interval [CI], 1.01-1.12) for any vascular event to 1.18 for peripheral vascular disease (HR, 1.18; 95% CI, 1.01-1.38). For women with gout, the risk was even higher for any vascular event (HR, 1.25; 95% CI, 1.15-1.35), coronary heart disease (1.25; 95% CI, 1.12-1.39), and peripheral vascular disease (HR, 1.89; 95% CI, 1.50-2.38). Both men and women with gout are at increased risk of incident vascular events. It is currently unclear why women with gout had higher risk, and more research is needed to better understand these mechanisms. Clinical management of gout is often suboptimal, and more efforts need to be focused on screening all patients with gout for cardiovascular risk factors.

J. Barton, MD

12 Chronic Juvenile Arthritis

Choosing Wisely: The American College of Rheumatology's Top 5 for Pediatric Rheumatology

Rouster-Stevens KA, for the American College of Rheumatology Pediatric Rheumatology Core Membership Group (Emory Univ School of Medicine, Atlanta, GA; et al)

Arthritis Care Res 66:649-657, 2014

Objective.—To create a pediatric rheumatology Top 5 list as part of the American Board of Internal Medicine Foundation's Choosing Wisely campaign.

Methods.—Delphi surveys of a core group of representative pediatric rheumatology providers from across North America generated candidate Top 5 items. Items with high content agreement and perceived to be of prevalent use and of high impact were included in a survey of all American College of Rheumatology (ACR) members who identified themselves as providing care to pediatric patients. Items with the highest ratings were subjected to literature review and further evaluation.

Results.—A total of 121 candidate items were proposed in the initial Delphi survey and were reduced to 28 items in subsequent surveys. These 28 items were sent to 1,198 rheumatology providers who care for pediatric patients, and 397 (33%) responded. Based upon survey data and literature review, the Top 5 items were identified. These items focused on testing for antinuclear antibodies, autoantibody panels, Lyme disease, methotrexate toxicity monitoring, and use of routine radiographs.

Conclusion.—The ACR pediatric rheumatology Top 5 is one of the first pediatric subspecialty–specific Choosing Wisely Top 5 lists and provides an opportunity for patients and providers to discuss appropriate use of health care in pediatric rheumatology (Table 2).

▶ High-quality, low-cost care has become a priority in the delivery of health care in the United States. In an effort to reduce unnecessary spending, the American Board of Internal Medicine Foundation started the Choosing Wisely campaign, which put out a call to medical specialties to identify a Top 5 list of tests, treatments, or services commonly used by specialties but that were costly and without a strong evidence base. The American College of Rheumatology (ACR) created a Top 5 list for adult rheumatology that was published in March

TABLE 2.—The American College of Rheumatology Pediatric Rheumatology Top 5 list*

Do not order autoantibody panels unless positive ANAs and evidence of rheumatic disease.†

There is no evidence that autoantibody testing (including ANA and autoantibody panels) enhances the diagnosis of children with musculoskeletal pain in the absence of evidence of rheumatic disease as determined by a careful history and physical examination.

Do not test for Lyme disease as a cause of musculoskeletal symptoms without an exposure history and appropriate examination findings.

Musculoskeletal manifestations of Lyme disease include acute arthralgias or intermittent or persistent episodes of oligoarthritis, usually including the knee. Lyme testing without these clinical features increases the likelihood of false-positive results, leading to unnecessary antibiotic exposure and unnecessary clinic visits. Chronic diffuse arthralgias or myalgias are not suggestive of Lyme disease.

Do not routinely perform surveillance joint radiographs to monitor JIA disease activity.

No available data suggest that routinely obtaining surveillance joint radiographs to monitor for the development or progression of erosive changes in children with JIA improves outcomes. Therefore, obtaining routine joint radiographs would lead to radiation exposure without any clear benefit.

Do not perform methotrexate toxicity labs more often than every 12 weeks when patients are on stable doses.

Laboratory abnormalities in children taking methotrexate are usually mild and rarely prompt significant changes in management. Screening low-risk children every 1–2 months may lead to unnecessary interruptions in treatment and contributes to higher cost of care. More frequent monitoring is required in the first 6 months after methotrexate initiation, following dose escalation, and in the long term in patients with risk factors for toxicity (obesity, diabetes mellitus, renal disease, systemic JIA, macrophage activation syndrome, Down syndrome, alcohol use, or concomitant use of hepatotoxic or myelosuppressive medications).

Do not repeat a confirmed positive ANA in patients with established JIA or SLE.

ANA positivity is important in SLE diagnosis and positivity guides frequency of slit-lamp examination for JIA uveitis screening. Beyond this, there is no evidence that ANA testing is valuable in the ongoing management of either disease. It is recommended that following diagnosis of SLE or JIA, ANA should not be repeated unless a child with JIA has symptoms suggestive of an evolving ANA-associated autoimmune disease.

*ANA = antinuclear antibody; JIA = juvenile idiopathic arthritis; SLE = systemic lupus erythematosus.

†Several laboratories offer rheumatology or autoantibody panels, including extractable nuclear antigens, which may include anti-Sm, anti-RNP, anticentromere, anti–Scl-70, anti-SSA/Ro, anti-SSB/La, anti–Jo-1, anti–PM-1, as well as testing for anti–double-stranded DNA and antihistone antibodies. We chose the term "autoantibody panel" to encompass all possible batteries of multiple autoantibody tests employed for the evaluation of ANA-associated rheumatic disease.

Reprinted from Rouster-Stevens KA, for the American College of Rheumatology Pediatric Rheumatology Core Membership Group. Choosing wisely: the American college of rheumatology's top 5 for pediatric rheumatology. *Arthritis Care Res.* 2014;66:649-657, with permission from American College of Rheumatology.

2013. More recently, pediatric rheumatologists followed a multistep process that included surveys, consensus techniques, and literature reviews to create a Top 5 list for pediatric rheumatology. As shown in Table 2, there are many similarities to the adult rheumatology Top 5 ("do not order autoantibody panels unless positive antinuclear antibody's (ANAs) and evidence of rheumatic disease") but also focused items for pediatric rheumatology ("do not perform methotrexate toxicity labs more often than every 12 weeks when patients are on stable doses" or "Do not repeat a confirmed positive ANA in patients with established juvenile idiopathic arthritis or systemic lupus erythematosus"). The steps taken to create the Top 5 lists in rheumatology were rigorous and inclusive of members of the ACR. The intent of the Top 5 is to encourage exchange of evidence-based information between patients, parents, and providers to result in the best quality of care while optimizing cost. The authors do note that the Top 5 are not meant to dictate or replace clinical judgment, rather, they promote open dialogue and appropriate use of health care among pediatric rheumatology patients.

J. Barton, MD

PART TWO

INFECTIOUS DISEASE

NANCY M. KHARDORI, MD, PhD

Preface

During the past year, the Ebola outbreak in West Africa and its documented importation to few other countries remained in the news for a few months. Two areas that I believe did not get much attention are the role of routine aggressive supportive care in improving survival and the true risk associated with travelers from the affected areas. It seemed prudent to include these two aspects of EBV disease in the 2015 YEAR BOOK OF MEDICINE. The ongoing and increasing antimicrobial resistance in common human pathogens has led to statements like "Pre 1940's" and "end of the antibiotic era" since we have not seen new classes of antibiotics or antibiotics with newer mechanisms of action. The emergence of resistance of *Acinetobacter baumannii* to colistin does mean the end of the line. A new antibiotic without detectable resistance was described using a novel technology to harvest antibiotic-producing bacteria from the soil. This antibiotic, teixobactin, has excellent activity against gram-positive pathogens (including drug- resistant strains) like *Staphylococcus aureus*, *Clostridium difficile*, *Bacillus anthracis*, and mycobacterium tuberculosis. Hopefully, the further use of this technology will lead to more antibiotics especially those with activity against gram-negative pathogens. New types of pharmacotherapy and bacteriotherapy against *C. difficile* based on the role of bile acids in its germination and survival are truly exciting. On the vaccine front, there has been significant progress with the improvement of available vaccines like meningococcal B vaccine and 9-valent HPV vaccine, as well as studies on new vaccines including long-term efficacy of Hepatitis E vaccine, dengue virus vaccine, and aerosolized measles vaccine. A novel antibody - driven design of a human CMV subunit vaccine has been shown to select potent neutralizing antibodies. Further follow-up of the perinatally-infected child has shown a reappearance of HIV after it was reported to have been cleared, pointing to early and continuous treatment of HIV infection. The point of care testing for diagnosis of infectious diseases continues to evolve with whole genome sequencing and MALDI-TOF MS coming to the forefront. I found the idea of an enteric virus replacing the beneficial function of commensal bacteria in the gut thrilling and full of promise, given the involvement of gut dysbiosis in infectious diseases and non-infectious diseases like diabetes and obesity. The association shown between prehospital vitamin D status and hospital-acquired *Clostridium difficile* infection may finally give us an evidence-based example of vitamins preventing infections.

I wish to gratefully ackonwledge the assistance of Ms Doris B Murray in getting my submitted materials ready for print.

Nancy M. Khardori, MD, PhD

13 Bacterial Infections

Antibiotic Treatment Strategies for Community-Acquired Pneumonia in Adults

Postma DF, for the CAP-START Study Group (Univ Med Ctr Utrecht, Netherlands; et al)

N Engl J Med 372:1312-1323, 2015

Background.—The choice of empirical antibiotic treatment for patients with clinically suspected community-acquired pneumonia (CAP) who are admitted to non-intensive care unit (ICU) hospital wards is complicated by the limited availability of evidence. We compared strategies of empirical treatment (allowing deviations for medical reasons) with beta-lactam monotherapy, beta-lactam–macrolide combination therapy, or fluoroquinolone monotherapy.

Methods.—In a cluster-randomized, crossover trial with strategies rotated in 4-month periods, we tested the noninferiority of the beta-lactam strategy to the beta-lactam–macrolide and fluoroquinolone strategies with respect to 90-day mortality, in an intention-to-treat analysis, using a noninferiority margin of 3 percentage points and a two-sided 90% confidence interval.

Results.—A total of 656 patients were included during the beta-lactam strategy periods, 739 during the beta-lactam–macrolide strategy periods, and 888 during the fluoroquinolone strategy periods, with rates of adherence to the strategy of 93.0%, 88.0%, and 92.7%, respectively. The median age of the patients was 70 years. The crude 90-day mortality was 9.0% (59 patients), 11.1% (82 patients), and 8.8% (78 patients), respectively, during these strategy periods. In the intention-to-treat analysis, the risk of death was higher by 1.9 percentage points (90% confidence interval [CI], −0.6 to 4.4) with the beta-lactam–macrolide strategy than with the beta-lactam strategy and lower by 0.6 percentage points (90% CI, −2.8 to 1.9) with the fluoroquinolone strategy than with the beta-lactam strategy. These results indicated noninferiority of the beta-lactam strategy. The median length of hospital stay was 6 days for all strategies, and the median time to starting oral treatment was 3 days (interquartile range, 0 to 4) with the fluoroquinolone strategy and 4 days (interquartile range, 3 to 5) with the other strategies.

Conclusions.—Among patients with clinically suspected CAP admitted to non-ICU wards, a strategy of preferred empirical treatment with beta-lactam monotherapy was noninferior to strategies with a beta-lactam–macrolide combination or fluoroquinolone monotherapy with regard to 90-day mortality.

▶ Community-acquired pneumonia (CAP) remains a leading cause of hospitalization and mortality worldwide.[1,2] Multiple guidelines exist recommending that antibiotic treatment be based on the severity of disease at presentation. The antibiotic guidelines for initial treatment of pneumonia in patients admitted to a non-intensive care ward recommend combination of a beta-lactam plus a macrolide or ciprofloxacin or monotherapy with moxifloxacin or levofloxacin. The evidence supporting these recommendations is limited, but the use of macrolides and fluoroquinolones has increased, with associated increase in resistance development.

This cluster-randomized crossover trial with strategies rotated in 4-month periods tests whether a preferred empirical treatment with beta-lactam monotherapy is noninferior to either preferred beta-lactam macrolide combination therapy or preferred fluoroquinolone monotherapy. The endpoint is 90-day all-cause mortality among adults with clinical diagnosis of CAP admitted to non-intensive care wards using 656, 793, and 888 patients for the 3 arms. Empirical treatment with beta-lactam monotherapy that allowed for deviations for medical reasons was noninferior to the other 2 strategies. The beta-lactam monotherapy arm was not associated with a longer length of hospital stay or a higher incidence of complications. Figure 1 in the original article illustrates the patient inclusion, adherence, and mortality among a total of 3325 eligible patients. The generalizability of these findings should be seen in the context of regional differences in microbial causes of pneumonia. The resistance of *Streptococcus pneumoniae* to penicillin is low in Netherlands.[3,4]

N. Khardori, MD

References

1. Welte T, Torres A, Nathwani D. Clinical and economic burden of community-acquired pneumonia among adults in Europe. *Thorax*. 2012;67:71-79.
2. Yu H, Rubin J, Dunning S, Li S, Sato R. Clinical and economic burden of community-acquired pneumonia in the Medicare fee-for-service population. *J Am Geriatr Soc*. 2012;60:2137-2143.
3. Antimicrobial resistance surveillance in Europe: annual report of the European Antimicrobial Resistance Surveillance Network (EARS-Net). Stockholm: European Centre for Disease Prevention and Control, 2012. http://www.ecdc.europa.eu/en/publications/antimicrobial-resistance-surveillance-europe-2011.pdf. Accessed June 12, 2015.
4. Klugman KP. Bacteriological evidence of antibiotic failure in pneumococcal lower respiratory tract infections. *Eur Respir K Suppl*. 2002;36:3s-8s.

Chronic Coinfections in Patients Diagnosed with Chronic Lyme Disease: A Systematic Review

Lantos PM, Wormser GP (Duke Univ School of Medicine, Durham, NC; New York Med College, Valhalla)

Am J Med 127:1105-1110, 2014

Purpose.—Often, the controversial diagnosis of chronic Lyme disease is given to patients with prolonged, medically unexplained physical symptoms. Many such patients also are treated for chronic coinfections with *Babesia*, *Anaplasma*, or *Bartonella* in the absence of typical presentations, objective clinical findings, or laboratory confirmation of active infection. We have undertaken a systematic review of the literature to evaluate several aspects of this practice.

Methods.—Five systematic literature searches were performed using Boolean operators and the PubMed search engine.

Results.—The literature searches did not demonstrate convincing evidence of: 1) chronic anaplasmosis infection; 2) treatment-responsive symptomatic chronic babesiosis in immunocompetent persons in the absence of fever, laboratory abnormalities, and detectable parasitemia; 3) either geographically widespread or treatment-responsive symptomatic chronic infection with *Babesia duncani* in the absence of fever, laboratory abnormalities, and detectable parasitemia; 4) tick-borne transmission of *Bartonella* species; or 5) simultaneous Lyme disease and *Bartonella* infection.

Conclusions.—The medical literature does not support the diagnosis of chronic, atypical tick-borne coinfections in patients with chronic, nonspecific illnesses.

▶ *Ixodes* spp. ticks transmit a number of human pathogens other than *Borrelia burgdorferi*, which causes Lyme disease. *Ixodes* ticks may transmit *Babesia microti* or other human *Babesia* species, *Anaplasma phagocytophilium*, tick-borne encephalitis virus, *Powassan* virus, and *Borrelia miyamotoi*. These agents may be transmitted individually or in combinations.

The considerably controversial diagnosis of "chronic Lyme disease," which is ill-defined, is given to patients with medically unexplained symptom complexes. Often these patients are also diagnosed with chronic coinfection with *Anaplasma*, *Babesia*, or *Bartonella* in the absence of typical presentations or objective clinical findings and laboratory confirmation.

In this systematic review, the authors address a number of major questions relevant to the diagnosis of coinfections in patients with a diagnosis of chronic Lyme disease. The results based on 5 systematic literature searches show that there is no evidence that *Ixodes* spp. tick is a natural or even plausible mode of transmission for *Bartonella* spp. and no literature exists to support Lyme disease/Bartonella coinfection. For the pathogens that are transmitted by *Ixodes* ticks, infections produce defined clinical syndromes corroborated by objective clinical and laboratory findings. In the absence of these, practitioners who frequently offer the diagnosis of chronic Lyme disease also give spurious diagnoses of chronic anaplasmosis, babesiosis, and bartonellosis.[1] Diagnosis and treatment of such chronic coinfections is clearly not justifiable in the absence of objective evidence.

N. Khardori, MD

Reference

1. MacDonald KL, Osterholm MT, LeDell KH, et al. A case-control study to assess possible triggers and cofactors in chronic fatigue syndrome. *Am J Med.* 1996;100: 548-554.

Cellulitis Recurrence Score: A tool for predicting recurrence of lower limb cellulitis

Tay EY, Fook-Chong S, Oh CC, et al (Natl Skin Centre, Singapore; Singapore General Hosp)

J Am Acad Dermatol 72:140-145, 2015

Background.—Cellulitis is the most common skin and soft tissue infection and is associated with frequent recurrences.

Objectives.—An objective of our study was to identify factors for recurrence in patients who present with a first episode of lower-limb cellulitis. A secondary aim was to formulate a score based on observed clinical risk factors that might predict recurrence within a year.

Methods.—Dermatology referral forms and national computerized records were reviewed from 2003 to 2012. Demographics, coexistent dermatoses, local factors, and comorbidities were reviewed.

Results.—A total of 102 (45.3%) of 225 patients had recurrence. Multivariate analysis showed that lymphedema ($P < .0005$), chronic venous insufficiency ($P < .0005$), peripheral vascular disease ($P = .002$), and deep vein thrombosis ($P = .008$) predicted for recurrence. The Cellulitis Recurrence Score (CRS) was constructed based on these factors. CRS ≥2 was associated with a positive predictive value of 83.6% and negative predictive value of 67.5%. Model performance was good (Hosmer-Lemeshow statistic, $P = .753$).

Limitations.—This is a retrospective study limited to an inpatient cohort.

Conclusion.—Lymphedema, chronic venous insufficiency, peripheral vascular disease, and deep vein thrombosis were risk factors. CRS is reliable for predicting recurrence, and early interventions should be considered in patients with CRS ≥2 (Table 3).

► Cellulitis with an incidence of 16.4% to 24.6 per 1000 person-years is the most common skin infection.[1,2] All-cause mortality for patients hospitalized for cellulitis is 7.2%. Blood, aspirate, and skin biopsy cultures grow various groups of streptococci in 75% to 90% of cases. Recurrence rates are 8% to 20% per year. The initial

TABLE 3.—Results from Multivariate Analysis of Risk Factors for Recurrent Lower Extremity Cellulitis and the Corresponding Score Assigned for Each Significant Factor

Covariate	Odds Ratio (95% CI)	*P* Value	B Coefficient	Score
Chronic venous insufficiency*	3.45 (1.79-6.66)	<.0005	1.2	1
Ipsilateral deep vein thrombosis†	3.81 (1.41-10.31)	.008	1.3	1
Lymphedema*,†	9.18 (3.22-26.16)	<.0005	2.2	2
Peripheral vascular disease	26.90 (3.30-218.92)	.002	3.3	3

*Kappa measurement of agreement between chronic venous insufficiency and lymphedema = 0.159.
†Kappa measurement of agreement between ipsilateral deep vein thrombosis and lymphedema = 0.253.

episode of cellulitis contributes to postcellulitic edema, which further predisposes to recurrences.[3] Use of long-term prophylactic antibiotics[4] and reduction of modifiable risk factors have been shown to decrease the rate of recurrence.

This study was conducted on patients referred to the inpatient dermatology service at a 1500-bed tertiary hospital in Singapore. A retrospective review of inpatient consultation and national computerized medical records for the period of March 2003 to March 2012 were reviewed by an independent doctor. Recurrence was defined as a second episode of cellulitis occurring in the same limb within 1 year of the first episode with documented resolution of cellulitis between episodes. Of the 225 patients referred for inpatient dermatology consultation, 102 (45.3%) developed a recurrence. A cellulitis recurrence score (CRS) was used to identify major risk factors. Table 3 shows the results of multivariate analysis of risk factors and the corresponding assigned score for each significant factor. A CRS of ≥2 was associated with recurrent cellulitis. Peripheral vascular disease had the highest odds ratio at 26.90 followed by lymphedema, ipsilateral deep vein thrombosis, and chronic venous insufficiency. Establishing the CRS at the time of initial episode would allow selection of those with CRS ≥2 for close follow-up and treatment of concomitant risk factors such as intertrigo and tinea pedis, in addition of those included in the scoring system and other interventions to reduce the incidence of recurrence.

N. Khardori, MD

References

1. Swartz MN. Cellulitis. *N Engl J Med.* 2004;350:904-912.
2. Figtree M, Konecny P, Jennings Z, Goh C, Krillis SA, Miyakis S. Risk stratification and outcome of cellulitis admitted to hospital. *J Infect.* 2010;60:431-439.
3. Cox NH. Oedema as a risk factor for multiple episodes of cellulitis/erysipelas of the lower leg: a series with community follow-up. *Br J Dermatol.* 2006;155: 947-950.
4. Thomas KS, Crook AM, Nunn AJ, et al. Penicillin to prevent recurrent leg cellulitis. *N Engl J Med.* 2013;368:1695-1703.

Clindamycin versus Trimethoprim–Sulfamethoxazole for Uncomplicated Skin Infections

Miller LG, Daum RS, Creech CB, et al (Univ of California, Los Angeles; Univ of Chicago, IL; Vanderbilt Univ, Nashville, TN; et al)
N Engl J Med 372:1093-1103, 2015

Background.—Skin and skin-structure infections are common in ambulatory settings. However, the efficacy of various antibiotic regimens in the era of community-acquired methicillin-resistant *Staphylococcus aureus* (MRSA) is unclear.

Methods.—We enrolled outpatients with uncomplicated skin infections who had cellulitis, abscesses larger than 5 cm in diameter (smaller for younger children), or both. Patients were enrolled at four study sites. All abscesses underwent incision and drainage. Patients were randomly assigned in a 1:1 ratio to receive either clindamycin or trimethoprim–sulfamethoxazole

(TMP-SMX) for 10 days. Patients and investigators were unaware of the treatment assignments and microbiologic test results. The primary outcome was clinical cure 7 to 10 days after the end of treatment.

Results.—A total of 524 patients were enrolled (264 in the clindamycin group and 260 in the TMP-SMX group), including 155 children (29.6%). One hundred sixty patients (30.5%) had an abscess, 280 (53.4%) had cellulitis, and 82 (15.6%) had mixed infection, defined as at least one abscess lesion and one cellulitis lesion. *S. aureus* was isolated from the lesions of 217 patients (41.4%); the isolates in 167 (77.0%) of these patients were MRSA. The proportion of patients cured was similar in the two treatment groups in the intention-to-treat population (80.3% in the clindamycin group and 77.7% in the TMP-SMX group; difference, −2.6 percentage points; 95% confidence interval [CI], −10.2 to 4.9; $P = 0.52$) and in the populations of patients who could be evaluated (466 patients; 89.5% in the clindamycin group and 88.2% in the TMP-SMX group; difference, −1.2 percentage points; 95% CI, −7.6 to 5.1; $P = 0.77$). Cure rates did not differ significantly between the two treatments in the subgroups of children, adults, and patients with abscess versus cellulitis. The proportion of patients with adverse events was similar in the two groups.

Conclusions.—We found no significant difference between clindamycin and TMP-SMX, with respect to either efficacy or side-effect profile, for the treatment of uncomplicated skin infections, including both cellulitis and abscesses.

▶ Skin and skin structure infections account for 14.2 million outpatient visits and 850 000 hospital admissions every year in the United States.[1] Complications of skin infections include bacteremia, metastatic infections, hospitalizations, surgical procedures, and death. Most skin infections in the United States are caused by methicillin-resistant *Staphylococcus aureus* (MRSA). Based on the bacteriology and on cost-effectiveness, either clindamycin or trimethoprim–sulfamethoxazole (TMP-SMX) is recommended for treatment. Few comparative data exist on the efficacy and safety of these 2 antibacterial agents.

This is a double-blind randomized clinical trial comparing clindamycin and TMP-SMX for treatment of uncomplicated skin infections at 4 US medical centers in areas where community-associated MRSA is endemic. Patients with uncomplicated skin infections with cellulitis, abscesses, or both were enrolled in a 1:1 randomized study to receive either clindamycin or TMP-SMX for 10 days. There was no significant difference in cure rates, and the adverse event rates were similar in the 2 groups. Incision and drainage was performed on all patiens with abscesses. All patients who underwent drainage had abscesses larger than 5 cm in diameter (smaller for young children). As in previous studies, 80% of cellulitis lesions could not be cultured because skin was intact. From the other 20%, 11.4% had MRSA, 0.4% had *Streptococcus pyogenes*, and 0.4% had group B *Streptococcus*. Expert opinion suggests that cellulitis is most commonly caused by *S pyogenes*.[2] TMP-SMX has not been considered an optimal choice for empirical treatment of cellulitis. Recent in vitro data show that if low concentration thymidine agar is used for testing, *S pyogenes* strains may be susceptible to

TMP-SMX. The results of this trial showing equal efficacy of clindamycin and TMP-SMX in cellulitis are consistent with this in vitro data.

N. Khardori, MD

References

1. Hersh AL, Chambers HF, Maselli JH, Gonzales R. National trends in ambulatory visits and antibiotic prescribing for skin and soft-tissue infections. *Arch Intern Med.* 2008;168:1585-1591.
2. Stevens DL, Bisno AL, Chambers HF, et al. Practice guidelines for the diagnosis and management of skin and soft-tissue infections. *Clin Infect Dis.* 2005;41: 1373-1406.

Antibiotic treatment for 6 weeks versus 12 weeks in patients with pyogenic vertebral osteomyelitis: an open-label, non-inferiority, randomised, controlled trial

Bernard L, on behalf of the Duration of Treatment for Spondylodiscitis (DTS) study group (Univ Hosp Bretonneau, Tours, France; Univ Hosp Raymond Poincaré, Garches, France; Univ Hosp Ambroise Paré, Boulogne, France)

Lancet 385:875-882, 2015

Background.—Duration of treatment for patients with vertebral osteomyelitis is mainly based on expert recommendation rather than evidence. We aimed to establish whether 6 weeks of antibiotic treatment is non-inferior to 12 weeks in patients with pyogenic vertebral osteomyelitis.

Methods.—In this open-label, non-inferiority, randomised controlled trial, we enrolled patients aged 18 years or older with microbiologically confirmed pyogenic vertebral osteomyelitis and typical radiological features from 71 medical care centres across France. Patients were randomly assigned to either 6 weeks or 12 weeks of antibiotic treatment (physician's choice in accordance with French guidelines) by a computer-generated randomisation list of permuted blocks, stratified by centre. The primary endpoint was the proportion of patients who were classified as cured at 1 year by a masked independent validation committee, analysed by intention to treat. Non-inferiority would be declared if the proportion of cured patients assigned to 6 weeks of treatment was not less than the proportion of cured patients assigned to 12 weeks of treatment, within statistical variability, by an absolute margin of 10%. This trial is registered with EudraCT, number 2006-000951-18, and ClinicalTrials.gov, number NCT00764114.

Findings.—Between Nov 15, 2006, and March 15, 2011, 359 patients were randomly assigned, of whom six in the 6-week group and two in the 12-week group were excluded after randomisation. 176 patients assigned to the 6-week treatment regimen and 175 to the 12-week treatment regimen were analysed by intention to treat. 160 (90·9%) of 176 patients in the 6-week group and 159 (90·9%) of 175 of those in the 12-week group met the criteria for clinical cure. The difference between the groups (0·05%, 95% CI −6·2 to 6·3) showed the non-inferiority of the 6-week regimen when compared with the 12-week regimen. 50 patients in the 6-week group and 51 in the 12-week group had adverse events, the most common being death (14 [8%] in the 6-week group vs 12 [7%] in the 12-week group), antibiotic intolerance (12 [7%] *vs* 9 [5%]), cardiorespiratory failure (7 [4%] *vs* 12 [7%]), and neurological complications (7 [4%] *vs* 3 [2%]).

Interpretation.—6 weeks of antibiotic treatment is not inferior to 12 weeks of antibiotic treatment with respect to the proportion of patients with pyogenic vertebral osteomyelitis cured at 1 year, which suggests that the standard antibiotic treatment duration for patients with this disease could be reduced to 6 weeks (Table 4).

▶ The incidence of pyogenic osteomyelitis of the vertebral spine has increased in recent years. The estimated incidence is 2.5 per 100 000 inhabitants per year in high-income countries.[1,2] Although not evidence-based, most guidelines recommend 6 to 12 weeks of antibiotic treatment as the standard of care.[3]

This multicenter, open-label, noninferiority randomized controlled trial conducted between 2000 and 2011 aimed at establishing whether 6 weeks of antibiotic treatment is noninferior to 12 weeks in patients with microbiologically and radiographically documented pyogenic osteomyelitis. The end point was the proportion of patients cured at 1 year. The definition of confirmed cure was a sustained absence of fever, pain, and inflammatory syndrome (C-reactive protein <10 mg/L) and absence of osteomyelitis 12 months after the end of treatment. Table 4 shows the duration and type of antibiotics used in the study. Overall results showed the noninferiority of a 6-week treatment regimen versus a 12-week regimen for patients with pyrogenic vertebral osteomyelitis meeting strict microbiological criteria and receiving culture-based appropriate antibiotic therapy. Noninferiority of the efficacy of 6-week treatment could not be demonstrated

TABLE 4.—Duration and Type of Antibiotics Used in the Study

	6-week Regimen (n = 176)	12-week Regimen (n = 175)	Total (n = 351)	*p* Value
Treatment duration, weeks	6 (6–6·6)	12·1 (12–13)	9·3 (6–12·1)	··
Oral fluoroquinolone and rifampicin	76 (43%)	79 (45%)	155 (44%)	0·793
Other combinations				··
Rifampicin and aminoglycoside	22 (13%)	25 (14%)	47 (13%)	··
Rifampicin and amoxicillin	3 (2%)	4 (2%)	7 (2%)	··
Fluoroquinolone and aminoglycoside	14 (8%)	11 (6%)	25 (7%)	··
Fluoroquinolone and meticillin	4 (2%)	3 (2%)	7 (2%)	··
Fluoroquinolone and cephalosporin	6 (3%)	6 (3%)	12 (3%)	··
Amoxicillin and aminoglycoside	15 (9%)	17 (10%)	32 (9%)	··
Cephalosporin and aminoglycoside	4 (2%)	3 (2%)	7 (2%)	··
Meticillin and aminoglycoside	2 (1%)	0	2 (1%)	··
Other	30 (17%)	27 (15%)	57 (16%)	··
Intravenous treatment duration, weeks	15 (7·0–28·0)	14 (6·5–26·5)	14 (7·0–27)	0·579

Data are median (IQR) or number (%) unless otherwise specified.

in subgroups (age 75 years or older, immunosuppression, diabetes mellitus, endocarditis, neurologic signs) likely because the size of these subgroups did not provide sufficient statistical power. An age of 75 years or older and *Staphylococcus aureus* infection were associated with a decreased chance of treatment success. The treatment duration exceeded planned duration by at least 1 week in 44 patients equally distributed between the 2 groups. The distribution of antibiotics did not differ between the 2 groups for any of the organisms. Median duration of intravenous administration was 15 days in the 6-week group and 14 days in the 12-week group. Intravenous treatment was far less than 14 days in 49% to 54% of patients. An earlier study had postulated that 4 to 6 weeks of parenteral therapy was the minimum acceptable duration for a favorable outcome in patients with pyogenic vertebral osteomyelitis.[4] In this study, 52% of patients received less than 14 days of intravenous therapy. No significant difference was shown in the proportion of patients with treatment failure between patients given intravenous treatment for > 1 week compared with those given intravenous treatment for less than 1 week. In addition to no clinical advantage of 12 weeks of antibiotics versus 6 weeks, the shorter duration of intravenous treatment would be expected to reduce the complications associated with the use of central venous access solely for the purpose of antibiotic therapy. In this study, 92% of patients were given antibiotics with a higher oral bioavailability. Perhaps the acute vertebral osteomyelitis in adults needs to be viewed differently from the contiguous chronic osteomyelitis secondary to trauma, nonhealing ulcers, and presence of hardware.

N. Khardori, MD

References

1. Grammatico L, Baron S, Rusch E, et al. Epidemiology of vertebralosteoyelitis (VO) in France: analysis of hospital-discharge data 2002–2003. *Epidemiol Infect.* 2008;136:653-660.
2. Grammatico-Guillon L, Baron S, Gettner S, et al. Bone and joint infections in hospitalized patients in France, 2008: clinical and economic outcomes. *J Hosp Infect.* 2012;82:4-48.
3. Zimmerli W. Clinical practice. Vertebral osteomyelitis. *N. Engl J Med.* 2010;362: 1022-1029.
4. McHenry MC, Easly KA, Locker GA. Vertebral Osteomyelitis: long term outcome for 253 patients from 7 Cleveland area hospitals. *Clin Infec Dis.* 2002;34: 1342-1350.

14 Vaccines

Legislative Prescriptions for Controlling Nonmedical Vaccine Exemptions

Yang YT, Silverman RD (George Mason Univ, Fairfax, VA; Indiana Univ, Indianapolis)

JAMA 313:247-248, 2015

Background.—Significant, largely avoidable outbreaks of vaccine-preventable illnesses (VPIs) occurred in several communities during 2014. Most were associated with more families actively declining to have their children immunized against these diseases. Although states can require that families submit documents proving their children have received all mandatory vaccinations before they are allowed to attend school, there are also exemptions based on medical and nonmedical grounds. Strict rules on vaccination against VPIs may avoid outbreaks similar to those seen in 2014. The protection afforded by current state childhood vaccination exemption law was assessed based on type of exemptions, populations affected, documentation and filing processes required, and the review process in place, including appeals and penalties allowed.

Exemptions.—All states permit medical exemptions based on compromised immune systems, previous adverse reactions, etc. Most also offer nonmedical exemptions that can involve family religious beliefs or philosophical or moral reasons.

Populations.—Laws that apply only to public school students are less protective. Often students in the process of obtaining their full set of vaccinations are permitted to attend school. More restrictive laws may exclude children from attending child care classes, preschool, kindergarten, or elementary school during an outbreak if they have received an exemption from the vaccination or if parents cannot prove the child was vaccinated.

Application Process.—Some states provide standardized forms that are readily available and easily filed, others must be notarized, some apply only to certain vaccinations whereas others cover all vaccinations, and some must be refiled annually. Parents should be given educational information about exemption-related risks, and some states require that they sign a form indicating they have read such information. A recent approach includes an "informed refusal" process that compels parents who want an exemption to speak with a health care practitioner about the benefits and risks of immunization or to take an online course on vaccine benefits and risks. Such an approach is expected to change parents' minds about opting for an exemption.

Review Process.—Whether parents can file an exemption without official review and whether they can claim a religious exemption without being cross-examined about the sincerity or content of their specific beliefs also affects how the law protects against VPIs. An appeals process may be in place, and criminal or civil penalties may be levied in some cases.

Conclusions.—The US incidence rates of VPIs is low, but international travel can include exposure to these diseases in other parts of the world. As a result, US populations may be exposed to the disease, which is dangerous for those who are not vaccinated against it. Politically it is unlikely that philosophical or religious exemptions will be eliminated. However, to guard against more outbreaks, more rigorous policies may be needed.

▶ Outbreaks of vaccine-preventable illnesses (VPIs; eg, measles, mumps, and pertussis) continue to occur in the United States, the most recent being the multistate measles outbreak that started in California.[1] There is an association between these outbreaks and increasing numbers of families actively declining immunizations against VPIs for their children.[2] The state vaccination laws routinely include conditions under which families may apply for exemptions on medical or nonmedical grounds. Many legislative initiatives have been focused on expanding exemptions, even though stricter rules on exemptions may help reduce VPIs. The 5 broad groups of exemption characteristics are shown in the accompanying Box in the original article on legislative options. Based on these characteristics, Mississippi and West Virginia, with no religious or philosophical exemptions, have the most restrictive, and the state of Vermont is among the most lenient. Importation of a case through international travel leading to a case in a community is more likely to result in an outbreak when opportunity exists to pass the infection to additional unprotected, vulnerable members in the community. This viewpoint offers ideas about legislative interventions to guard against VPIs. The ideas include implementing a combination of various, more vigorous policies from having to submit annual exemption requests, to completing education requirements, to extending vaccination requirements to private schools.

N. Khardori, MD

References

1. Centers for Disease Control and Prevention (CDC). CDC Current Outbreak List. CDC website. http://www.cdc.gov/outbreaks/. Accessed July 28, 2014.
2. Gastanaduy PA, Redd SB, Fiebelkorn AP, et al. Division of Viral Disease, National Center for immunization and Respiratory Diseases, CDC. Measles-United States, January 1-May 23, 2014. *MMWR Morb Mortal Wkly Rep*. 2014;63:496-499.

Long-Term Efficacy of a Hepatitis E Vaccine

Zhang J, Zhang X-F, Huang S-J, et al (Xiamen Univ, China; Jiangsu Provincial Ctr for Disease Control and Prevention, Nanjing, China; et al)
N Engl J Med 372:914-922, 2015

Background.—Hepatitis E virus (HEV) is a leading cause of acute hepatitis. The long-term efficacy of a hepatitis E vaccine needs to be determined.

Methods.—In an initial efficacy study, we randomly assigned healthy adults 16 to 65 years of age to receive three doses of either a hepatitis E vaccine (vaccine group; 56,302 participants) or a hepatitis B vaccine (control group; 56,302 participants). The vaccines were administered at 0, 1, and 6 months, and the participants were followed for 19 months. In this extended follow-up study, the treatment assignments of all participants remained double-blinded, and follow-up assessments of efficacy, immunogenicity, and safety were continued for up to 4.5 years.

Results.—During the 4.5-year study period, 60 cases of hepatitis E were identified; 7 cases were confirmed in the vaccine group (0.3 cases per 10,000 person-years), and 53 cases in the control group (2.1 cases per 10,000 person-years), representing a vaccine efficacy of 86.8% (95% confidence interval, 71 to 94) in the modified intention-to-treat analysis. Of the participants who were assessed for immunogenicity and were seronegative at baseline, 87% of those who received three doses of the hepatitis E vaccine maintained antibodies against HEV for at least 4.5 years; HEV antibody titers developed in 9% in the control group. The rate of adverse events was similar in the two groups.

Conclusions.—Immunization with this hepatitis E vaccine induced antibodies against HEV and provided protection against hepatitis E for up to 4.5 years.

▶ Hepatitis E virus (HEV) has a worldwide distribution and a wide spectrum of clinical manifestations.[1,2] Waterborne infections caused by genotype 1 or 2 occur mostly in resource-limited countries as outbreaks as well as sporadic cases with high mortality in pregnant women. Transmission from humans and animals is caused by HEV genotype 3 or 4 and occurs in developed as well as resource-limited countries. Understandably, water and other basic sanitation are critical to control HEV infection. However, they are sometimes not feasible and/or may not prevent additional infections. The knowledge that all major genotypes of HEV in humans belong to the same serotype has facilitated the development of vaccines against HEV. Two genotype 1 recombinant HEV vaccines have been shown to have short-term efficacy in clinical trials.

This article reports on the extended follow-up of the 112 604 healthy adults enrolled in a phase 3 trial in 2007.[3] Based on the short efficacy at 19 months of the study, the vaccine was licensed in China where it has been in use since 2012.

In the current study, follow-up assessments of efficacy, immunogenicity, and safety were continued for up to 4.5 years while all the participants remained double-blinded. The antibody level induced by the vaccine decreased quickly in the first 2 years after vaccination followed by a slow decrease, but detectable levels remained up to 4.5 years after first vaccination. Three doses of vaccine-induced slightly higher antibody levels than 2 doses. The persistent immunity was associated with sustained vaccine efficacy.

N. Khardori, MD

References

1. Kamar N, Bendall R, Legrand-Abravanel F, et al. Hepatitis E. *Lancet.* 2012;379: 2477-2488.
2. Krain LJ, Nelson KE, Labrique AB. Host immune status and response to hepatitis E virus infection. *Clin Microbiol Rev.* 2014;27:139-165.
3. Zhu FC, Zhang J, Zhang XF, et al. Efficacy and safety of a recombinant hepatitis E vaccine in healthy adults: a large-scale, randomized, double-blind placebo controlled, phase 3 trial. *Lancet.* 2010;376:895-902.

A Case-Control Study to Estimate the Effectiveness of Maternal Pertussis Vaccination in Protecting Newborn Infants in England and Wales, 2012–2013

Dabrera G, Amirthalingam G, Andrews N, et al (Public Health England, London, UK; et al)
Clin Infect Dis 60:333-337, 2015

Background.—Infants with pertussis infection are at risk of severe clinical illness and death. Several countries, including the United Kingdom, have introduced maternal pertussis vaccination during pregnancy to protect infants from infection following national increases in pertussis notifications. The objective of this study was to estimate the effectiveness of maternal pertussis vaccination in protecting infants against laboratory-confirmed pertussis infection.

Methods.—A case-control study was undertaken in England and Wales between October 2012 and July 2013. Cases were infants aged <8 weeks at onset with pertussis infection tested by real-time polymerase chain reaction or culture. Family doctors of each case were asked to identify healthy infants born consecutively after the case in each practice, to act as controls. Fifty-eight cases and 55 controls were included in this study. Odds ratios (ORs) were calculated for the association between maternal vaccination and infant pertussis infection. The vaccine effectiveness (VE) was calculated as 1 − OR. This was adjusted for sex, geographical region, and birth period.

Results.—Mothers of 10 cases (17%) and 39 controls (71%) received pertussis vaccine in pregnancy. This gave an unadjusted VE of 91% (95% confidence interval [CI], 77%–97%). Adjusted VE was 93% (95% CI, 81%–97%).

Conclusions.—Maternal pertussis vaccination is effective in preventing pertussis infection in infants aged <8 weeks and may be considered in other countries experiencing high levels of pertussis notifications.

▶ Increase in cases of pertussis has been reported from many parts of the world despite sustained periods of high vaccine coverage. The most recent peak activity occurred in England and Wales in 2011, continued to increase into 2012, and extended to all age groups including infants less than 3 months old. The latter group is at the highest risk of severe complications and showed an incidence of 240 cases per 100 000 with 14 deaths among 429 infected infants.

The UK Department of Health is recommending that pregnant women be offered a single dose of acellular pertussis vaccine between 28 and 38 weeks' gestation. This measure has been recommended in the United States and is now recommended in New Zealand, Belgium, and Israel. The rationale for the approach is that a dose of pertussis vaccine during pregnancy boosts antibody levels in the mother and should provide passive protection to the newborn in the first 2 months of life before the initiation of infant vaccination schedule at 8 weeks.[1] The transplacental transfer of maternal antibodies is maximal from 34 weeks' gestation.[2] The added benefit is the protection of mothers against pertussis since mothers are a frequent source of infection for infants.

This first case-control study was conducted on infants in England and Wales between October 2012 and July 2013. The diagnosis of confirmed cases was made by qualitative polymerase chain reaction or culture and included infants less than 8 weeks old. The vaccine effectiveness from this intervention was 93%. This study provides evidence of the effectiveness of the measure that was initially based on a theoretical assumption. The observed effectiveness is likely to be a combination of the direct effect of transplacental antibody transfer and indirect effect on mothers to infant transmission of pertussis.

N. Khardori, MD

References

1. Van Rie A, Wendelboe AM, Englund JA. Role of maternal pertussis antibodies infants. *Pediatr Infect Dis J.* 2005;24:S62-S65.
2. Healy CM. Vaccines in pregnant women and research initiatives. *Clin Obstet Gynecol.* 2012;55:474-486.

Antibody-driven design of a human cytomegalovirus gHgLpUL128L subunit vaccine that selectively elicits potent neutralizing antibodies

Kabanova A, Perez L, Lilleri D, et al (Università della Svizzera Italiana, Bellinzona; et al)

Proc Natl Acad Sci U S A 111:17965-17970, 2014

The use of neutralizing antibodies to identify the most effective antigen has been proposed as a strategy to design vaccines capable of eliciting protective B-cell immunity. In this study, we analyzed the human antibody response to cytomegalovirus (human cytomegalovirus, HCMV) infection and found that antibodies to glycoprotein (g)B, a surface glycoprotein that has been developed as a HCMV vaccine, were primarily nonneutralizing. In contrast, most of the antibodies to the complex formed by gH, gL, protein (p)UL128, pUL130, and pUL131 (the gHgLpUL128L pentamer) neutralized HCMV infection with high potency. Based on this analysis, we developed a single polycistronic vector encoding the five pentamer genes separated by "self-cleaving" 2A peptides to generate a stably transfected CHO cell line constitutively secreting high levels of recombinant pentamer that displayed the functional antigenic sites targeted by human neutralizing antibodies. Immunization of mice with the pentamer formulated with different adjuvants elicited HCMV neutralizing antibody titers that persisted to high levels over time and that were a hundred- to thousand-fold higher than those found in individuals that recovered from primary HCMV infection. Sera from mice immunized with the pentamer vaccine neutralized infection of both epithelial cells and fibroblasts and prevented cell-to-cell spread and viral dissemination from endothelial cells to leukocytes. Neutralizing monoclonal antibodies from immunized mice showed the same potency as human antibodies and targeted the same as well as additional sites on the pentamer. These results illustrate with a relevant example a general and practical approach of analytic vaccinology for the development of subunit vaccines against complex pathogens.

▶ Human cytomegalovirus (HCMV), a ubiquitous member of Herpes virus family establishes a lifelong infection. Primary infection during pregnancy with an overall incidence of 0.6% is the most frequent cause of congenital birth defects.[1] Severe infection with HCMV also develops in patients with immunocompromising illness and/or therapies. HCMV has been associated with immune senescence and atherosclerosis. Patients requiring organ transplant who are seronegative for HCMV are at risk for life-threatening HCMV disease when transplanted from a HCMV seropositive donor. HCMV is a complex pathogen that exploits multiple glycoprotein complexes on the virion for binding and fusion to a broad range of host cells.

The work presented here represents a novel concept for development of subunit vaccines against complex pathogens using HCMV as the model. The researchers analyzed the human antibody response to HCMV infection and found that antibodies to glycoprotein (g)B, a surface glycoprotein that has been developed as a HCMV vaccine, are primarily nonneutralizing.[2] On the other hand, most of the antibodies to a pentamer complex formed by 2 other glycoproteins and 3 proteins neutralized HCMV infection efficiently. They developed a vector encoding the 5 pentamer genes to generate a stably infected cell line. The cell line constitutively secrets high levels of recombinant pentamer and displays the antigenic sites targeted by human neutralizing antibody. Mice immunized with this vaccine produced neutralizing HCMV antibodies much higher than those found in individuals recovering from primary infection. Immune sera from these mice neutralized HCMV infection of both epithelial cells and fibroblasts. The in vivo protective role of these antibodies is demonstrated by the finding from the same research group that the early production of antipentamer antibodies in pregnant women correlates with protection of the fetus.[3] This concept and technology illustrates a general approach to develop subunit vaccines against complex pathogens.

N. Khardori, MD

References

1. Griffiths P, Plotkin S, Mocarski E, et al. Desirability and feasibility of a vaccine against cytomegalovirus. *Vaccine*. 2013;31:B197-B203.

2. Plotkin SA, Smiley ML, Friedman HM, et al. Towne-vaccine-induced prevention of cytomegalovirus disease after renal transplants. *Lancet.* 1984;1:528-530.
3. Lilleri D, Kabanova A, Revello MG, et al. Fetal human cytomegalovirus transmission correlates with delayed maternal antibodies to gH/gL/pUL128–130-131 complex during primary infection. *PLoS One.* 2013;8:e59863.

A Randomized, Controlled Trial of an Aerosolized Vaccine against Measles

Low N, Bavdekar A, Jeyaseelan L, et al (Univ of Bern, Switzerland; King Edward Memorial Hosp Research Centre, Pune, India; Christian Med College, Vellore, India; et al)
N Engl J Med 372:1519-1529, 2015

Background.—Aerosolized vaccine can be used as a needle-free method of immunization against measles, a disease that remains a major cause of illness and death. Data on the immunogenicity of aerosolized vaccine against measles in children are inconsistent.

Methods.—We conducted an open-label noninferiority trial involving children 9.0 to 11.9 months of age in India who were eligible to receive a first dose of measles vaccine. Children were randomly assigned to receive a single dose of vaccine by means of either aerosol inhalation or a subcutaneous injection. The primary end points were seropositivity for antibodies against measles and adverse events 91 days after vaccination. The noninferiority margin was 5 percentage points.

Results.—A total of 1001 children were assigned to receive aerosolized vaccine, and 1003 children were assigned to receive subcutaneous vaccine; 1956 of all the children (97.6%) were followed to day 91, but outcome data were missing for 331 children because of thawed specimens. In the per-protocol population, data on 1560 of 2004 children (77.8%) could be evaluated. At day 91, a total of 662 of 775 children (85.4%; 95% confidence interval [CI], 82.5 to 88.0) in the aerosol group, as compared with 743 of 785 children (94.6%; 95% CI, 92.7 to 96.1) in the subcutaneous group, were seropositive, a difference of −9.2 percentage points (95% CI, −12.2 to −6.3). Findings were similar in the full-analysis set (673 of 788 children in the aerosol group [85.4%] and 754 of 796 children in the subcutaneous group [94.7%] were seropositive at day 91, a difference of −9.3 percentage points [95% CI, −12.3 to −6.4]) and after multiple imputation of missing results. No serious adverse events were attributable to measles vaccination. Adverse-event profiles were similar in the two groups.

Conclusions.—Aerosolized vaccine against measles was immunogenic, but, at the prespecified margin, the aerosolized vaccine was inferior to the subcutaneous vaccine with respect to the rate of seropositivity.

▶ Through its Global Vaccine Action Plan, the World Health Organization aims to eliminate measles by 2020 in at least 5 regions.[1] The availability of a safe and effective injectable measles vaccine since 1963 and intensified vaccination effort between 2000 and 2010 have reduced measles deaths by 74%.[2] However, major outbreaks have continued, particularly in resource-poor countries with low immunization coverage. An alternate delivery vaccine may increase coverage if it can be administered by people without clinical training and does not cause injection-associated infections. An aerosolized measles vaccine developed in Mexico has been used in that country since 1980.[3] The aerosolized vaccine delivered to the site of natural infection has been shown to induce measles-specific antibodies and cell-mediated immunity. The data about the clinical efficacy of this aerosolized vaccine in children are inconsistent.

This is an open-label noninferiority trial involving children in India (aged 9-11.9 months old). Children eligible to receive first dose of measles vaccine were randomized to receive by aerosol inhalation or subcutaneous injection. Aerosolized vaccine resulted in statistically inferior levels of seropositivity at 91 days. Adverse events associated with the vaccine were rare and the profiles were similar in the 2 groups. Aerosolized measles vaccine has been shown to induce higher and more sustained levels of serologic protection than subcutaneous vaccine in school-age children in Africa when administered as a second dose. There are no data to evaluate the efficacy and cost-effectiveness of aerosolized measles vaccine for primary vaccination in children older than 12 months and as a second dose in children younger than 5 years.

N. Khardori, MD

References

1. *Global Vaccine Action Plan 2011–2020*. Geneva, Switzerland: World Health Organization; 2013. http://www.who.int/immunizations/global_vaccine_action_plan/GVAP_doc_2011_2020/en. Accessed May 26, 2015.
2. Simons E, Ferrari M, Fricks J, et al. Assessment of the 2010 global measles mortality reduction goal: results from a model of surveillance data. *Lancet*. 2012;379: 2173-2178.
3. Wong-Chew RM, Islas-Romero R, Garcia-Garcia Mde L, et al. Immunogenicity of aerosol measles vaccine given as the primary measles immunization to nine-month-old Mexican children. *Vaccine*. 2006;24:683-690.

Clinical efficacy and safety of a novel tetravalent dengue vaccine in healthy children in Asia: a phase 3, randomised, observer-masked, placebo-controlled trial

Capeding MR, the CYD14 Study Group (Research Inst for Tropical Medicine, Alabang, Philippines; et al)
Lancet 384:1358-1365, 2014

Background.—An estimated 100 million people have symptomatic dengue infection every year. This is the first report of a phase 3 vaccine efficacy trial of a candidate dengue vaccine. We aimed to assess the efficacy of the CYD dengue vaccine against symptomatic, virologically confirmed dengue in children.

Methods.—We did an observer-masked, randomised controlled, multicentre, phase 3 trial in five countries in the Asia-Pacific region. Between June 3, and Dec 1, 2011, healthy children aged 2–14 years were randomly assigned (2:1), by computer-generated permuted blocks of six with an interactive voice or web response system, to receive three injections of a recombinant, live, attenuated, tetravalent dengue vaccine (CYD-TDV), or placebo, at months 0, 6, and 12. Randomisation was stratified by age and site. Participants were followed up until month 25. Trial staff responsible for the preparation and administration of injections were unmasked to group allocation, but were not included in the follow-up of the participants; allocation was concealed from the study sponsor, investigators, and parents and guardians. Our primary objective was to assess protective efficacy against symptomatic, virologically confirmed dengue, irrespective of disease severity or serotype, that took place more than 28 days after the third injection. The primary endpoint was for the lower bound of the 95% CI of vaccine efficacy to be greater than 25%. Analysis was by intention to treat and per protocol. This trial is registered with ClinicalTrials.gov, number NCT01373281.

Findings.—We randomly assigned 10 275 children to receive either vaccine (n = 6851) or placebo (n = 3424), of whom 6710 (98%) and 3350 (98%), respectively, were included in the primary analysis. 250 cases of virologically confirmed dengue took place more than 28 days after the third injection (117 [47%] in the vaccine group and 133 [53%] in the control group). The primary endpoint was achieved with 56·5% (95% CI 43·8–66·4) efficacy. We recorded 647 serious adverse events (402 [62%] in the vaccine group and 245 [38%] in the control group). 54 (1%) children in the vaccine group and 33 (1%) of those in the control group had serious adverse events that happened within 28 days of vaccination. Serious adverse events were consistent with medical disorders in this age group and were mainly infections and injuries.

Interpretation.—Our findings show that dengue vaccine is efficacious when given as three injections at months 0, 6, and 12 to children aged 2–14 years in endemic areas in Asia, and has a good safety profile. Vaccination could reduce the incidence of symptomatic infection and hospital admission and has the potential to provide an important public health benefit.

▶ Of the estimated 390 million dengue virus infections every year, about 100 million people have symptomatic clinically apparent disease.[1] No specific drugs are available for prevention or treatment. Results of a randomized, controlled phase 2b trial of the recombinant live attenuated, CYD tetravalent dengue vaccine (CYD-TDV) in Thai schoolchildren published in 2012 did not meet its primary outcome.[2]

This is multicenter observer-masked randomized controlled multicenter phase 3 trial done in the Asia-Pacific region—Indonesia, Malaysia, Philippines, Thailand, and Vietnam. A total of 10 275 healthy children aged 2 to 14 years were randomized into vaccine or placebo groups. The primary endpoint of overall vaccine efficacy was 56.5% after 3 injections at months 0, 6, and 12, and the safety profile was good. Despite moderate overall efficacy, the vaccination prevented

80% of cases of dengue hemorrhagic fevers and reductions in hospital admissions. It was noted that CYD-TDV vaccine prevented more than 75% of serotype 3 and 4 infection and 50% of those caused by serotype 1. The vaccine efficacy was 35% against serotype 2, higher than that seen in the first trial,[2] likely because of the lower incidence of serotype 2 in the present trial. Further studies are being done to investigate the serotype-specific efficacy profiles. This trial, done over more than 3 years in Asia, which has 70% of the global dengue burden, points to a substantial effect of the vaccine on severe disease manifestations. A second phase 3 clinical trial in 5 Latin American countries enrolling 2000 children and adolescents (aged 9-16 years) has been concluded.

N. Khardori, MD

References

1. World Health Organization. Dengue: Guidelines for Diagnosis, Treatment, Prevention and Control. New ed. 2009. http://www.who.int/tdr/publications/documents/dengue-diagnosis:pdf. Accessed June 7, 2014.
2. Sabchareon A, Wallace D, Sirivichayakul C, et al. Protective efficacy of the recombinant, live-attenuated, CYD tetravalent dengue vaccine in Thai schoolchildren: a randomised, controlled phase 2b trial. *Lancet.* 2012;380:1559-1567.

15 Viral Infections

Chikungunya Virus Transmission Found in the United States: US Health Authorities Brace for Wider Spread
Kuehn BM
JAMA 312:776-777, 2014

Background.—The first two cases of locally transmitted chikungunya virus were confirmed in Florida, signalling the movement of the virus from the Caribbean and Central and South America to North America. Infection with chikungunya virus spread rapidly in the Caribbean between December 2013 and July 2014, with an estimated 12% of the population of French Saint Margin infected. US travelers become infected during travel, so it was only a matter of time until cases would be transmitted locally in the United States.

Virus Facts.—Chikungunya virus is transmitted by the *Aedes aegypti* and *Aedes albopictus* mosquitoes, both of which are established in the southeastern United States and parts of the Southwest. *A. albopictus* is also found in the Mid-Atlantic and lower Midwest states. Dengue virus infection is spread by the same vectors, but chikungunya infections cause symptomatic disease in 80% of those infected, whereas dengue produces many mild or asymptomatic cases. Patients can have nonspecific flu-like symptoms but physicians should suspect the virus if they report a history of travel to an area where the disease is spreading. Chikungunya infection hallmarks are the abrupt onset of a fever over 102°F and severe pain or swelling in multiple joints. Doctors may also see rash, muscle pain, or headache typically 3 to 5 days after exposure but sometimes within 1 to 12 days.

During the last major outbreak of chikungunya infection in Africa and Southeast Asia, a single mutation caused a change that allowed more efficient transmission by *A. albopictus*. A similar mutation in the current strain would increase the US risk.

Prevention and Identification.—Prevention consists of taking steps to prevent mosquito bites by using repellent, wearing long sleeves, and ensuring window and door screens are intact. Both of the mosquitoes are active during the day, so repellant should be used during daytime hours. Those living where these mosquitos are common should eliminate standing water from boat covers, pots, and other places to destroy breeding sites.

Physicians in suspected areas should have a heightened awareness of chikungunya virus infection as a possibility. Patient samples should be tested for both the virus and antibodies to the virus.

Treatment.—Until a diagnosis is made, patients should receive treatment as if they had dengue infection. Care for chikungunya is usually supportive care plus pain management. Nonsteroidal anti-inflammatory drugs can worsen dengue-associated bleeding in patients but can help in chikungunya. A vaccine is being developed.

▶ Chikungunya virus, a mosquito-borne Alphavirus, circulates in the forested regions of sub-Saharan Africa in transmission cycles involving nonhuman primate hosts.[1] Between 1879 and 1956, a member of the eastern, central, and southern African (ECSA) enzootic lineage was introduced into Asia. This strain, called the Asian lineage, has caused outbreaks in India and Southeast Asia and continues to circulate in Southeast Asia. Another ECSA lineage progenitor caused an outbreak in coastal Kenya in 2004 and subsequently spread to Indian Ocean islands and India. Explosive epidemics involving millions of people occurred. Infected air travelers took the disease to Europe, Asia, and the Americas. This was followed by local transmission in Italy, France, and countries in South and Southeast Asia. Now *Aedes albopictus*, in addition to *Aedes aegypti*, serves as a second chikungunya virus vector. The first local transmission of chikungunya virus in the Western Hemisphere was reported in December 2013 (Caribbean) by the World Health Organization. The disease spread quickly through the Caribbean and Central and South America, exceeding 400 000 cases in July 2014. The first 2 cases of transmission within the continental United States were reported by the Florida Department of Health in July 2014. Both *A. aegypti* and *A. albopictus* mosquitoes are established in the continental United States. They both live in the Southeastern United States and parts of the Southwest. *A. albopictus* is also found in the Mid-Atlantic states and lower Midwest. The spread of chikungunya virus in the United States is expected to be similar to that of dengue virus, which has same vectors, rather than following the pattern of its spread in the Caribbean and other parts of the Americas.

N. Khardori, MD

Reference

1. Weaver SC, Lecuit M. Chikungunya virus and the global spread of a mosquito-borne disease. *N Engl J Med.* 2015;372:1231-1239.

Viremic Relapse after HIV-1 Remission in a Perinatally Infected Child

Luzuriaga K, Gay H, Ziemniak C, et al (Univ of Massachusetts Med School, Worcester; Univ of Mississippi Med Ctr, Jackson; Johns Hopkins Univ School of Medicine Baltimore, MD; et al)

N Engl J Med 372:786-788, 2015

Background.—A perinatally infected child was reported to have achieved remission of human immunodeficiency virus type 1 (HIV-1) infection after receiving antiretroviral therapy (ART) between ages 30 hours and 18 months. The child had persistently undetectable plasma HIV-1 viremia for 12 months and no HIV-1-n-specific immune responses.

The child also had persistently undetectable plasma HIV-1 RNA levels as revealed by normal standard clinical assays. Plasma viremia was undetectable through 21.9 months after discontinuing ART. Subsequent changes in the child's condition were reported.

Update.—A routine clinical follow-up evaluation at age 46.4 months, or 27.6 months after ART was discontinued, revealed the plasma viral load had rebounded although the child had no symptoms or signs of illness and had not received any vaccines. ART was reinitiated and plasma viral load dropped within 72 hours. In addition, circulating CD4+ T-cell levels increased to 43% and the ratio of CD4+ T cells to CD8+ T cells normalized. HIV-1-n-specific antibody and cell-mediated immune responses were detected at viremic rebound as well.

Analysis.—Before the rebound, sequencing attempts were unsuccessful. However, the sequence identity obtained by single-genome amplification and sequencing directly from rebounding plasma virus showed 98.6% sequence identity to maternal plasma viral sequences obtained 24 months after the child was born. The return to HIV-1 viremia after a quiescent period is consistent with the model of HIV-1 latency in which long-lived resting memory CD4+ T cells are generated during routine immunologic memory formation. Whether ART should have been initiated earlier or continued longer to achieve an extended period of remission is unclear.

Conclusions.—Studies are under way to determine whether very early treatment restricts or eliminates HIV-1 reservoirs and to determine if ART alone will extend remission times. Until these studies are completed, ART should be initiated as early as possible in infants and continued without interruption.

▶ In 2013, remission of human immunodeficiency virus type 1 (HIV-1) in a perinatally infected child called the "Mississippi Child" was reported. The child had received antiretroviral therapy (ART) between 30 hours and 18 months of age. He had remained persistently undetectable for HIV viremia for 12 months without HIV-specific immune responses.[1] HIV viremia remained undetectable at 21.9 months after the discontinuation of ART. However, at 27.6 months after discontinuation of ART and at age 46.4 months, the plasma viral load rebounded to 16 750 copies per milliliter. No acute retroviral or incident viral syndrome or vaccination had occured during this time. Epidemiological risk factors for reinfection were also absent. The HIV load dropped to 2658 copies 72 hours after the reinitiation of ART. The CD4 T cell increased to 43% and the CD4 to CD8 T-cell ratio normalized. At the time of viremic rebound, HIV-specific immune response was detected by enzyme-linked immunosorbent assay and Western blot testing. The return of HIV-1 viremia after a substantial period of quiescence is consistent with the development of long-lived resting memory CD4 T cells, leading to virologic latency. As has been reported before, early treatment may restrict, but not eradicate, HIV-1 reservoirs and continuation of treatment without interruption is prudent.[2]

N. Khardori, MD

References

1. Persaud D, Gay H, Ziemniak C, et al. Absence of detectable HIV-1 viremia after treatment cessation in an infant. *N Engl J Med.* 2013;369:1828-1835.
2. Rainwater-Lovett K, Luzuriaga K, Persaud D. Very early combination antiretroviral therapy in infants: prospects for cure. *Curr Opin HIV AIDS.* 2015;10:4-11.

A Case of Severe Ebola Virus Infection Complicated by Gram-Negative Septicemia

Kreuels B, Wichmann D, Emmerich P, et al (Inst for Clinical Chemistry and Laboratory Medicine, Hamburg, Germany; World Health Organization Collaborating Ctr for Arbovirus and Hemorrhagic Fever Reference and Research, Hamburg, Germany; et al)

N Engl J Med 371:2394-2401, 2014

Ebola virus disease (EVD) developed in a patient who contracted the disease in Sierra Leone and was airlifted to an isolation facility in Hamburg, Germany, for treatment. During the course of the illness, he had numerous complications, including septicemia, respiratory failure, and encephalopathy. Intensive supportive treatment consisting of high-volume fluid resuscitation (approximately 10 liters per day in the first 72 hours), broad-spectrum antibiotic therapy, and ventilatory support resulted in full recovery without the use of experimental therapies. Discharge was delayed owing to the detection of viral RNA in urine (day 30) and sweat (at the last assessment on day 40) by means of polymerase-chain-reaction (PCR) assay, but the last positive culture was identified in plasma on day 14 and in urine on day 26. This case shows the challenges in the management of EVD and suggests that even severe EVD can be treated effectively with routine intensive care.

▶ A Zaire Ebola virus (EBOV) epidemic of unprecedented scale in West Africa has been going on since December 2013. The public health emergency in the region has been augmented by high rates of infection among health care personnel, resulting in a substantial number of fatal cases.[1]

This article reports on a World Health Organization epidemiologist working in Sierra Leone who was airlifted to the unit for the treatment of highly contagious infections (UTHCI) in Hamburg, Germany, on day 10 of his illness. The measures of infection control in this unit are similar to those used in biosafety level 4 laboratories. The patient had received supportive care and antimicrobial therapy during the 10 days and was clinically stable at the time of transfer on day 10. On day 13, he developed fever, hypoxemia, tachycardia, shortness of breath, and abdominal pain suggestive of concomitant secondary peritonitis and sepsis related to gastrointestinal mucosal translocation of bacteria. The new severe systemic symptoms developed while the EBOV RNA load was declining. Blood cultures grew a Gram-negative organism that could not be further identified under the conditions of the UTHCI. Based on in vitro susceptibility, the patient was treated with meropenem. The patient developed multiple organ dysfunction including encephalopathy. He slowly improved and was transferred out of

UTHCI on day 28 and discharged home on day 40 after viral cultures of EBOV polymerase chain reaction–positive samples of body fluids had been free of infectious virus particles for 20 days. This patient did not receive any experimental therapies for EBOV and demonstrates successful treatment of severe EBOV disease with serious complications by general intensive care measures in the absence of new EBOV-specific therapies. Figure 3 in the original article gives detailed insight into the host-pathogen interactions in this patient.

N. Khardori, MD

Reference

1. Lamontagne F, Clement C, Fletcher T, Jacob ST, Fischer WA II, Fowler RA. Doing today's work superbly well—treating Ebola with current tools. *N Engl J Med.* 2014;371:1565-1566.

Assessment of the potential for international dissemination of Ebola virus via commercial air travel during the 2014 west African outbreak

Bogoch II, Creatore MI, Cetron MS, et al (Univ of Toronto, Ontario, Canada; St Michael's Hosp, Toronto, Ontario, Canada; Ctrs for Disease Control and Prevention, Atlanta, GA; et al)

Lancet 385:29-35, 2015

Background.—The WHO declared the 2014 west African Ebola epidemic a public health emergency of international concern in view of its potential for further international spread. Decision makers worldwide are in need of empirical data to inform and implement emergency response measures. Our aim was to assess the potential for Ebola virus to spread across international borders via commercial air travel and assess the relative efficiency of exit versus entry screening of travellers at commercial airports.

Methods.—We analysed International Air Transport Association data for worldwide flight schedules between Sept 1, 2014, and Dec 31, 2014, and historic traveller flight itinerary data from 2013 to describe expected global population movements via commercial air travel out of Guinea, Liberia, and Sierra Leone. Coupled with Ebola virus surveillance data, we modelled the expected number of internationally exported Ebola virus infections, the potential effect of air travel restrictions, and the efficiency of airport-based traveller screening at international ports of entry and exit. We deemed individuals initiating travel from any domestic or international airport within these three countries to have possible exposure to Ebola virus. We deemed all other travellers to have no significant risk of exposure to Ebola virus.

Findings.—Based on epidemic conditions and international flight restrictions to and from Guinea, Liberia, and Sierra Leone as of Sept 1, 2014 (reductions in passenger seats by 51% for Liberia, 66% for Guinea, and 85% for Sierra Leone), our model projects 2·8 travellers infected with Ebola virus departing the above three countries via commercial flights, on average, every month. 91 547 (64%) of all air travellers departing Guinea, Liberia, and Sierra Leone had expected destinations in low-income and lower-middle-income countries. Screening international travellers departing three airports would enable health assessments of all travellers at highest risk of exposure to Ebola virus infection.

Interpretation.—Decision makers must carefully balance the potential harms from travel restrictions imposed on countries that have Ebola virus activity against any potential reductions in risk from Ebola virus importations. Exit screening of travellers at airports in Guinea, Liberia, and Sierra Leone would be the most efficient frontier at which to assess the health status of travellers at risk of Ebola virus exposure, however, this intervention might require international support to implement effectively (Table 3).

▶ For only the third time in its history, the World Health Organization (WHO) declared a public health emergency of international concern (PHEIC) on August 8, 2014. The declaration was based on the unprecedented scale and

TABLE 3.—Top 20 Final Destination Countries of Individuals Initiating Air Travel from Within Guinea, Liberia, and Sierra Leone and Corresponding Indicators of Health System Capacity

			Health-System Capacity Measures (Global Rank Out of 191 Countries)			
	Traveller Volume*	Proportion of Total Volume (%)	Health-Care Expenditure per Head, US$†	Physicians per 1000 People†	Nurses and Midwives per 1000 People†	Hospital Beds per 1000 People†
Ghana	25 272	17·5%	83 (149)	0·1 (135)	0·9 (116)	0·9 (142)
Senegals	20 818	14·4%	51 (158)	0·1 (135)	0·4 (140)	0·3 (165)
UK	12 493	8·7%	3647 (20)	2·8 (42)	8·8 (23)	2·9 (69)
France	10 292	7·1%	4690 (14)	3·2 (31)	9·3 (19)	6·4 (15)
Gambia	9849	6·8%	26 (177)	0 (152)	0·6 (130)	1·1 (134)
Côte d'Ivoire	8266	5·7%	88 (147)	0·1 (135)	0·5 (136)	NA
Morocco	7574	5·2%	190 (119)	0·6 (104)	0·9 (116)	0·9 (142)
Belgium	5541	3·8%	4711 (13)	3 (34)	15·8 (4)	6·5 (13)
Nigeria	4182	2·9%	94 (144)	0·4 (110)	1·6 (100)	NA
China	4090	2·8%	322 (100)	1·9 (67)	1·9 (92)	3·8 (49)
Mali	3680	2·5%	42 (164)	0·1 (135)	0·4 (140)	0·1 (168)
USA	2927	2·0%	8895 (3)	2·5 (52)	9·8 (18)	2·9 (69)
India	2466	1·7%	61 (153)	0·7 (102)	1·7 (96)	0·7 (149)
Kenya	2392	1·7%	45 (162)	0·2 (122)	0·8 (121)	1·4 (123)
Germany	1825	1·3%	4683 (15)	3·8 (14)	11·5 (12)	8·2 (6)
Lebanon	1706	1·2%	675 (62)	3·2 (31)	2·7 (81)	3·5 (55)
South Africa	1558	1·1%	645 (64)	0·8 (99)	4·9 (55)	NA
Guinea-Bissau	1340	0·9%	30 (175)	0 (152)	0·6 (130)	1 (139)
Canada	1299	0·9%	5741 (8)	2·1 (61)	9·3 (19)	2·7 (75)
Italy	1293	0·9%	3032 (23)	4·1 (9)	0·3 (145)	3·4 (60)

NA = No data available.
*From Sept 1, 2013, to Dec 31, 2013.
†2007–12 estimates from World Bank.
Reprinted from Bogoch II, Creatore MI, Cetron MS, et al. Assessment of the potential for international dissemination of Ebola virus via commercial air travel during the 2014 west African outbreak. *Lancet.* 2015;385:29-35, with permission from Bogoch et al.

geographic range of the Ebola virus (EBV) epidemic in West Africa, the constrained public health infrastructure of affected countries, high fatality ratio and observed international spread to Nigeria, the most populous country in Africa. Alongside coordinated international action to control the epidemic at its source, uncoordinated unilateral actions have emerged, including controversial measures that ban travel and trade to and from affected countries.[1] The 2005 WHO International Health Regulations are to "prevent, protect against, control, and provide a public health response to the international spread of disease in ways that are commensurate with and restricted to public health risks and which avoid unnecessary interference with international traffic and trade." These are the guiding principles by which 196 participating countries are bound when responding to a PHEIC.

This study reports on the patterns of commercial air travel out of Guinea, Liberia, and Sierra Leone starting September 1, 2014, the areas deemed the most likely sources of exported EBV infections. Two complementary data sets from the International Air Transport Association were used for travel analyses. Table 3 shows the top 20 final destination countries of individuals initiating air travel from within Guinea, Libera, and Sierra Leone and corresponding indicators of health system capacity. The volume of international air traffic departing from these 3 countries was low. The model used in this study projects an average of 2.8 travelers infected with EBV departing from the 3 countries via commercial flights every month. The analyses presented show that exit screening at international points of departure would offer greater efficiency and might be simpler to operationalize than entry screening of all flights arriving from the affected countries directly. In contrast, entry screening at international airports to which no direct flights are arriving from affected countries is highly inefficient, especially if authorities are unable to easily identify which travelers originated from countries currently experiencing community-based EBV transmission. Based on the benefits of interconnectedness and the risks of interdependence that are deeply intertwined, public health intervention to global threats made by individual countries must use the best available evidence to be "commensurate with and restricted to public health risks and avoid unnecessary interference with international traffic and trade."

N. Khardori, MD

Reference

1. York G. *World Moves to Cut Off West Africa as Ebola Panic Intensifies.* Toronto (Ontario): Globe and Mail; 2014, http://www.theglobeandmail.com/life/health-and-fitness/health/ebola-hysteria-sweeps-africa/article20072025/. Accessed August 20, 2014.

16 Tuberculosis

Acquired Rifampicin Resistance in Thrice-Weekly Antituberculosis Therapy: Impact of HIV and Antiretroviral Therapy

Narendran G, Menon PA, Venkatesan P, et al (Natl Inst for Research in Tuberculosis (formerly Tuberculosis Research Centre), Chetpet, Chennai, India; et al)

Clin Infect Dis 59:1798-1804, 2014

Background.—Risk factors for acquired rifampicin resistance (ARR) in human immunodeficiency virus (HIV)/tuberculosis coinfection, in the highly active antiretroviral therapy (HAART) era, needs evaluation. We studied the impact of HIV and HAART on ARR among patients taking thrice-weekly antituberculosis therapy.

Methods.—This cross-protocol analysis included patients with newly diagnosed, rifampicin-susceptible pulmonary tuberculosis, with and without HIV, enrolled in clinical trials (who took >80% of medication) at the National Institute for Research in Tuberculosis between 1999 and 2013. All patients received rifampicin and isoniazid for 6 months reinforced with pyrazinamide and ethambutol in the first 2 months, given thrice-weekly throughout the study along with HAART in one of the groups. Outcomes were categorized and multivariate logistic regression analysis performed to identify risk factors for ARR.

Results.—The per-protocol results included patients with tuberculosis: 246 HIV-uninfected patients ($HIV^{-}TB^{+}$), 212 HIV patients not on HAART (non-HAART), and 116 HIV-infected patients on HAART. Median CD4 counts of the latter 2 groups were 150 and 93 cells/μL, respectively, and the median viral loads were 147 000 and 266 000 copies/mL, respectively. Compared with $HIV^{-}TB^{+}$, the relative risks (RRs) for an unfavorable response in the coinfected, non-HAART and HAART groups were 2.1 (95% confidence interval [CI], 1.7–14.8; $P < .0001$) and 2.1 (95% CI, .9–5.2; $P = .3$), whereas for ARR, the RRs were 21.1 (95% CI, 2.6–184; $P < .001$) and 8.2 (95% CI, .6–104; $P = .07$), respectively

Conclusions.—HIV-infected patients with tuberculosis treated with a thrice-weekly antituberculosis regimen are at a higher risk of ARR, compared with HIV-uninfected patients, in the presence of baseline isoniazid resistance. HAART reduces but does not eliminate the risk of ARR.

▶ The management of human immunodeficiency virus (HIV) disease in many parts of the world is complicated by the coexisting high prevalence of tuberculosis. The development of drug resistance in *Mycobacterium tuberculosis* is a major concern, especially in developing parts of the world.[1] In immunosuppressed AIDS patients, tuberculosis treatment regimens without rifampicin have shown inferior cure rates.[2] Because of the ability of rifampicin to destroy intracellular and intermittently growing *M. tuberculosis*, it is an indispensable part of treatment of HIV-associated tuberculosis despite drug-drug interaction with concomitant HIV therapy.

This cross-protocol analysis from southern India included patients with newly diagnosed rifampicin-susceptible pulmonary tuberculosis with and without HIV with 78% of adherence to medication enrolled in clinical trials between 1999 and 2013. All patients received rifampicin and isoniazid for 6 months with pyrazinamide and ethambutol in the first 2 months administered 3 times a week. A multivariate logistic regression analysis was performed to identify risk factors for acquired rifampicin resistance. This is a unique comparison of tuberculosis treatment outcomes from 3 groups of patients: HIV and MTB coinfection on highly active antiretroviral therapy (HAART), HIV, and MTB coinfection not on HAART and MTB without HIV coinfection. All 3 groups of patients were treated with an identical 3 times weekly antituberculosis therapy in the same setting. The study concludes that patients with HIV and MTB coinfection are at a higher risk of acquired resistance to rifampicin than the HIV-uninfected patients with tuberculosis while on a 3 times a week regimen for MTB infection especially in the presence of baseline isoniazid resistance. Everyday tuberculosis treatment regimens along with early diagnosis and treatment of HIV infection would be preferable in this cohort of patients to prevent amplification of drug resistance. The logistic challenges to everyday directly observed therapy are insurmountable and lead to the "compromise" alternate tuberculosis treatment regimens.

N. Khardori, MD

References

1. World Health Organization. *Global Tuberculosis Report 2013*. WHO; 2013, http://apps.who.int/iris/bistream/10665/91355/1/9789241564656_eng.pdf. Accessed January 31, 2014.
2. O'Donnel MM, Carvalho SS, Gadelha AJ, et al. Poor response to tuberculosis treatment with regimens without rifampicin in immunosuppressed AIDS in patients. *Braz J Infect Dis*. 2002;6:272-275.

Prevention of Anti–Tumor Necrosis Factor–Associated Tuberculosis: A 10-Year Longitudinal Cohort Study

Muñoz L, for the Prevention of Anti-TNF–Associated Tuberculosis Study Team of Bellvitge University Hospital (Bellvitge Univ Hospital–Institut d'investigació biomèdica de Bellvitge (IDIBELL), Barcelona, Spain; et al)
Clin Infect Dis 60:349-356, 2015

Background.—The extent to which anti–tumor necrosis factor (TNF)–associated tuberculosis can be prevented is unclear, and there is no established guidance on the optimal screening strategy for latent tuberculosis (LTBI) in patients about to start anti-TNF therapy. We aimed to determine the effectiveness of a comprehensive program for the prevention of anti-TNF–associated tuberculosis, and to evaluate 3 LTBI screening strategies and the need for retesting patients with negative results at baseline.

Methods.—In total, 726 patients were screened prior to anti-TNF therapy using 1 of 3 diagnostic strategies over 3 consecutive periods: first, a 2-step tuberculin skin test (TST); second, a 2-step TST plus QuantiFERON-TB Gold In-Tube test (QFT-GIT) (2-step TST/QFT); and third, a single-step TST plus QFT-GIT (TST/QFT). Infected patients were offered preventive therapy. We assessed differences in the incidence of tuberculosis between anti-TNF exposed and nonexposed patients, and between the 3 study periods.

Results.—Tuberculosis developed during the first year in 2.85 per 1000 exposed patient-years (3/1052 patient years) and 1.77 per 1000 nonexposed patient-years (1/566 patient-years). No cases occurred beyond the first year of treatment. LTBI diagnoses decreased with the single-step TST/QFT (26.5%) compared with the 2-step TST (42.5%; $P < .001$) and 2-step TST/QFT (38.5%; $P = .02$); the incidence of tuberculosis among exposed patients did not change significantly across the 3 periods (2.63/1000, 3.91/1000, and 2.4/1000 patient-years, respectively).

Conclusions.—Although anti-TNF–associated tuberculosis can be reduced, some risk remains during the first year of therapy. Neither the 2-step TST nor systematic retesting after negative baseline testing is justified.

► Biological response modifiers, especially tumor necrosis factor antagonists (anti-TNF), have improved the course of chronic immune-mediated inflammatory diseases (IMIDs). Their use, however, has been associated with an increase in the risk of granulomatous infectious disease such as tuberculosis and histoplasmosis. The risk of tuberculosis differs in various parts of the world depending on tuberculosis burden of each region.[1,2] The reported incidence is 522 cases per 100 000 in Spain compared with 24.6 cases per 100 000 in the United States. The monoclonal antibodies infliximab and adalimumab pose a higher risk than other agents. Tuberculosis associated with anti-TNF therapy is mostly due to reactivation of latent TB injection (LTBI) and can be prevented by screening and treatment prior to initiating treatment.

This is a 10-year prospective longitudinal observational cohost study conducted in Spain between 2003 and 2013 to define the role of comprehensive LTBI screening and treatment program in prevention, to determine the most optimal approach to diagnosis of LTBI, and to determine whether systematic retesting is necessary for patients with negative baseline LTBI screening. The findings show that anti-TNF—associated tuberculosis can be greatly reduced, but a small risk remains during the first year of treatment. The optimal testing approach in this study was the single-step tuberculin skin test (TST) plus QuantiFERON-TB Gold In-Tube test. Two-step TST approach is therefore no longer justified. Systematic periodic retesting for LTBI in patients with negative test results before anti-TNF therapy offered no benefit.

N. Khardori, MD

References

1. Keane J, Gershon S, Wise RP, et al. Tuberculosis associated with infliximab, a tumor necrosis factor alpha-neutralizing agent. *N Engl J Med.* 2001;345: 1098-1104.
2. Wallis RS, Broder MS, Wong JY, Hanson ME, Beenhouwer DO. Granulomatous infectious diseases associated with tumor necrosis factor antagonist. *Clin Infect Dis.* 2004;38:1261-1265.

Whole genome sequencing: A new paradigm in the surveillance and control of human tuberculosis

Hasnain SE, O'Toole RF, Grover S, et al (Indian Inst of Technology (IIT), Hauz Khas, New Delhi, India; Trinity College, Dublin, Ireland; et al)
Tuberculosis 95:91-94, 2015

Whole Genome Sequencing (WGS) is emerging as a very powerful tool for the management, outbreak analyses, surveillance and determining drug resistance of human infectious pathogens including *Mycobacterium tuberculosis* and MRSA. WGS can also discriminate relapse TB from re-infection and the resolution provided by WGS has no comparison to conventional technologies. With current cost coming down to <£70 per bacterial genome, WGS has emerged as an alternative to all the existing technologies put together. We discuss the advantage and disadvantages of WGS and whether it can become a point of care tool in not just developed countries but also in developing countries which have a huge TB burden. The likely utility of WGS for other pathogens and also in characterizing holobionts is also discussed (Box 1).

▶ Molecular techniques in diagnostic microbiology have made a significant impact on the early and specific diagnosis of infectious diseases. Unlike the methods that depend on in vitro cultivation, the turn around time is much faster, resulting in point of care testing. The genotypic methods are able to detect a microbial species and trace its epidemiology and also detect virulent genes and resistance genes. XpertMTB/RIF, a cartridge-based nucleic acid amplification assay provides simultaneous detection of *Mycobacterium tuberculosis* and rifampicin resistance directly from sputum in less than 2 hours. For the molecular typing of clinical isolates of *M. tuberculosis* complex, techniques used include restrictive fragment length polymorphism (RFLP), clustered regularly interspaced short palindromic repeats (CRISPR), and mycobacterial interspersed repetitive units (MIRU)—variable number tandem repeats (VNTR). The later method is considered the gold standard. However, all methods possess a number of intrinsic limitations.[1] Whole genome sequencing (WGS) overcomes many of these limitations. It was used for the first time with the dual purpose of ascertaining clustering of tuberculosis cases and quantification of active transmission. This review presents a discussion on the recent applications of WGS to diagnosis, treatment, and epidemiology of tuberculosis. It offers the capability to distinguish a tuberculosis relapse from reinfection, maps community outbreaks

Box 1: Advantages of WGS Over the Existing Most Powerful Genotyping Method

Technique Parameter	Diagnosis Time	Cost	Markers Covered	Detection of Specific Strains Diversity	Detection of Micro-Evolution During Outbreak	Drug Resistance Detection	Transmission and Tracking Bacterial Pathogen	Resolution of Relapse and Re-Infection Cases	Clustering	Genome Coverage
WGS	Few hours	<£70	Unlimited	More accurate	Provided	Yes	Real Time	High	Low	Whole genome
Traditional genotype method (MIRUVNTR)	2-3 days	<£135	Limited	Less accurate	Not provided	No	N/A	Low	High	Limited to variable region of genome

Reprinted from Hasnain SE, O'Toole RF, Grover S, et al. Whole genome sequencing: a new paradigm in the surveillance and control of human tuberculosis. *Tuberculosis* 2015;95:91-94, with permission from Elsevier.

of tuberculosis, and detects resistance to anti-tuberculosis drugs. Box 1 lists advantages of WGS over the existing genotyping methods. With the cost of WGS down to $100 per bacterial genome, it has the potential of becoming a point-of-care test in less resourceful countries, which carry a huge burden of tuberculosis. The authors also discuss present limitations in this technology, including the upfront cost of next-generation sequencing equipment. Once the limitations are addressed, WGS is likely to become multipurpose point-of-care cost-effective method of diagnosing and managing infectious diseases.

N. Khardori, MD

Reference

1. Comas I, Homolka S, Niemann S, Gagneux S. Genotyping of genetically monomorphic bacteria: DNA sequencing in mycobacterium tuberculosis highlights the limitations of current methodologies. *PLoS One*. 2009;4:e7815.

17 Clinical Diagnostics

MALDI-TOF MS for the Diagnosis of Infectious Diseases

Patel R (Mayo Clinic, Rochester, MN)

Clin Chem 61:100-111, 2015

Background.—First introduced into clinical microbiology laboratories in Europe, MALDI-TOF MS is being rapidly embraced by laboratories around the globe. Although it has multiple applications, its widespread adoption in clinical microbiology relates to its use as an inexpensive, easy, fast, and accurate method for identification of grown bacteria and fungi based on automated analysis of the mass distribution of bacterial proteins.

Content.—This review provides a historical perspective on this new technology. Modern applications in the clinical microbiology laboratory are reviewed with a focus on the most recent publications in the field. Identification of aerobic and anaerobic bacteria, mycobacteria, and fungi are discussed, as are applications for testing urine and positive blood culture bottles. The strengths and limitations of MALDI-TOF MS applications in clinical microbiology are also addressed.

Summary.—MALDI-TOF MS is a tool for rapid, accurate, and cost-effective identification of cultured bacteria and fungi in clinical microbiology. The technology is automated, high throughput, and applicable to a broad range of common as well as esoteric bacteria and fungi. MALDI-TOF MS is an incontrovertibly beneficial technology for the clinical microbiology laboratory.

► In parallel with advances in genomic diagnosis of infectious diseases, attempts to reduce the time to identification of bacteria and fungi have resulted in the use of proteomics technology. The possibility of using mass spectrometry for identification of bacteria was introduced in 1975.[1] Once the technology for the analysis of intact proteins was invented in 1980, it became more feasible to identify bacteria by this technology. Koichi Tanaka described a "soft desorption ionization" method for mass spectroscopic analysis of biological macromolecules in 1985 for which he was awarded the Nobel Prize in Chemistry.[2] The term "matrix-assisted laser desorption ionization" (MALDI) was coined when an organic compound matrix was used for soft desorption ionization. The development of well-validated comprehensive databases of mass spectra representing different types of bacteria and fungi allowed automation of MALDI-TOF MS, at which point it became a tool for the clinical microbiology laboratory. This extensive review takes the reader from historical perspective to the actual methodology and its performance in identification of aerobic bacteria, anaerobic bacteria, mycobacteria, and fungi. In addition, the laboratory workflow, cost-effectiveness, antimicrobial susceptibility testing, testing of positive blood culture bottles, and direct testing of clinical samples is reviewed. The review ends with current limitations and future prospects. Currently, the US Food and Drug Administration–cleared list of organisms that can be identified by this technology is limited to Gram-negative bacteria.

N. Khardori, MD

References

1. Anhalt J, Fenselau C. Identification of bacteria using mass spectrometry. *Anal Chem.* 1975;47:219-225.
2. Tanaka K. The origin of macromolecule ionization by laser irradiation (Lecture). In: Frangsmyr T, ed. *The Nobel Prizes 2002.* Stockholm, Sweden: Nobel Foundation; 2003.

A Comparison of Lyme Disease Serologic Test Results From 4 Laboratories in Patients With Persistent Symptoms After Antibiotic Treatment

Fallon BA, Pavlicova M, Coffino SW, et al (Columbia Univ, Palisades, NY)
Clin Infect Dis 59:1705-1710, 2014

Background.—As the incidence of Lyme disease (LD) has increased, a number of "Lyme specialty laboratories" have emerged, claiming singular expertise in LD testing. We investigated the degree of interlaboratory variability of several LD serologic tests—whole cell sonicate (WCS) enzyme-linked immunosorbent assay (ELISA), immunoglobulin M (IgM) and immunoglobulin G (IgG) Western blots (WBs), and an ELISA based on the conserved sixth region of variable major protein–like sequence expressed (C6)—that were performed at 1 university laboratory, 1 commercial laboratory, and 2 laboratories that specialize in LD testing.

Methods.—Serum samples from 37 patients with posttreatment Lyme syndrome, as well as 40 medically healthy controls without prior LD, were tested independently at the 4 laboratories.

Results.—In general, there was little difference among the laboratories in the percentage of positive test results on the ELISAs and IgG WBs, although the number of discordant results was often high. When in-house criteria for positivity were used at the 2 specialty laboratories, specificity at 1 laboratory declined considerably on both the IgM and IgG WBs. The Centers for Disease Control and Prevention (CDC) 2-tiered criteria improved overall concordance. At the 2 laboratories that performed the C6 ELISA, the percentage of positive tests was comparable to that of the WCS ELISA while providing higher specificity. The IgM WB performed poorly in our patient population of individuals with later-stage illness, a result consistent with previous studies.

Conclusions.—Although there was surprisingly little difference among the laboratories in percentage of positive results on most assays using

TABLE 1.—Number and Percentage of Positive Serologic Test Results and Discordant Pairs for 37 Posttreatment Lyme Syndrome Patients (University Reference Laboratory Versus Commercial and Lyme Specialty Laboratories)

Test	University Reference Laboratory	Commercial Laboratory			Specialty Laboratory A			Specialty Laboratory B		
	No. Positive[a] (%)	No. Positive[a] (%)	*P* Value	Discordant Pairs	No. Positive[b] (%)	*P* Value	Disc Pairs	No. Positive[c] (%)	*P* Value	Disc Pairs
?/+ ELISA	23 (62.2)	25 (67.6)	.773	12	25 (67.6)	.789	14	25 (67.6)	.724	8
C6 ELISA	...	...	...	...	25 (67.6)	...	...	23 (62.2)	...	...
WB IgM (CDC)	8 (21.6)	6 (16.2)	.724	8	1 (2.7)	.016	7	16 (43.2)	.027	10
WB IgM (laboratory)	...	...	...	...	1 (2.7)	.016	7[d]	23 (62.2)	<.001	15[d]
WB IgG (CDC)	21 (56.8)	16 (43.2)	.074	5	16 (43.2)	.074	5	18 (48.6)	.250	3
WB IgG (laboratory)	...	...	...	...	14 (37.8)	.016	7[d]	26 (70.3)	.131	7[d]
2-tier: ?/+ ELISA & WB IgG	18 (48.6)	15 (40.5)	.250	3	14 (37.8)	.220	6	16 (43.2)	.688	6
2-tier: C6 ELISA & WB IgG	...	...	...	...	15 (40.5)	...	...	17 (45.9)	...	...
2-tier: ?/+ ELISA & C6 ELISA	...	...	...	...	22 (59.5)	...	...	18 (48.6)	...	...

Abbreviations: ?/+, indeterminate/positive; CDC, Centers for Disease Control and Prevention; ELISA, enzyme-linked immunosorbent assay; IgG, immunoglobulin G; IgM, immunoglobulin M; WB, Western blot.

[a]The university-based reference laboratory and commercial laboratory used CDC criteria for all WB tests. Criteria for a positive IgM WB were ≥2 of the following bands: Osp C, 39, 41. Criteria for a positive IgG WB were ≥5 of the following bands: 18, Osp C, 28, 30, 39, 41, 45, 58, 66, 93.

[b]In-house laboratory criteria for a positive IgM WB at Specialty Laboratory Awere ≥2 of the following bands: 23, 39, 41, 83/93. Criteria for a positive IgG WB were ≥3 of the following bands: 20, 23, 31, 34, 35, 39, 83/93.

[c]In-house laboratory criteria for a positive IgM WB at Specialty Laboratory B were ≥2 of the following bands: 23–25, 31, 34, 39, 41, 83/93. Criteria for a positive IgG WB were ≥2 of the following bands: 23–25, 31, 34, 39, 41, 83/93.

[d]Results using in-house criteria at Specialty Laboratories A and B were compared with results using CDC criteria at the university-based reference laboratory.

Reprinted from Fallon BA, Pavlicova M, Coffino SW, et al. A comparison of lyme disease serologic test results from 4 laboratories in patients with persistent symptoms after antibiotic treatment. *Clin Infect Dis.* 2014;59:1705-1710, with permission from The Author.

TABLE 2.—Number and Percentage of False-Positive Serologic Test Results and Discordant Pairs for 40 Medically Healthy Controls (University Reference Laboratory Versus Commercial and Lyme Specialty Laboratories)

Test	University Reference Laboratory No. Positive[a] (%)	Commercial Laboratory No. Positive[a] (%)	Commercial Laboratory *P* Value	Commercial Laboratory Disc Pairs	Specialty Laboratory A No. Positive[a] (%)	Specialty Laboratory A *P* Value	Specialty Laboratory A Disc Pairs	Specialty Laboratory B No. Positive[a] (%)	Specialty Laboratory B *P* Value	Specialty Laboratory B Disc Pairs
?/+ ELISA	5 (12.5)	3 (7.5)	.683	6	1 (2.5)	.125	4	3 (7.5)	.683	6
C6 ELISA	...	...	...	...	0	...	...	0	...	...
WB IgM (CDC)	5 (12.5)	0	.074	5	1 (2.5)	.125	4	8 (20.0)	.505	9
WB IgM (laboratory)	...	...	...	...	1 (2.5)	.125[b]	4	15 (37.5)	.024	16[b]
WB IgG (CDC)	1 (2.5)	0	1.00	1	0	1.00	1	3 (7.5)	.480	2
WB IgG (laboratory)	...	...	...	...	0	1.00[b]	1	11 (27.5)	.004	10[b]
2-tier: ?/+ ELISA & WB IgG	0	0	...	0	0	...	0	1 (2.5)	1.000	1
2-tier: C6 ELISA & WB IgG	...	...	...	...	0	...	...	0	...	...
2-tier: ?/+ ELISA & C6 ELISA	...	...	...	...	0	...	...	0	...	...
+ WB IgM or IgG (CDC)	5 (12.5)	0	.074	5	1 (2.5)	.133	4	10 (25.0)	.182	9
+WB IgM or IgG (laboratory)					1 (2.5)	.133	4	23 (57.5)	<.001	22

Abbreviations: ?/+, indeterminate/positive; CDC, Centers for Disease Control and Prevention; Disc pairs, discordant pairs; ELISA, enzyme-linked immunosorbent assay; IgG, immunoglobulin G; IgM, immunoglobulin M; WB, Western blot.

[a]Criteria for a positive test are given in Table 1.

[b]Results using in-house criteria at Specialty Laboratories A and B were compared with results using CDC criteria at the university-based reference laboratory.

Reprinted from Fallon BA, Pavlicova M, Coffino SW, et al. A comparison of lyme disease serologic test results from 4 laboratories in patients with persistent symptoms after antibiotic treatment. *Clin Infect Dis.* 2014;59:1705-1710, with permission from The Author.

CDC criteria, interlaboratory variability was considerable and remains a problem in LD testing (Tables 1 and 2).

▶ The Centers for Disease Control and Prevention in collaboration with a group of university-based researchers, established a paradigm in 1995 as the standard for performing and interpreting Lyme disease serologies in the United States.[1] This 2-tier system of enzyme-linked immunosorbent assay followed by Western blot has a number of shortcomings, including the false impression that there is a delay in the human immune response to *Borrelia burgdorferi*. The fact is that the immune response to *B. burgdorferi* is similar to that of other infections. A specific immunoglobulin (Ig) M response is detectable within 7 days of infection, and IgG response is a few days later.[2] Based on the use of whole cultured *B. burgdorferi* recombinant proteins or single-peptide antigens, fundamental issues of sensitivity and specificity of all current Lyme disease serological tests remain problematic. In the meantime, a number of "Lyme specialty laboratories" have emerged.

In this study, serum samples from 37 patients with posttreatment Lyme syndrome and 40 healthy controls were tested independently at a general commercial laboratory and 2 laboratories that specialize in Lyme disease testing. Based on the results shown in Table 1 and Table 2, the level of discordance is high among laboratories. For a select group of patients, the clinicians may consider sending patient serum samples to a second laboratory if Lyme disease is highly suspected. It is important to remember that the positive predictive value of a test declines when specificity is poor, clinical history is not consistent with Lyme disease, and there is no exposure to a Lyme-endemic area.[3]

N. Khardori, MD

References

1. Centers for Disease Control and Prevention. Recommendations for test performance and interpretation from the second national conference on serologic diagnosis of Lyme disease. *MMWR Morb Mortal Wkly Rep.* 1995;44:590-591.
2. Augero-Rosenfeld ME, Nowakowski J, Bittker S, Cooper D, Nadelman RB, Wormser GP. Evolution of the serologic response to Borrelia Burgdorferi in treated patients with culture-confirmed erythema migrans. *J Clin Microbiol.* 1996;34:1-9.
3. Wormser GP, Carbonato C, Miller S, et al. A limitation of 2-stage serological testing for Lyme disease: enzyme immunoassay and immunoblot assay are not independent test. *Clin Infect Dis.* 2000;30:545-548.

18 Health Care Associated Infections

Toward a True Bacteriotherapy for *Clostridium difficile* Infection

Rupnik M (Univ of Maribor, Slovenia; et al)

N Engl J Med 372:1566-1568, 2015

Background.—*Clostridium difficile* is a common pathogen reported in nosocomial infections and is associated with disturbed intestinal microbial status. Research into how the microbiota changes during *C. difficile* infection has sought to define changes in species diversity and to identify the mechanisms underlying microbiota-associated protection against such an infection. Advances have been made in these areas.

Microbiota Changes.—Healthy gut microbiota contain many microorganisms, many different species, and higher levels of some types than of others. Disrupting these features can alter gut status from healthy to dysfunctional. As a result *C. difficile* infection can occur, eventually producing toxins that cause intestinal and inflammatory symptoms. Different antibiotics affect bacteria in different ways.

Protective Mechanisms.—Protective mechanisms are not linked to high or low bacterial diversity. In tests conducted in humans and mice, some bacteria conveyed resistance only in mice, some only in humans, and some to both. The four bacterial species with the strongest associations with resistance to infection in one study were tested individually or combined to determine their performance. The combination of the four protected animals from *C. difficile* and all the animals survived. One of the four, *C. scindens*, provided slightly inferior protection compared to that produced by the combination.

To identify the mechanism by which *C. scindens* provides protection, research focused on the life cycle and requirements of *C. difficile*. The effects of various bile acids on spore germination differ, with just a small proportion of gut bacteria, including *C. scindens*, able to convert stimulatory combinations of bile acids into inhibitory combinations of bile acid. This is likely to be the mechanism by which *C. scindens* produces resistance to infection.

Conclusions.—Analysis of the research to date indicates that combining different species of bacteria with various modes of action against *C. difficile* is probably a more effective strategy than relying on a single species to provide resistance to infection. This approach may further the use of

bacteriotherapy, in which fecal matter from a healthy donor is suspended in solution and injected into the patient's intestinal tract.

▶ The restoration of gut microbiota is now an accepted method of treating patients with multiple relapses of *Clostridium difficile* infection.[1] The procedure is called by multiple names, including fecal transplantation, fecal replacement, fecal microbiota transplantation, and bacteriotherapy. Scientific attempts have been made to define changes in species diversity and understand the mechanism leading to microbiota-associated protection against *C. difficile* infection.

The article describes clinical implications of basic research published recently that represents an advance on both fronts.[2] The authors in this study analyzed gut microbiota in both mice and humans. Disruption of any of the 3 features of gut microbiota results in increased growth of *C. difficile*. Once the vegetative cells of *C. difficile* reach a large number, they produce toxins A and B, resulting in symptomatic *C. difficile* infection. Bile acids in the gut signal the spore that it is in the anaerobic conditions of the intestinal tract resulting in germination of the spore. Various antibiotic classes have different effects on the composition of the gut microbiota, but the actual numbers of bacterial cell do not change in antibiotic-treated mice. By combining mathematical modeling approaches with data on composition of gut microbiota in humans and mice with established toxin-induced *C. difficile* disease, they found 3 bacterial species were associated with resistance to *C. difficile* infection in both humans and mice, and others had the same effect in only humans or mice. They tested 4 bacterial species individually or in combination in a mouse model for their protective activity against *C. difficile*. One of the species, *Clostridium scindens*, provided protection only slightly inferior to that provided by the combination. A few species in the microbiota, including *C. scindens*, can convert stimulatory combinations of bile acids into inhibitory combinations, which may be mechanism through which *C. scindens* mediates resistance to *C. difficile* infection in mice. Combining different species of bacteria with differing modes of action may be better if these data are duplicated in humans.

N. Khardori, MD

References

1. Adamu BO, Lawley TD. Bacteriotherapy for the treatment of intestinal dysbiosis caused by *Clostridium difficile* infection. *Curr Opin Microbiol*. 2013;16:596-601.
2. Buffie CG, Bucci V, Stein RR, et al. Precision microbiome reconstitution restores bile acid mediated resistance to *Clostridium difficile*. *Nature*. 2015;517:205-208.

Association Between Prehospital Vitamin D Status and Hospital-Acquired *Clostridium difficile* Infections

Quraishi SA, Litonjua AA, Moromizato T, et al (Massachusetts General Hosp, Boston; Brigham and Women's Hosp, Boston, MA; et al)
JPEN J Parenter Enteral Nutr 39:47-55, 2015

Objective.—To investigate whether preadmission 25-hydroxyvitamin D (25(OH)D) levels are associated with the risk of hospital-acquired Clostridium difficile infection (HACDI).

Materials and Methods.—Our retrospective cohort study focused on 568 adult patients from 2 Boston teaching hospitals between August 1993 and November 2006. All patients had 25(OH)D levels measured before hospitalization and were at risk for HACDI (defined as the presence of C difficile toxin A or B in stool samples obtained >48 hours after hospitalization). We performed multivariable regression analyses to test the association of prehospital 25(OH)D levels with HACDI while adjusting for clinically relevant covariates.

Results.—In these 568 patients, mean (SD) 25(OH)D level was 19 (12) ng/mL, and 11% of patients met criteria for incident HACDI. Following adjustment for age, sex, race (nonwhite vs white), patient type (medical vs surgical), and Deyo-Charlson index, patients with 25(OH)D levels <10 ng/mL had higher odds of HACDI (odds ratio [OR], 2.90; 95% confidence interval [CI], 1.01–8.34) compared with patients with 25(OH)D levels ≥30 ng/mL. When patients with HACDI were analyzed relative to a larger patient cohort without HACDI (n = 5047), those with 25(OH)D levels <10 ng/mL (OR, 4.96; 95% CI, 1.84–13.38) and 10–19.9 ng/mL (OR, 3.36; 95% CI, 1.28–8.85) had higher adjusted odds of HACDI compared with patients with 25(OH)D levels ≥30 ng/mL.

Conclusions.—In our cohort of adult patients, vitamin D status before hospital admission was inversely associated with the risk of developing HACDI. These data support the need for randomized, controlled trials to test the role of vitamin D supplementation to prevent HACDI.

▶ The past decade has seen a 3-fold increase in the incidence of hospital-acquired *Clostridium difficile* infections (HACDIs) in the United States. In addition to excess annual health care expenditure and increased average length of stay, 15 000 potentially avoidable deaths occur each year among the 350 000 new cases.[1,2] National guidelines for prevention of transmission, conventional and newer treatment modalities including fecal transplantation have not decreased the incidence. Known risk factors include systemic antibiotic exposure, older age, and procedures involving the gastrointestinal tract. There is controversial evidence about the role of H2 blockers and proton pump inhibitors through their acid suppressant effects. The role of common immunomodulatory factors is unknown. Recent evidence suggests that vitamin D levels may play an important role in susceptibility to hospital-acquired infections through its regulatory effect on innate and adaptive immunity.[3,4] The prevalence of suboptimal levels of 25-hydroxyvitamin D is high in the general population.

This 2-center retrospective cohort study of hospitalized adult patients reports on the association of developing HACDIs and vitamin D levels. Patients in whom vitamin D level was measured within 1 year of hospitalization (1993-2006) at 2 acute care hospitals were included. Research Patient Data Registry, a computerized registry that serves as a central data warehouse for all inpatient and outpatient records at the 2 hospitals, was used. Figure 1 in the original article shows the vitamin D status vs risk of HACDI. The authors hypothesize that 25(OH)D levels > 30 ng/mL may attenuate the effect of barrier site disruption characteristic of HACDI through optimal expression of endogenous antimicrobial peptides.

N. Khardori, MD

References

1. Dubberke E. *Clostridium difficile* infection: the scope of the problem. *J Hosp Med.* 2012;7:S1-S4.
2. Centers for Disease Control and Prevention (CDC). Vital signs: preventing *Clostridium difficile* infections. *MMWR Morb Mortal Wkly Rep.* 2012;6:157-162.
3. Adams JS, Hewison M. Unexpected actions of vitamin D: new perspectives on the regulation of innate and adaptive immunity. *Nat Clin Pract Endocrinol Metab.* 2008;4:80-90.
4. Youssef DA, Ranasinghe T, Grant WB, Peiris AN. Vitamin D's potential to reduce the risk of hospital-acquired infections. *Dermatoendocrinol.* 2012;4:167-175.

Colonization With Toxinogenic *C. difficile* Upon Hospital Admission, and Risk of Infection: A Systematic Review and Meta-Analysis

Zacharioudakis IM, Zervou FN, Pliakos EE, et al (Warren Alpert Med School of Brown Univ, Providence, RI)

Am J Gastroenterol 110:381-390, 2015

Objectives.—It has been suggested that colonization with *C. difficile* protects from infection. Nevertheless, the association between carriage of toxinogenic strains and ensuing *C. difficile* infections (CDIs) has not been studied.

Methods.—We searched PubMed and EMBASE databases up to 20 June 2014, using the term "difficile". Our primary outcomes of interest included the prevalence of isolation of toxinogenic *C. difficile* or its toxins from asymptomatic patients on hospital admission through stool or rectal swab testing and the risk of ensuing infection among colonized and noncolonized patients. Data on previous hospitalization, antibiotic, and proton pump inhibitor (PPI) use and prior CDIs among colonized and noncolonized patients were also extracted.

Results.—Nineteen out of 26,081 studies on 8,725 patients were included. The pooled prevalence of toxinogenic *C. difficile* colonization was 8.1% (95% confidence interval (CI) 5.7−11.1%), with an increasing trend over time ($P = 0.003$), and 10.0% (95% CI 7.1−13.4%) among North American studies. Patients colonized upon hospital admission had a 5.9 times higher risk of subsequent CDIs compared with noncolonized patients (relative risk (RR) 5.86; 95% CI 4.21−8.16). The risk of CDI for colonized patients was 21.8% (95% CI 7.9−40.1%), which was significantly higher than that of noncolonized patients (3.4%; 95% CI 1.5−6.0%; $P = 0.03$), with an attributable risk of 18.4%. History of hospitalization during the previous 3 months was associated with a higher risk of colonization (RR 1.63; 95% CI 1.13−2.34), as opposed to previous antibiotic (RR 1.07; 95% CI 0.75−1.53) and PPI use (RR 1.44; 95% CI

0.94–2.23), as well as history of CDI (RR 1.45; 95% CI 0.66–3.18) that had no impact.

Conclusions.—Over 8% of admitted patients are carriers of toxinogenic *C. difficile* with an almost 6 times higher risk of infection. These findings update current knowledge regarding the contribution of colonization in CDI epidemiology and stress the importance of preventive measures toward colonized patients.

▶ *Clostridium difficile* surveillance is included in the Center for Disease Control and Prevention's (CDC's) emerging infections program (EIP). The CDC performed an active population and laboratory-based surveillance in 2011 across 10 geographic areas in the United States to identify cases of *C. difficile* infection.[1] The surveillance was conducted at 10 EIP sites across 34 counties (population approximately 11.2 million) for the entire calendar year. All *C. difficile*–positive test results from 88 inpatient and 33 outpatient laboratories serving residents in surveillance areas were identified. A case was defined as a positive result on a *C. difficile* toxin or molecular assay of a stool specimen obtained from a resident at least 1 year of age who had not had a positive assay in the previous 8 weeks (to exclude incident infection). This active surveillance estimated that about half a million infections occurred in the United States in 2011.[2] An estimated 29 000 died and 83 000 had a recurrence. The findings also support the growing evidence that *C. difficile* is no longer restricted to acute care settings. The incidence was higher among females, whites, and persons aged 65 years or older. Only 24% of cases occurred in hospital settings, and an estimated 345 000 occurred outside the hospitals. Although roughly 46.2% of outside the hospital cases were community-associated by definition, 82% reported that they had visited outpatient health care settings such as doctors or dentists offices in the 12 weeks before collection of the positive stool specimen.

This study reports on the role of asymptomatic carriers of toxigenic strains admitted to the hospital who are not targeted by infection control policies. This systematic review and meta-analysis shows that a significant and increasing burden of toxinogenic *C. difficile* is imported into the hospitals. Toxinogenic *C. difficile* colonization was demonstrated in 8.1% overall and 10% among North American studies with a 6 times higher risk of subsequent infection. The only factor that was found to confer risk for carriage is exposure to the hospital environment within the previous 3 months, providing a high-risk population for potential screening programs. The findings support the hypothesis that the use of antibiotics and PPIs does not contribute to the establishment of colonization but to the progression from carrier state to infection. Given the association between carriage and infection in the epidemiology of *C. difficile*, the identification of carriers on admission and implementation of infection control policies targeted to this population is indicated. The colonization status had a significant association with hospitalization during the preceding 3 months and therefore would serve as a screening tool.

N. Khardori, MD

References

1. Lessa FC, Mu Y, Bamberg WM, et al. Burden of *Clostridium difficile* infection in the United States. *N Engl J Med.* 2015;372:825-834.
2. Chitnis AS, Holzbaur SM, Belflower RM, et al. Epidemiology of community-associated *Clostridium difficile* infection, 2009 through 2011. *JAMA Intern Med.* 2013;173:1359-1367.

19 New Antibiotics

A new antibiotic kills pathogens without detectable resistance
Ling LL, Schneider T, Peoples AJ, et al (NovoBiotic Pharmaceuticals, Cambridge, MA; Univ of Bonn, Germany; et al)
Nature 517:455-459, 2015

Antibiotic resistance is spreading faster than the introduction of new compounds into clinical practice, causing a public health crisis. Most antibiotics were produced by screening soil microorganisms, but this limited resource of cultivable bacteria was overmined by the 1960s. Synthetic approaches to produce antibiotics have been unable to replace this platform. Uncultured bacteria make up approximately 99% of all species in external environments, and are an untapped source of new antibiotics. We developed several methods to grow uncultured organisms by cultivation *in situ* or by using specific growth factors. Here we report a new antibiotic that we term teixobactin, discovered in a screen of uncultured bacteria. Teixobactin inhibits cell wall synthesis by binding to a highly conserved motif of lipid II (precursor of peptidoglycan) and lipid III (precursor of cell wall teichoic acid). We did not obtain any mutants of *Staphylococcus aureus* or *Mycobacterium tuberculosis* resistant to teixobactin. The properties of this compound suggest a path towards developing antibiotics that are likely to avoid development of resistance (Table 1).

► It is difficult to imagine the continuation and success of recent advances in medicine without the contribution of antimicrobial agents. The emergence of antibiotic resistance threatens what has already been accomplished as well as further advances. The most revealing way of describing the impact of antibiotic resistance on human health is to say that the toll of antibiotic-resistant infections is much greater than the toll of epidemic diseases such as human immunodeficiency virus infection or Ebola virus disease. The highly successful era of mid-20th-century screening cultures of soil-derived organisms such as *Streptomyces* for inhibitory/killing activity against other bacteria led to the development of antibiotics against various classes of bacteria. With antibiotic resistance increasing by the 1990s and soil-derived sources exhausting, alternate methodology for antibiotic discovery programs was sought. The use of genomics, high-tech chemical approaches, and high-throughput screening proved expensive and inefficient.

This basic science research goes back to harvesting soil bacteria to screen them for antibiotic production. However, the method of cultivation is drastically different from the conventional in vitro plate culture. The methodology is based on the

TABLE 1.—Activity of Teixobactin Against Pathogenic Microorganisms

Organism and Genotype	Teixobactin MIC ($\mu g\ ml^{-1}$)
S. aureus (MSSA)	0.25
S. aureus +10% serum	0.25
S. aureus (MRSA)	0.25
Enterococcus faecalis (VRE)	0.5
Enterococcus faecium (VRE)	0.5
Streptococcus pneumoniae (penicillin^R)	≤0.03
Streptococcus pyogenes	0.06
Streptococcus agalactiae	0.12
Viridans group streptococci	0.12
B. anthracis	≤0.06
Clostridium difficile	0.005
Propionibacterium acnes	0.08
M. tuberculosis H37Rv	0.125
Haemophilus influenzae	4
Moraxella catarrhalis	2
Escherichia coli	25
Escherichia coli (asmB1)	2.5
Pseudomonas aeruginosa	>32
Klebsiella pneumoniae	>32

The MIC was determined by broth microdilution. MSSA, methicillin-sensitive *S. aureus*; VRE, vancomycin-resistant enterococci.

Reprinted from Ling LL, Schneider T, Peoples AJ, et al. A new antibiotic kills pathogens without detectable resistance. *Nature*. 2015;517:455-459, with permission from Macmillan Publishers Limited.

fact that 99% of all species in the external environment do not grow under laboratory conditions.[1] The investigators have previously developed several methods to propagate these uncultivable bacteria through cultivation in their natural environments. In this study, they report the use of a multichannel device, the iChip, to simultaneously isolate and grow unculturable bacteria.[2] In the process, they describe a new genus related to *Aquabacterium* (Gram-negative organism) that produce a new cell wall inhibitor, teixobactin. Teixobactin has broad-spectrum activity against Gram-positive pathogens including antibiotic resistant strains (Table 1) with low minimum inhibitory concentrations (MICs). The susceptible organisms include *Staphylococci, Streptococci, Enterococci, Clostridium difficile, Bacillus anthracis*, and *Mycobacterium tuberculosis*. Resistance to teixobactin could not be induced in *Streptococcus aureus* or *Mycobacterium tuberculosus* after serial passage in the presence of sub-MIC levels of the drug. No toxicity was demonstrated against 2 mammalian cell lines at the highest dose tested. Even though the current clinical need is for antibiotics against resistant Gram-negative bacteria, this technology and report brings a ray of light to otherwise grim prospect of continuing antibiotic resistance.

N. Khardori, MD

References

1. Lewis K. Platforms for antibiotic discovery. *Natue Rev Drug Discov.* 2013;12: 371-387.
2. Nichols D, Cahoon N, Trakhtenberg EM, et al. Use of iChip for high throughput in situ cultivation of "uncultivable" microbial species. *Appl Environ Microbiol.* 2010;76:2445-2450.

20 Miscellaneous

An enteric virus can replace the beneficial function of commensal bacteria

Kernbauer E, Ding Y, Cadwell K (New York Univ School of Medicine; New York Presbyterian Hosp; et al)

Nature 516:94-98, 2015

Intestinal microbial communities have profound effects on host physiology. Whereas the symbiotic contribution of commensal bacteria is well established, the role of eukaryotic viruses that are present in the gastrointestinal tract under homeostatic conditions is undefined. Here we demonstrate that a common enteric RNA virus can replace the beneficial function of commensal bacteria in the intestine. Murine norovirus (MNV) infection of germ-free or antibiotic treated mice restored intestinal morphology and lymphocyte function without inducing overt inflammation and disease. The presence of MNV also suppressed an expansion of group 2 innate lymphoid cells observed in the absence of bacteria, and induced transcriptional changes in the intestine associated with immune development and type I interferon (IFN) signalling. Consistent with this observation, the IFN-a receptor was essential for the ability of MNV to compensate for bacterial depletion. Importantly, MNV infection offset the deleterious effect of treatment with antibiotics in models of intestinal injury and pathogenic bacterial infection. These data indicate that eukaryotic viruses have the capacity to support intestinal homeostasis and shape mucosal immunity, similarly to commensal bacteria.

► The role of symbiotic commensal (resident) bacteria in the gastrointestinal tract in maintaining host physiology is well established.[1] However, the role of eukaryotic viruses present in the gastrointestinal tract under homeostatic conditions is undefined.[2,3] Recent deep sequencing efforts reveal the existence of a complex enteric virome.[4] The viral component of the microbiome could include pathogens such as noroviruses that continue to persist after the disease is resolved. Members of the *Anelloviridae* and *Circoviridae* families are ubiquitously detected in healthy individuals as are uncharacterized viruses that display little sequence identify with known viruses. Murine norovirus (MNV) of the *Calciviridae* family is endemic in mouse facilities, displays tropism for myeloid cells and can establish persistent infection without obvious disease in immunocompetent mice. The observation that MNV induces inflammatory pathologies in mice genetically susceptible to inflammatory bowel disease resembles the effects of commensal bacteria. The bacterial component of the microbiota, however, provides considerable benefit to the host by generating metabolites, promoting the development of mucosal immune system and preventing colonization by pathogenic bacteria. Whether eukaryotic viruses in the gastrointestinal tract interact with the host in an analogous symbiotic manner is not known.

This study has used a germ-free mouse model to determine whether infection with MNV can provide developmental cues similar to those attributed to the bacteria. The findings provide evidence that the presence of known or unidentified viruses may be beneficial during periods after the administration of antibacterials as well as during development or recovery stages when the immune system and the intestinal microbiota are vulnerable.

N. Khardori, MD

References

1. Honda K, Littman DR. The microbiome in infectious disease and inflammation. *Annu Rev Immunol.* 2012;30:759-795.
2. Duerkop BA, Hooper LV. Resident viruses and their interactions with the immune system. *Nature Immunol.* 2013;14:654-659.
3. Virgin HW. The virome in mammalian physiology and disease. *Cell.* 2014;157: 142-150.
4. Norman JM, Handley SA, Virgin HW. Kingdom-agnostic metagenomics and the importance of complete characterization of enteric microbial communities. *Gastroenterology.* 2014;146:1459-1469.

Do Human Extraintestinal *Escherichia coli* Infections Resistant to Expanded-Spectrum Cephalosporins Originate From Food-Producing Animals? A Systematic Review

Lazarus B, Paterson DL, Mollinger JL, et al (The Univ of Queensland, Herston, Australia; Biosecurity Sciences Laboratory, Coopers Plains, Queensland, Australia; et al)

Clin Infect Dis 60:439-452, 2015

To find out whether food-producing animals (FPAs) are a source of extraintestinal expanded-spectrum cephalosporin-resistant *Escherichia coli* (ESCR-EC) infections in humans, Medline, Embase, and the Cochrane Database of Systematic Reviews were systematically reviewed. Thirty-four original, peer-reviewed publications were identified for inclusion. Six molecular epidemiology studies supported the transfer of resistance via whole bacterium transmission (WBT), which was best characterized among poultry in the Netherlands. Thirteen molecular epidemiology studies supported transmission of resistance via mobile genetic elements, which demonstrated greater diversity of geography and host FPA. Seventeen molecular epidemiology studies did not support WBT and two did not support mobile genetic element–mediated transmission. Four observational epidemiology studies were consistent with zoonotic transmission. Overall, there is evidence that a proportion of human extraintestinal ESCR-EC infections originate from FPAs. Poultry, in particular, is probably a source, but the quantitative and geographical extent of the problem is unclear and requires further investigation.

▶ A number of studies have suggested that the use of antibiotics in food-producing animals (FPAs) directly correlates to the emergence of extended-spectrum cephalosporin-resistant *Escherichia coli* (ESCR-EC) within animal populations.[1] The past decade has seen global spread, rapidly rising incidence, and increased mortality associated with infections caused by ESCR-EC along with a shift from healthcare associated to community acquired infections. The source of ESCR-EC for human infections has been controversial.[2] Ingestion of contaminated meat has been hypothesized to lead to widespread transmission of resistant bacteria between FPAs and humans.

This is a systematic review of published literature on the role of FPAs in human infections caused by ESCR-EC. Molecular epidemiology studies were reviewed to determine the transfer of resistance via whole bacterium transmission (WBT), mobile genetic elements-mediated transmission, and zoonotic transmission. This extensive review of worldwide research concludes that there is evidence for a proportion of human extraintestinal ESCR-EC infection originating from FPAs. It is more likely that the source appears to be poultry compared with other FPAs. Transmission occurs by both whole bacteria and mobile genetic elements, but the specific parameters, magnitude, and geographic extent of the problem are not clear at this point. Whole-genome sequencing may be the most sound and cost-effective method of conducting molecular epidemiological analysis. A broader sampling including environmental and human commensal samples would add to the applicability of the database.

N. Khardori, MD

References

1. Cavaco LM, Abatih E, Aarestrup FM, Guardabassi L. Selection and persistence of CTX-M producing Escherichia coli in the intestinal flora of pigs treated with amoxicillin, ceftiofur, or cefquinome. *Antimicrob Agents Chemother.* 2008;52:3612-3616.
2. Ewers C, Bethe A, Semmler T, Guenther S, Wieler LH. Extended spectrum beta-lactamase-producing and AmpC-producing *Escherichia coli* from livestock and companion animals, and their putative impact on public health: a global perspective. *Clin Microbiol Infect.* 2012;18:646-655.

Decolonization of Children After Incision and Drainage for MRSA Abscess: A Retrospective Cohort Study

Finnell SME, Rosenman MB, Christenson JC, et al (Indiana Univ School of Medicine, Indianapolis; et al)

Clin Pediatr 54:445-450, 2015

Background/Purpose.—Whether decolonization following incision and drainage (I&D) for methicillin-resistant *Staphylococcus aureus* (MRSA) abscess decreases repeat I&D and MRSA-positive cultures in children is unknown.

Materials/Methods.—Referral to the Pediatric Infectious Disease Service (PIDS) for decolonization was determined for eligible children (2003-2010), with outcomes studied over 12 months.

Results.—We identified 653 children; 54 had been seen by PIDS. In the PIDS group, no patients (0/54, 0%) had a repeat I&D. In the no PIDS group 36/599 (6%) had a repeat I&D, $P = .06$. Logistic regression modeling for repeat I&D showed no significant effect, odds ratio = 0.29; 95% confidence interval = 0.04-2.15; $P = .23$. In the PIDS group, 3 patients (3/54, 5.6%) had a repeat MRSA-positive culture. In the no PIDS group, 58/599 (9.7%) had a positive repeat culture, $P = .46$. Logistic regression modeling for positive culture showed no significant effect (odds ratio = 0.55; 95% confidence interval = 0.17-1.81; $P = .32$).

Conclusions.—We detected no statistically significant association between decolonization and repeat I&D or MRSA-positive culture.

► In the United States, the incidence of hospitalizations for skin/skin structure infection (SSTI) caused by methicillin-resistant *Staphylococcus aureus* (MRSA) is estimated to be greater than 45 per 100 000 children.[1] Many of these hospitalized children require incision and drainage. Recurrence rates of SSTIs are reported to be as high as 70% in select studies.[2] Various decolonization protocols developed to decrease recurrence include general hygiene advice, regular bleach baths, or chlorhexidine body washes and/or daily nasal antibiotic application. A recent randomized controlled trial in children showed a lasting effect (12 months) of decolonization in the group in which the whole household received the decolonization protocol compared with the index care only.[3] Other studies have shown a trend toward a positive effect of the decolonization but have failed to demonstrate a statistically significant effect on longer-term outcomes.

This is a retrospective cohort study based on the hypothesis that a consult or visit to a pediatric infectious disease service (PIDS) for MRSA decolonization intervention after an incision and drainage for culture-documented abscess would affect the rate of repeat surgical procedure and subsequent MRSA culture positivity. Tables 2 and 3 in the original article show the effects of intervention on repeat surgical procedure and repeat culture positivity, respectively. No statistically significant association was seen between referral to PIDS for decolonization and the outcomes. However, the rates of both repeat procedure and subsequent positive culture were low in this study.

N. Khardori, MD

References

1. Lautz TB, Raval MV, Barsness KA. Increasing national burden of hospitalizations for skin and soft tissue infections in children. *J Pediatr Surg*. 2011;46:1935-1941.
2. Fritz SA, Camins BC, Eisenstein KD, et al. Effectiveness of measures to eradicate Staphylocossus aureus carriage in patients with community-associated skin and soft-tissue infections: a randomized trial. *Infect Control Hosp Epidemiol*. 2011; 32:872-880.
3. Fritz SA, Hogan PG, Hayek G, et al. Household versus individual approaches to eradication of community-associated *Staphylococcus aureus* in children: a randomized trial. *Clin Infect Dis*. 2012;54:743-751.

Efficacy and Safety of the Mosquitocidal Drug Ivermectin to Prevent Malaria Transmission After Treatment: A Double-Blind, Randomized, Clinical Trial

Ouédraogo AL, Bastiaens GJH, Tiono AB, et al (Centre Natl de Recherche et de Formation sur le Paludisme, Ouagadougou, Burkina Faso; Radboud Univ Med Ctr, Nijmegen, The Netherlands; et al)

Clin Infect Dis 60:357-365, 2015

Background.—Artemisinin combination therapy effectively clears asexual malaria parasites and immature gametocytes but does not prevent posttreatment malaria transmission. Ivermectin (IVM) may reduce malaria transmission by killing mosquitoes that take blood meals from IVM-treated humans.

Methods.—In this double-blind, placebo-controlled trial, 120 asymptomatic *Plasmodium falciparum* parasite carriers were randomized to receive artemether-lumefantrine (AL) plus placebo or AL plus a single or repeated dose (200 μg/kg) of ivermectin (AL-IVM1 and AL-IVM2, respectively). Mosquito membrane feeding was performed 1, 3, and 7 days after initiation of treatment to determine *Anopheles gambiae* and *Anopheles funestus* survival and infection rates.

Results.—The AL-IVM combination was well tolerated. IVM resulted in a 4- to 7-fold increased mortality in mosquitoes feeding 1 day after IVM ($P < .001$). Day 7 IVM plasma levels were positively associated with body mass index ($r = 0.57$, $P < .001$) and were higher in female participants ($P = .003$), for whom *An. gambiae* mosquito mortality was increased until 7 days after a single dose of IVM (hazard rate ratio, 1.34 [95% confidence interval, 1.07–1.69]; $P = .012$). Although we found no evidence that IVM reduced *Plasmodium* infection rates among surviving mosquitoes, the mosquitocidal effect of AL-IVM1 and AL-IVM2 resulted in 27% and 35% reductions, respectively, in estimated malaria transmission potential during the first week after initiation of treatment.

Conclusions.—We conclude that IVM can be safely given in combination with AL and can reduce the likelihood of malaria transmission by reducing the life span of feeding mosquitoes.

Clinical Trials Registration.—NCT0160325.

► The critical factor in the epidemiology of malaria is the transmission of mature gametocytes of *Plasmodium* from humans to mosquitoes. Mosquitoes become infectious within 11 to 16 days after a blood meal.[1] The current first live treatment for uncomplicated falciparum malaria is Artemisinin combination therapy (ACT), which clears asexual parasites and developing gametocytes but leaves mature *P falciparum* gametocytes mostly unaffected. This leads to a proportion of patients potentially able to transmit malaria to mosquitoes after successful ACT treatment.[2] The attempts to prevent malaria transmission after ACT have focused on supplementation with gametocytocidal compounds. An alternative approach is to reduce the likelihood of the mosquitoes surviving long enough after a blood meal to be able to transmit malaria to other humans. By causing flaccid muscle paralysis, Ivermectin (IVM) has been shown to reduce the life span of *Anopheles* mosquitoes. Given its excellent safety profile in humans, IVM has been used in mass drug administration campaigns to reduce the burden of onchocerciasis and filariasis in Africa.

This is a randomized, double-blind placebo-controlled clinical trial to determine the safety and impact of coadministration of IVM with antimalarial therapy. A single or repeated dose of IVM was given in combination with artemether-lumefantrine (AL) to study the survival of mosquitoes long enough to complete the sporogonic cycle of malaria. The AL-IVM was safe and significantly reduced the survival of 2 major malaria vectors in sub-Saharan Africa. The mosquitocidal effect of IVM in *Anopheles gambiae* and *Anopheles funestus* was apparent 3 to 7 days after a single dose. The mosquitocidal effect was not complete. *P falciparum* parasites were detected in a small number of mosquitoes surviving until day 10. The authors estimate that single and repeated doses of IVM may lead to 27% and 35% reduction in posttreatment malaria transmission from symptomatic malaria patients in the first week after effective antimalarial treatment.

N. Khardori, MD

References

1. Meis JF, Wismans PG, Jap PH, Lensen AH, Ponnudurai T. A scanning electron microscopic study of the sporogonic development of *Plasmodium falciparum* in *Anopheles stephensi*. *Acta Trop*. 1992;50:227-236.
2. Sawa P, Shekalaghe SA, Drakeley CJ, et al. Malaria transmission after artemether-lumefantrine and dihydroartemisinin-piperaquine: a randomized trial. *J Infect Dis*. 2013;207:1637-1645.

Effect of Biofilms on Recalcitrance of Staphylococcal Joint Infection to Antibiotic Treatment

Dastgheyb S, Parvizi J, Shapiro IM, et al (Natl Insts of Health, Bethesda, MD; Thomas Jefferson Univ, Philadelphia, PA; The Rothman Inst, Philadelphia, PA)
J Infect Dis 211:641-650, 2015

The pathogenesis of joint infections is not well understood. In particular, we do not know why these infections respond poorly to antibiotic treatment. Here we show that methicillin-resistant *Staphylococcus aureus*, a major cause of joint infections, forms exceptionally strong biofilmlike aggregates in human synovial fluid (SF), to an extent significantly exceeding biofilm formation observed in growth medium or serum. Screening a transposon bank identified bacterial fibronectin- and fibrinogen-binding proteins as important for the formation of macroscopic clumps in SF, suggesting an important role of fibrin-containing clots in the formation of bacterial aggregates during joint infection. Pretreatment of SF with plasmin led to a strongly reduced formation of aggregates and increased susceptibility to antibiotics. These results give important insight into the pathogenesis of staphylococcal joint infection and the mechanisms underlying resistance to treatment. Furthermore, they point toward a potential novel approach for treating joint infections.

▶ Biofilm formation has been speculated to play a key role in the pathogenesis of joint infections.[1] The role of synovial fluid against the infecting bacteria has been described as both antimicrobial and as reduced killing by neutrophils.[2,3] Studies of biofilm formation in vitro are limited by the artificially created environment with selected growth conditions. It is difficult to correlate the data from animal models of biofilms in joint infections to human disease.

This study uses an ex vivo approach to systematically investigate the bacterial behavior in synovial fluid during joint infection. The synovial fluid aspirated from human subjects during total knee arthroplasty or arthrocentesis was used to replace serum (in vivo) and growth media (in vitro). Community-acquired methicillin-resistant *Staphylococcus aureus*, clone USA300 strain LAC, was used as the bacterial inoculum. This strain is a skin infection isolate and the background strain for the Nebraska transposon bank. A number of other well-characterized studies of *S aureus* were also used for comparison. The studies included growth measurement by colony-forming unit determination or quantitative polymerase chain reaction, scanning electron microscopy, confocal microscopy, antibiotic exposure, and measurement of aggregate size distribution. The results show that the synovial fluid environment leads to strong aggregation (biofilm formation) of *S aureus* across various types of strains of methicillin-resistant and methicillin-sensitive *S aureus*. Extensive aggregation was not demonstrated only by a strain lacking adhesion to fibrinogen and fibronectin. Fibrin and fibronectin-binding proteins form the molecular basis of the observed aggregation. Conversely, plasmin treatment prevented aggregation. The formation of aggregates explains the common culture negativity of aspirate joint fluids, difficulty of neutrophils to phagocytise aggregates, and resistance to host defenses and antimicrobial agents.

N. Khardori, MD

References

1. Arnold WV, Shirtliff ME, Stoodley P. Bacterial biofilms and periprosthetic infections. *Instr Course Lect.* 2014;63:385-391.
2. Simon GL, Miller HG, Borenstein DG. Synovial fluid inhibits killing of *Staphylococcus aureus* by neutrophils. *Infect Immun.* 1983;4:1004-1010.
3. Gruber BF, Miller BS, Onnen J, Welling RD, Wojtys EM. Antibacterial properties of synovial fluid in the knee. *J Knee Surg.* 2008;21:180-185.

Association Between Hospitalization for Pneumonia and Subsequent Risk of Cardiovascular Disease

Corrales-Medina VF, Alvarez KN, Weissfeld LA, et al (Univ of Ottawa, Ontario, Canada; Univ of Pittsburgh, PA; et al)
JAMA 313:264-274, 2015

Importance.—The risk of cardiovascular disease (CVD) after infection is poorly understood.

Objective.—To determine whether hospitalization for pneumonia is associated with an increased short-term and long-term risk of CVD.

Design, Settings, and Participants.—We examined 2 community-based cohorts: the Cardiovascular Health Study (CHS, n = 5888; enrollment age, ≥65 years; enrollment period, 1989–1994) and the Atherosclerosis Risk in Communities study (ARIC, n = 15 792; enrollment age, 45-64 years; enrollment period, 1987–1989). Participants were followed up through December 31, 2010. We matched each participant hospitalized with pneumonia to 2 controls. Pneumonia cases and controls were followed for occurrence of CVD over 10 years after matching. We estimated hazard ratios (HRs) for CVD at different time intervals, adjusting for demographics, CVD risk factors, subclinical CVD, comorbidities, and functional status.

Exposures.—Hospitalization for pneumonia.

Main Outcomes and Measures.—Incident CVD (myocardial infarction, stroke, and fatal coronary heart disease).

Results.—Of 591 pneumonia cases in CHS, 206 had CVD events over 10 years after pneumonia hospitalization. Compared with controls, CVD risk among pneumonia cases was highest during the first year after hospitalization and remained significantly higher than among controls through 10 years. In ARIC, of 680 pneumonia cases, 112 had CVD events over 10 years after hospitalization. After the second year, CVD risk among pneumonia cases was not significantly higher than among controls.

	Pneumonia Cases	Controls	HR (95% CI)
CHS			
No. of participants	591	1182	
CVD events			
0-30 d	54	6	4.07 (2.86-5.27)
31-90 d	11	9	2.94 (2.18-3.70)
91 d-1 y	22	55	2.10 (1.59-2.60)
9-10 y	4	12	1.86 (1.18-2.55)
ARIC			
No. of participants	680	1360	
CVD events			
0-30 d	4	3	2.38 (1.12-3.63)
31-90 d	4	0	2.40 (1.23-3.47)
91 d-1 y	11	8	2.19 (1.20-3.19)
1-2 y	8	7	1.88 (1.10-2.66)

Conclusions and Relevance.—Hospitalization for pneumonia was associated with increased short-term and long-term risk of CVD, suggesting that pneumonia may be a risk factor for CVD.

▶ Characterization of risk factors for cardiovascular disease (CVD) is essential for designing preventive strategies. Infections through induction of demand ischemia, endothelial dysfunction, procoagulant changes in blood, and inflammatory changes in the atherosclerotic plaques can increase the short-term risk of cardiovascular disease.[1,2] The effect on CVD risk can extend to the long term because the heightened systemic inflammatory and procoagulant activity consequent to infection can persist long after the resolution of infection.[3,4] The increased short-term and long-term morbidity and mortality in patients with infectious could be explained by the increased risk for CVD. Respiratory tract infections have been shown to be associated with increased risk of CVD. Pneumonia is a well-characterized syndrome that affects 1.2% of the population in the Northern Hemisphere each year and is the most common diagnosis in the hospitalized patients in the United States.

This is a matched-cohort study involving 2 population-based, multicenter, observational cohorts followed for more than 21 years. The cohorts are in the Cardiovascular Health Study (CHS, n = 5888) and the Atherosclerosis Risk in Communities (ARIC, n = 15 792) databases. Figure 3 in the original article summarizes the adjusted failure plots to show the magnitude of risk increase for CVD that was associated with hospitalization for pneumonia in CHS and ARIC. Hospitalization with pneumonia in older adults was associated with subsequent increase in the risk of CVD. The highest risk (4-fold increase) was in the first 30 days after pneumonia with a progressive decline during the first year. The risk remained approximately 1.5-fold higher in subsequent years. The association persisted after adjusting for other known factors contributing to risk of CVD. The results were validated in a cohort of younger adults, using robust sensitivity analysis with different controls and stringent definitions for pneumonia hospitalization. The risk was similar or higher than that associated with smoking, diabetes, and hypertension.

N. Khardori, MD

References

1. Corrales-Medina VF, Madjid M, Musher DM. Role of acute infection in triggering acute coronary syndromes. *Lancet Infect Dis.* 2010;10:83-92.
2. Corrales-Medina VF, Musher DM, Shachkina S, Chirinoa JA. Acute pneumonia and the cardiovascular system. *Lancet.* 2013;381:496-505.
3. Yende S, D'Angelo G, Kellum JA, et al. GenIMS Investigators. Inflammatory markers at hospital discharge predict subsequent mortality after pneumonia and sepsis. *Am J Respir Crit Care Med.* 2008;177:1242-1247.
4. Yende S, D'Angelo G, Mayr F, et al. GenIMS Investigators. Elevated hemostasis markers after pneumonia increases 1-year risk of all cause and cardiovascular deaths. *PLoS One.* 2011;6:e22847.

PART THREE

HEMATOLOGY AND ONCOLOGY

COLLEEN A. LAWTON, MD

21 Supportive Care

A Personalized Approach to Assessing and Managing Pain in Patients With Cancer

Hui D, Bruera E (The Univ of Texas MD Anderson Cancer Ctr, Houston)

J Clin Oncol 32:1640-1646, 2014

Pain is one of the most common and distressing symptoms in patients with cancer. In this review, we discuss an evidence-based approach to personalized pain assessment and management. Recent insights into the pain expression pathway have led to a paradigm shift in pain management, allowing clinicians to deliver personalized treatments tailored to the individual's needs. Personalized pain management begins with systematic screening, followed by comprehensive pain assessment. Impeccable characterization of pain informs its etiology and the mechanism to guide treatment choices. Identification of modulators of pain expression such as psychological distress, alcoholism, substance use, and delirium allow clinicians to further tailor treatment recommendations. Documentation of a personalized pain goal provides an individualized response criterion. A multidimensional treatment plan is then formulated targeting the pain mechanism, etiologic factors, and modulators. Finally, longitudinal monitoring customized to the individual's needs allows clinicians to improve adherence and, ultimately, to optimize pain control over time.

► Cancer pain exists for patients who have curable disease and those with metastatic or otherwise incurable disease. Today with advances in pain management, cancer pain should be fairly easily controlled. Yet one of the top concerns of many cancer patients is whether they will suffer from uncontrolled pain.

Once pain occurs, if it is not well addressed, it is clear that it will take increased doses of analgesics/narcotics to get the pain under control compared with pain addressed early. In addition, uncontrolled or poorly controlled pain is a major cause of depression in cancer patients, thus, affecting quality of life in a dramatic way. So any improvement that can be made to help control pain is worth serious consideration.

Thinking about pain management in a personalized way as these authors have done makes sense just as personalized cancer treatment does. The number of issues that can affect pain management are lengthy; thus, characterizing a patient's individual pain story is critical in providing the best chance of good pain control.

We can all learn a great deal from this personalized approach to cancer pain control starting with and most importantly using a systematic and complete cancer pain history.

C. A. Lawton, MD

Supportive and palliative radiation oncology service: Impact of a dedicated service on palliative cancer care

Tseng YD, Krishnan MS, Jones JA, et al (Harvard Radiation Oncology Program, Boston, MA; Brigham and Women's Hosp, Boston, MA; Univ of Pennsylvania, Philadelphia; et al)

Pract Radiat Oncol 4:247-253, 2014

Purpose.—The American Society of Clinical Oncology has recommended tailoring palliative cancer care (PCC) to the distinct and complex needs of advanced cancer patients. The Supportive and Palliative Radiation Oncology (SPRO) service was initiated July 2011 to provide dedicated palliative radiation oncology (RO) care to cancer patients. We used care providers' ratings to assess SPRO's impact on the quality of PCC and compared perceptions of PCC delivery among physicians practicing with and without a dedicated palliative RO service.

Methods and Materials.—An online survey was sent to 117 RO care providers working at 4 Boston area academic centers. Physicians and nurses at the SPRO-affiliated center rated the impact of the SPRO service on 8 PCC quality measures (7-point scale, "very unfavorably" to "very favorably"). Physicians at all sites rated their department's performance on 10 measures of PCC (7-point scale, "very poorly" to "very well").

Results.—Among 102 RO care providers who responded (response rate, 89% for physicians; 83% for nurses), large majorities believed that SPRO improved the following PCC quality measures: overall quality of care (physician/nurse, 98%/92%); communication with patients and families (95%/96%); staff experience (93%/84%); time spent on technical aspects of PCC (eg, reviewing imaging) (88%/56%); appropriateness of treatment recommendations (85%/84%); appropriateness of dose/fractionation (78%/60%); and patient follow-up (64%/68%). Compared with physicians practicing in departments without a dedicated palliative RO service, physicians at the SPRO-affiliated department rated the overall quality of their department's PCC more highly ($P = .02$).

Conclusions.—Clinicians indicated that SPRO improved the quality of PCC. Physicians practicing within this dedicated service rated their department's overall PCC quality higher than physicians practicing at academic centers without a dedicated service. These findings point to dedicated palliative RO services as a promising means of improving PCC quality.

▶ Palliative care is an emerging area of medicine that is showing great promise. Whereas in the past decade palliative care was really only considered at the very end of life, there are now data showing a benefit to improving in both quality of life and overall survival with the input of palliative care earlier at least on the oncology treatment continuum.

Exactly how to execute the best palliative care program remains to be defined, but these data looking at a dedicated radiation oncology supportive and palliative care service suggest that it improves palliative care at least from the perspective of physicians and other health care providers who have access to this dedicated service. The providers rated the dedicated supportive palliative care radiation service as better than the standard palliative care service without the dedicated radiation oncology service in overall quality of care, communication with patients and families, appropriateness of treatment recommendations, dose fractionation, and follow-up among other measures of a palliative care service.

Taken as a whole, these data certainly support the consideration of implementing a radiation oncology-specific palliative care service in many of our large hospitals to provide what appears to be an improved palliative care experience for our cancer patients.

C. A. Lawton, MD

Voice Quality After Treatment of Early Vocal Cord Cancer: A Randomized Trial Comparing Laser Surgery With Radiation Therapy

Aaltonen L-M, Rautiainen N, Sellman J, et al (Univ of Helsinki, Finland; et al)

Int J Radiat Oncol Biol Phys 90:255-260, 2014

Objective.—Early laryngeal cancer is usually treated with either transoral laser surgery or radiation therapy. The quality of voice achieved with these treatments has not been compared in a randomized trial.

Methods and Materials.—Male patients with carcinoma limited to 1 mobile vocal cord (T1aN0M0) were randomly assigned to receive either laser surgery (n = 32) or external beam radiation therapy (n = 28). Surgery consisted of tumor excision with a CO_2 laser with the patient under general anaesthesia. External beam radiation therapy to the larynx was delivered to a cumulative dose of 66 Gy in 2-Gy daily fractions over 6.5 weeks. Voice quality was assessed at baseline and 6 and 24 months after treatment. The main outcome measures were expert-rated voice quality on a grade, roughness, breathiness, asthenia, and strain (GRBAS) scale, videolaryngostroboscopic findings, and the patients' self-rated voice quality and its impact on activities of daily living.

Results.—Overall voice quality between the groups was rated similar, but voice was more breathy and the glottal gap was wider in patients treated with laser surgery than in those who received radiation therapy. Patients treated with radiation therapy reported less hoarseness-related inconvenience in daily living 2 years after treatment. Three patients in each group had local cancer recurrence within 2 years from randomization.

Conclusions.—Radiation therapy may be the treatment of choice for patients whose requirements for voice quality are demanding. Overall voice quality was similar in both treatment groups, however, indicating a need for careful consideration of patient-related factors in the choice of a treatment option.

▶ When patients are diagnosed with early-stage carcinoma of the vocal cord, the most important end point after treatment is, of course, control of their disease. Yet because the tumor is highly curable, issues of toxicity become extremely important. Voice change or, worse, voice loss is a devastating issue for patients so that voice quality after any curative procedure becomes paramount.

We in radiation oncology have touted our modality as offering a very high cure rate and excellent preservation of voice quality. Yet the otolaryngologists will make the same claim with their use of laser surgery for this malignancy. Thus, this randomized trial of radiation therapy versus laser surgery for early vocal cord cancer is important.

What the authors report is that both modalities resulted in high cure rates (approximately 90%). The question of voice quality revealed that both forms of treatment resulted in good voice quality, but that the radiation therapy-treated patients had less breathy and glottal gap issues compared to the laser group. These data certainly support the use of radiation therapy as an excellent treatment option for these patients and perhaps the best treatment option for many patients given that the overall voice quality was better for the radiation therapy group. Physician and patient input are always critical in selecting the best form of treatment, but certainly radiation therapy needs to be front and center in the discussion of treatment options for these patients.

C. A. Lawton, MD

Managing Body Image Difficulties of Adult Cancer Patients: Lessons From Available Research

Fingeret MC, Teo I, Epner DE (Univ of Texas MD Anderson Cancer Ctr, Houston)

Cancer 120:633-641, 2014

Background.—Body image is a critical psychosocial issue for patients with cancer because they often undergo significant changes to appearance and functioning. The primary purpose of this review article was to identify empirically-supported approaches to treat body image difficulties of adult cancer patients that can be incorporated into high-quality comprehensive cancer care.

Methods.—An overview was provided of theoretical models of body image relevant to cancer patients, and findings were presented from published literature on body image and cancer from 2003 to 2013. These data were integrated with information from the patient-doctor communication literature to delineate a practical approach for assessing and treating body image concerns of adult cancer patients.

Results.—Body image difficulties were found across patients with diverse cancer sites, and were most prevalent in the immediate postoperative and treatment period. Age, body mass index, and specific cancer treatments have been identified as potential risk factors for body image disturbance in cancer patients. Current evidence supports the use of time-limited cognitive-behavioral therapy interventions for addressing these difficulties. Other intervention strategies also show promise but require further study. Potential indicators of body image difficulties were identified to alert health care professionals when to refer patients for psychosocial care, and a framework was proposed for approaching conversations about body image that can be used by the oncologic treatment team.

Conclusions.—Body image issues affect a wide array of cancer patients. Providers can use available evidence combined with information from the health care communication literature to develop practical strategies for treating body image concerns of patients with cancer.

▶ When we as oncologists think of body image challenges for our cancer patients, we immediately think of breast cancer as the major oncologic disease process affecting body image. Yet as a genitourinary radiation oncologist, I have had many testicular cancer patients described having a testicle removed as the same devastating change as having a breast removed. We can also imagine devastating effects on body image for many other cancer patients, such as our melanoma patients, whose wide excisions can lead to significant scarring; our colorectal cancer patients, who can be left with colostomies; our head and neck cancer patients, who are often left with significant neck alterations from both lymph node dissection and radiation; and our sarcoma patients, who are often left with large surgical defects and beyond. Thus, changes in body image are a very important aspect for most if not all of our patients with cancer.

How best to address this huge quality-of-life issue for our patients is not well understood and needs attention so that we as oncologists can improve our patients' lives beyond "fixing" their cancer.

This article is an excellent review of the current state of research on this topic and summarizes well some practical recommendations for us as we try to assist our patients. Critical in the messaging from this article is the need for psychological support for our patients as they try to manage body image issues. Developing ways to insert support even before surgery (often the primary body-altering maneuver) is clearly worth considering and worth investigating.

C. A. Lawton, MD

Effect of Communication Skills Training Program for Oncologists Based on Patient Preferences for Communication When Receiving Bad News: A Randomized Controlled Trial

Fujimori M, Shirai Y, Asai M, et al (Natl Cancer Ctr Hosp East, Kashiwa; et al)

J Clin Oncol 32:2166-2172, 2014

Purpose.—The aim of this study was to identify the effects of a communication skills training (CST) program for oncologists, developed based on patient preferences regarding oncologists' communication.

Participants and Methods.—Thirty oncologists were randomly assigned to either an intervention group (IG; 2-day CST workshop) or control group (CG). Participants were assessed on their communication performance during simulated consultation and their confidence in communicating with patients at baseline and follow-up. A total of 1,192 patients (response rate, 84.6%) who had consultations with the participating oncologists at baseline and/or follow-up were assessed regarding their distress using the Hospital Anxiety and Depression Scale, satisfaction with the consultation, and trust in their oncologist after the consultation.

Results.—At the follow-up survey, the performance scores of the IG had improved significantly, in terms of their emotional support ($P = .011$), setting up a supportive environment ($P = .002$), and ability to deliver information ($P = .001$), compared with those of the CG. Oncologists in the IG were rated higher at follow-up than those in the CG in terms of their confidence in themselves ($P = .001$). Patients who met with oncologists after they had undergone the CST were significantly less depressed than those who met with oncologists in the CG ($P = .027$). However, the CST program did not affect patient satisfaction with oncologists' style of communication.

Conclusion.—A CST program based on patient preferences is effective for both oncologists and patients with cancer. Oncologists should consider CST as an approach to enhancing their communication skills.

▶ When a patient receives a diagnosis of "cancer," it is truly a life-changing moment. Fear, anxiety, and depression can and do set in quickly, and thus effective communication on the part of the oncologist (surgical, medical, or radiation) is critical. Yet most of us have little formal education in this area. Furthermore, given our busy practices it is hard to develop these skills as time is so precious.

Trying to understand the potential benefit of training to improve our communication skills is imperative to taking the time out of our practices to do so. Thus, this randomized controlled trial is exactly the type of data we need to push oncologists to get this focused training. The training amounted to a 2-day workshop with the majority of the time dedicated to "role playing" with standardized patients and focusing particularly on the reassurance aspect of communication. This reassurance aspect targets the patient's emotions and empathic responses to them. In addition, the facilitator and standardized patients all had years of experience in this area and thus the quality of this education was high.

In the end, these data showed a benefit to this focused education for oncologists in terms of increased emotional support for patients, better ability to set up a supportive environment, increased oncologists ability to deliver life-altering information, and less depression for the patients. We as oncologists need to make the effort to get this education, and we should push to be sure that it exists in our training programs.

C. A. Lawton, MD

Tadalafil for Prevention of Erectile Dysfunction After Radiotherapy for Prostate Cancer: The Radiation Therapy Oncology Group [0831] Randomized Clinical Trial

Pisansky TM, Pugh SL, Greenberg RE, et al (Mayo Clinic, Rochester, MN; Radiation Therapy Oncology Group, Philadelphia, PA; Fox Chase Cancer Ctr, Philadelphia, PA; et al)

JAMA 311:1300-1307, 2014

Importance.—Tadalafil is used to treat erectile dysfunction after prostate cancer treatment, but its role as a preventive agent is undefined.

Objectives.—To determine primarily whether tadalafil preserved erectile function in men treated with radiotherapy for prostate cancer, and secondarily to determine whether participant- or partner-reported overall sexual function and sexual and marital satisfaction were affected.

Design, Setting, and Participants.—Stratified, placebo-controlled, double-blind, parallel-group study with 1:1 randomization at 76 community-based and tertiary medical sites in the United States and Canada. Two hundred forty-two participants with intact erectile function scheduled to receive radiotherapy for prostate cancer were recruited between November 2009 and February 2012 with follow-up through March 2013.

Interventions.—One hundred twenty-one participants were assigned 5 mg of tadalafil daily and 121 were assigned placebo for 24 weeks starting with external radiotherapy (63%) or brachytherapy (37%). Participant-reported International Index of Erectile Function response before radiotherapy and at weeks 2 and 4, between weeks 20 and 24, between weeks 28 and 30, and 1 year thereafter. Participants and partners could respond also to the Sexual Adjustment Questionnaire and to the Locke Marital Adjustment Test before radiotherapy, between weeks 20 and 24 and weeks 28 and 30, and at 1 year.

Main Outcomes and Measures.—Primary outcome was off-drug spontaneous erectile function 28 to 30 weeks after radiotherapy started. Secondary end points were spontaneous erection at 1 year; overall sexual function and satisfaction; marital adjustment; and partner-reported satisfaction and marital adjustment at 28 to 30 weeks and 1 year, predictors of tadalafil response; and adverse events.

Results.—Among 221 evaluable participants, 80 (79%; 95% CI, 70%-88%) assigned to receive tadalafil retained erectile function between weeks 28 and 30 compared with 61 (74%; 95% CI, 63%-85%) assigned to receive placebo ($P = .49$); an absolute difference of 5% (95% CI, −9% to 19%). A significant difference was also not observed at 1 year (72%; 95% CI, 60%-84% vs 71%; 95% CI, 59%-84%; $P = .93$). Tadalafil was not associated with significantly improved overall sexual function or satisfaction; a significant difference was not observed in any domain subscale. Partners of men assigned tadalafil noted no significant effect on sexual satisfaction, and marital adjustment was not significantly improved in participants or partners.

Conclusions and Relevance.—Among men undergoing radiotherapy for prostate cancer, daily use of tadalafil compared with placebo did not result in improved erectile function. These findings do not support daily use of tadalafil to prevent erectile dysfunction in these patients.

Trial Registration.—clinicaltrials.gov Identifier: NCT00931528.

▶ Minimizing toxicity is an important goal in the treatment of localized prostate cancer, given the high likelihood of cure and resultant longevity. Toxicity related to definitive radiation comes in the form of gastrointestinal, genitourinary, and sexual changes. Fortunately, the toxicities related to gastrointestinal and genitourinary changes are modest, but sexual dysfunction is a much greater problem.

Upwards of 30% to 40% of patients with full "normal" sexual functioning before definitive radiation therapy for localized prostate cancer can have decreased sexual functioning. This of course is related to age and sexual activity. Therefore, methods to mitigate such dysfunction are worth studying. One of the simplest ways to potentially decrease this toxicity is the use of oral agents such as the phosphodiesterase-5-inhibitors. These agents are known to reduce endothelial dysfunction and thus improve cavernosal vasodilation and erectile dysfunction in the general male population. Thus, it is reasonable to hypothesize that these agents could help with sexual dysfunction after radiation therapy.

In a phase III double-blinded, placebo-controlled method, this trial studied the use of one of these agents. Considered the "gold standard" methodology to evaluate these drugs; unfortunately, no improvement was seen in sexual functioning at approximately 7 months after initiation of radiation therapy and the drug. Although this trial did not show a benefit to this medication and dosing schedule, the concept of continuing to evaluate this class of drugs and other agents and perhaps other dosing schedules is still warranted. We await these results and other trials to help decrease this life-altering toxicity for our prostate cancer patients treated with radiation therapy.

C. A. Lawton, MD

22 Geriatric Oncology

Radiation Treatment in Older Patients: A Framework for Clinical Decision Making

Smith GL, Smith BD (Univ of Texas MD Anderson Cancer Ctr, Houston)

J Clin Oncol 32:2669-2678, 2014

In older patients, radiation treatment plays a vital role in curative and palliative cancer therapy. Radiation treatment recommendations should be informed by a comprehensive, personalized risk-benefit assessment that evaluates treatment efficacy and toxicity. We review several clinical factors that distinctly affect efficacy and toxicity of radiation treatment in older patients. First, locoregional tumor behavior may be more indolent in older patients for some disease sites but more aggressive for other sites. Assessment of expected locoregional relapse risk informs the magnitude and timeframe of expected radiation treatment benefits. Second, assessment of the competing cancer versus noncancer mortality and morbidity risks contextualizes cancer treatment priorities holistically within patients' entire spectrum and time course of health needs. Third, assessment of functional reserve helps predict patients' acute treatment tolerance, differentiating those patients who are unlikely to benefit from treatment or who are at high risk for treatment complications. Potential radiation treatment options include immediate curative treatment, delayed curative treatment, and no treatment, with additional consideration given to altered radiation target, dose, or sequencing with chemotherapy and/or surgery. Finally, when cure is not feasible, palliative radiation therapy remains valuable for managing symptoms and achieving meaningful quality-of-life improvements. Our proposed decision-making framework integrates these factors to help radiation oncologists formulate strategic treatment recommendations within a multidisciplinary context. Future research is still needed to identify how advanced technologies can be judiciously applied in curative and palliative settings to enhance risk-benefit profiles of radiation treatment in older patients and more accurately quantify treatment efficacy in this group.

► Most cancers occur in the older (> 65 years) population, especially the common ones such as breast and prostate. Exactly how to treat older patients compared with a younger cohort is of significant interest in that multiple studies are showing both overtreatment and undertreatment in the elderly. Factoring in comorbidities and aggressiveness of the malignancy are 2 very significant features that need to be addressed so as to offer the best treatment for these patients. The above applies to all forms of oncologic treatment from surgery to chemotherapy and radiation therapy.

These authors looked specifically at the issue of radiation therapy, both curative and palliative, to try to develop some practical guidance in the correct use of this modality in older cancer patients. The factors that they have addressed include the behavior of the tumor locally/regionally and comorbidities, which could affect tolerances to treatment but also a competing risk for death. These factors are appropriate and helpful to the practicing radiation oncologists in making good decisions on the use of radiation therapy, which can be uniquely different in the older cancer patient depending on where they stand on features such as tumor aggressiveness and their comorbidities.

C. A. Lawton, MD

Receipt of Guideline-Concordant Treatment in Elderly Prostate Cancer Patients

Chen RC, Carpenter WR, Hendrix LH, et al (Univ of North Carolina at Chapel Hill)

Int J Radiat Oncol Biol Phys 88:332-338, 2014

Purpose.—To examine the proportion of elderly prostate cancer patients receiving guideline-concordant treatment, using the Surveillance, Epidemiology, and End Results (SEER)-Medicare linked database.

Methods and Materials.—A total of 29,001 men diagnosed in 2004-2007 with localized prostate cancer, aged 66 to 79 years, were included. We characterized the proportion of men who received treatment concordant with the National Comprehensive Cancer Network guidelines, stratified by risk group and age. Logistic regression was used to examine covariates associated with receipt of guideline-concordant management.

Results.—Guideline concordance was 79%-89% for patients with low- or intermediate-risk disease. Among high-risk patients, 66.6% of those aged 66-69 years received guideline-concordant management, compared with 51.9% of those aged 75-79 years. Discordance was mainly due to conservative management—no treatment or hormone therapy alone. Among the subgroup of patients aged ≤76 years with no measured comorbidity, findings were similar. On multivariable analysis, older age (75-79 vs 66-69 years, odds ratio 0.51, 95% confidence interval 0.50-0.57) was associated with a lower likelihood of guideline concordance for high-risk prostate cancer, but comorbidity was not.

Conclusions.—There is undertreatment of elderly but healthy patients with high-risk prostate cancer, the most aggressive form of this disease.

▶ Exactly how to treat or monitor patients with prostate cancer can be a difficult oncologic challenge, as we know that many prostate cancer patients will not die from their disease, especially those with low-risk malignancies. Patients young or old need to be made aware of this challenge. Yet, we also know that more than 30 000 US men will die of prostate cancer this year. Most of these patients will present with high-risk disease. Getting the above facts clear in the minds of both patients and their physician care givers is critical in applying the best course of treatment to each patient regardless of age.

These data showing relative undertreatment of healthy men older than 75 years is concerning and warrants serious contemplation by the patients and, more importantly, their oncologists. Level I data show the overall survival benefit of aggressive radiation and hormone therapy over hormone therapy alone. Many of these healthy older men are being given clearly inferior treatment.

C. A. Lawton, MD

23 Prostate Cancer

Dosimetric analysis of radiation therapy oncology group 0321: The importance of urethral dose

Hsu I-C, Hunt D, Straube W, et al (Univ of California San Francisco; RTOG Statistical Ctr, Philadelphia, PA; Image-Guided Therapy Ctr, St Louis, MO; et al)

Pract Radiat Oncol 4:27-34, 2014

Purpose.—Radiation Therapy Oncology Group 0321 is the first multi-institutional cooperative group high-dose-rate (HDR) prostate brachytherapy trial with complete digital brachytherapy dosimetry data. This is a descriptive report of the data and an analysis of toxicity.

Methods and Materials.—Patients are treated with external beam radiation therapy at 45 Gy and 1 HDR implant with 19 Gy in 2 fractions. Implants are done with transrectal ultrasound guidance, and computed tomography (CT)-compatible nonmetallic catheters. HDR planning is done on ≤3-mm-thick CT slices. The "mean DVH" (dose–volume histogram) of the planning target volume (PTV), implanted volume (IP), and organs at risk are calculated. This includes the mean and standard deviation (SD) of the volume at 10-percentage-point intervals from 10% to 200% of the prescribed dose. The conformal index (COIN), homogeneity index (HI), catheters per implant, and patients per institution are calculated. Multivariate analysis and hazard ratios calculation of all the variables against reported grade ≥2 (G2+) genitourinary (GU) adverse events (Common Terminology Criteria for Adverse Events, version 3) are performed.

Results.—Dosimetry data are based on 122 eligible patients from 14 institutions. The mean of PTV, IP, catheters per implant, and patients per institution are 54 cc, 63 cc, 19 and 9, respectively. The mean of % $V100_{PTV}$, $V80_{Bladder}$, $V80_{Rectum}$, and $V120_{Urethra}$ were 94%, 0.40 cc, 0.15 cc, and 0.25 cc, respectively. There are too few G2+ gastrointestinal adverse event (GI AE) for correlative analysis; thus, the analysis has been performed on the more common G2+ GU AE. There are positive correlations noted between both acute and late G2+ GU AE and urethral dose at multiple levels. Positive correlations with late AE are seen with PTV and IP at high-dose levels. A negative correlation is seen between HI and acute AE. A higher patient accrual rate is associated with a lower rate of G2+ acute and late AE.

Conclusions.—Higher urethral dose, larger high-dose volumes, and lower dose homogeneity are associated with greater toxicities. A mean dose–volume histogram comparison at all dose levels should be used for quality control and future research comparison.

▶ Using brachytherapy in the treatment of adenocarcinoma of the prostate dates back to approximately 1911 when radium needles were implanted transurethrally into the prostate in an effort to treat the disease. Complications were high, but with time, improvements were made, and radium needles were implanted transperineally.

Several investigators, including the group at Memorial Sloan Kettering, performed brachytherapy as an open technique using radioactive I-125 in the 1970s. Initially the procedure looked promising in terms of results, yet the nonuniformity of the implant often resulted in underdosing certain portions of the gland and overdosing others. This inhomogeneity resulted in poor cancer control and increased toxicity. Brachytherapy continued to evolve using available isotopes. Each step forward was an attempt to increase cancer control but keep toxicities low.

Low-dose-rate brachytherapy (LDR) evolved extensively in the late 1980s and early 1990s. Both radioactive palladium 103 and radioactive iodine 125 were used with reasonable results in terms of cancer control and morbidity. High-dose-rate (HDR) brachytherapy was also being developed at this time with the hope of the same goal.

Given the operator-dependent nature of brachytherapy (generally related to volume of procedures), the ability to carefully define a "good implant" via LDR or HDR was challenging. Our planning systems were not as well developed as they are today, so guidelines on how to achieve good results were difficult.

Therefore, data such as the analysis here on Radiation Therapy Oncology Group 03-21 are important as we try to improve outcomes for our prostate brachytherapy patients. Meticulous dose documentation is critical in all the organs at risk, including the urethra, bladder, and rectum, and needs to be monitored carefully to achieve the best results.

C. A. Lawton, MD

Short-term androgen suppression and radiotherapy versus intermediate-term androgen suppression and radiotherapy, with or without zoledronic acid, in men with locally advanced prostate cancer (TROG 03.04 RADAR): an open-label, randomised, phase 3 factorial trial

Denham JW, Joseph D, Lamb DS, et al (Univ of Newcastle, New South Wales, Australia; Sir Charles Gairdner Hosp, Perth, Australia; Wellington Cancer Centre, New Zealand; et al)

Lancet Oncol 15:1076-1089, 2014

Background.—We investigated whether 18 months of androgen suppression plus radiotherapy, with or without 18 months of zoledronic acid, is more effective than 6 months of neoadjuvant androgen suppression plus radiotherapy with or without zoledronic acid.

Methods.—We did an open-label, randomised, 2 × 2 factorial trial in men with locally advanced prostate cancer (either T2a N0 M0 prostatic adenocarcinomas with prostate-specific antigen [PSA] ≥10 μg/L and a Gleason score of ≥7, or T2b–4 N0 M0 tumours regardless of PSA and Gleason score). We randomly allocated patients by computer-generated minimisation—stratified by centre, baseline PSA, tumour stage, Gleason score, and use of a brachytherapy boost—to one of four groups in a 1:1:1:1 ratio. Patients in the control group were treated with neoadjuvant androgen suppression with leuprorelin (22·5 mg every 3 months, intramuscularly) for 6 months (short-term) and radiotherapy alone (designated STAS); this procedure was either followed by another 12 months of androgen suppression with leuprorelin (intermediate-term; ITAS) or accompanied by 18 months of zoledronic acid (4 mg every 3 months for 18 months, intravenously; STAS plus zoledronic acid) or by both (ITAS plus zoledronic acid). The primary endpoint was prostate cancer-specific mortality. This analysis represents the first, preplanned assessment of oncological endpoints, 5 years after treatment. Analysis was by intention-to-treat. This trial is registered with ClinicalTrials.gov, number NCT00193856.

Findings.—Between Oct 20, 2003, and Aug 15, 2007, 1071 men were randomly assigned to STAS (n = 268), STAS plus zoledronic acid (n = 268), ITAS (n = 268), and ITAS plus zoledronic acid (n = 267). Median follow-up was 7·4 years (IQR 6·5–8·4). Cumulative incidences of prostate cancer-specific mortality were 4·1% (95% CI 2·2–7·0) in the STAS group, 7·8% (4·9–11·5) in the STAS plus zoledronic acid group, 7·4% (4·6–11·0) in the ITAS group, and 4·3% (2·3–7·3) in the ITAS plus zoledronic acid group. Cumulative incidence of all-cause mortality was 17·0% (13·0–22·1), 18·9% (14·6–24·2), 19·4% (15·0–24·7), and 13·9% (10·3–18·8), respectively. Neither prostate cancer-specific mortality nor all-cause mortality differed between control and experimental groups. Cumulative incidence of PSA progression was 34·2% (28·6–39·9) in the STAS group, 39·6% (33·6–45·5) in the STAS plus zoledronic acid group, 29·2% (23·8–34·8) in the ITAS group, and 26·0% (20·8–31·4) in the ITAS plus zoledronic acid group. Compared with STAS, no difference was noted in PSA progression with ITAS or STAS plus zoledronic acid; however, ITAS plus zoledronic acid reduced PSA progression (sub-hazard ratio [SHR] 0·71, 95% CI 0·53–0·95; $p = 0{\cdot}021$). Cumulative incidence of local progression was 4·1% (2·2–7·0) in the STAS group, 6·1% (3·7–9·5) in the STAS plus zoledronic acid group, 1·5% (0·5–3·7) in the ITAS group, and 3·4% (1·7–6·1) in the ITAS plus zoledronic acid group; no differences were noted between groups. Cumulative incidences of bone progression were 7·5% (4·8–11·1), 14·6% (10·6–19·2), 8·4% (5·5–12·2), and 7·6% (4·8–11·2), respectively. Compared with STAS, STAS plus zoledronic acid increased the risk of bone progression (SHR 1·90, 95%

CI 1·14–3·17; $p = 0{\cdot}012$), but no differences were noted with the other two groups. Cumulative incidence of distant progression was 14·7% (10·7–19·2) in the STAS group, 17·3% (13·0–22·1) in the STAS plus zoledronic acid group, 14·2% (10·3–18·7) in the ITAS group, and 11·1% (7·6–15·2) in the ITAS plus zoledronic acid group; no differences were recorded between groups. Cumulative incidence of secondary therapeutic intervention was 25·6% (20·5–30·9), 28·9% (23·5–34·5), 20·7% (16·1–25·9), and 15·3% (11·3–20·0), respectively. Compared with STAS, ITAS plus zoledronic acid reduced the need for secondary therapeutic intervention (SHR 0·67, 95% CI 0·48–0·95; $p = 0{\cdot}024$); no differences were noted with the other two groups. An interaction between trial factors was recorded for Gleason score; therefore, we did pairwise comparisons between all groups. Post-hoc analyses suggested that the reductions in PSA progression and decreased need for secondary therapeutic intervention with ITAS plus zoledronic acid were restricted to tumours with a Gleason score of 8-10, and that ITAS was better than STAS in tumours with a Gleason score of 7 or lower. Long-term morbidity and quality-of-life scores were not affected adversely by 18 months of androgen suppression or zoledronic acid.

Interpretation.—Compared with STAS, ITAS plus zoledronic acid was more effective for treatment of prostate cancers with a Gleason score of 8–10, and ITAS alone was effective for tumours with a Gleason score of 7 or lower. Nevertheless, these findings are based on secondary endpoint data and post-hoc analyses and must be regarded cautiously. Long-term follow-up is necessary, as is external validation of the interaction between zoledronic acid and Gleason score. STAS plus zoledronic acid can be ruled out as a potential therapeutic option.

▶ It is well documented by multiple randomized clinical trials that patients with locally advanced prostate cancer (clinical T3 and T4N0M0) benefit from the addition of hormone therapy to definitive radiation therapy. Even as little as 4 months of androgen-deprivation therapy (ADT) and radiation therapy provides meaningful improvement in cancer control over radiation alone. Phase III randomized trials have also shown a clear benefit to longer ADT over shorter course such that the standard for such patients is 28 to 36 months of ADT in addition to radiation therapy. Yet recent data from Canada shows no improvement in cancer control in patients treated with 18 months of ADT versus 36 months. Clearly the longer those patients are on ADT, the more likely they are to suffer significant late effects of bone loss and muscle mass loss.

So the question of how short a course of ADT is possible while still achieving the best cancer control remains. One possible way to improve cancer control without increasing ADT duration is the addition of bisphosphonates, which have been shown to be effective in decreasing bony metastasis in patients with metastatic disease. Thus, these authors performed this 2 × 2 factorial trial to see if the addition of 18 months of zoledronic acid could help decrease the need for longer term ADT.

The addition of 18 months of zoledronic acid clearly did not replace the effect of long-term ADT and thus is not a way to decrease the need for long-term ADT. Whether 18 months of zoledronic acid will help provide a decrease in metastatic disease for patients on long-term ADT is still not known, but further maturation of this data will give us insights into this interesting question.

C. A. Lawton, MD

Low Rates of Adjuvant Radiation in Patients With Nonmetastatic Prostate Cancer With High-Risk Pathologic Features

Kalbasi A, Swisher-McClure S, Mitra N, et al (Perelman School of Medicine at the Univ of Pennsylvania, Philadelphia; et al)

Cancer 120:3089-3096, 2014

Background.—The 2013 American Urological Association/American Society for Radiation Oncology consensus guidelines recommend offering adjuvant radiotherapy (RT) after radical prostatectomy in patients with high-risk pathologic features for recurrence. In the current study, the authors examined practice patterns of adjuvant RT use in patients with elevated pathologic risk factors over a time period spanning the publication of supporting randomized evidence.

Methods.—Using the National Cancer Data Base, a total of 130,681 patients were identified who underwent surgical resection for prostate cancer between 2004 and 2011 with at least 1 of the following pathologic risk factors for early biochemical failure: pT3a disease or higher, positive surgical margins and/or lymph node-positive disease. Using multivariable logistic regression, the authors examined factors associated with adjuvant RT use including patient, clinical, demographic, and temporal characteristics.

Results.—Adjuvant RT was administered to 9.9% of the patients with at least 1 pathologic risk factor. Use of adjuvant RT did not change over the study period ($P = .23$). On multivariable analysis, we found that patients treated at high-volume surgical facilities were less likely to receive adjuvant RT (15.9% vs 7.8%; odds ratio, 0.58 [95% confidence interval, 0.50-0.65]; $P < .0001$). Older age, comorbidities, black race, lower income, and lower population density were also associated with lower rates of adjuvant RT.

Conclusions.—Use of adjuvant RT is uncommon and remained unchanged between 2004 and 2011. Patients treated at high-volume surgical facilities are less likely to receive adjuvant RT, irrespective of margin status.

► Prostate cancer is the second leading cause of cancer deaths in men in the United States behind lung cancer. It claims the lives of roughly 30 000 US men annually. Thus, effective treatment for prostate cancer is imperative.

In the United States, surgery is most often selected as the patient's up-front approach to this malignancy. Surgery alone is often successful, and no further treatment is required. But for many patients, surgery alone is not enough. This is especially true for patients with high-risk pathologic features such as T3 disease, positive margins, and/or detectable postoperative prostate-specific antigen. It is for these patients that additional therapy is warranted.

The good news is that we have multiple phase III randomized trials showing the benefit of postoperative radiation therapy for patients with these high-risk features. Because these data exist, both the American Urological Association and the American Society for Radiation Oncology have published a joint guideline recommending offering radiation therapy to these patients. The bad news is that the data reported in this article shows that despite level I data, there has not been an appropriate increase in the use of postoperative radiation therapy. This is a sad comment on the part of our referring urologists who need to start the postoperative radiation therapy conversation. Of course not all patients are good candidates for radiation, but that decision should reside in the hands of the radiation oncologists and the patient. My hope is that with time, these data and the guideline resulting from such will become more widely utilized. Another analysis like this in 3 to 5 years should be done.

C. A. Lawton, MD

RTOG 95-17, a Phase II trial to evaluate brachytherapy as the sole method of radiation therapy for Stage I and II breast carcinoma—year-5 toxicity and cosmesis

Rabinovitch R, Winter K, Kuske R, et al (Univ of Colorado Hosp, Aurora; Radiation Therapy Oncology Group, Philadelphia, PA; AZ Oncology Services, Scottsdale; et al)
Brachytherapy 13:17-22, 2014

Purpose.—Radiation Therapy Oncology Group (RTOG) 95-17, a Phase II trial to evaluate multicatheter brachytherapy (mCathBrachy) as the sole method of radiation therapy for Stage I–II breast cancer (BrCa), was the first cooperative group trial in North America to evaluate accelerated partial breast irradiation (APBI) and include patient-reported outcomes (PROs). This report presents the year-5 toxicity and cosmesis data.

Methods and Materials.—After lumpectomy and axillary dissection for invasive BrCa (tumor size <3 cm with zero to three positive lymph nodes), 100 patients (pts), 98 evaluable, were treated (txed) with mCathBrachy from 1997 to 2000 with 34 Gy administered twice daily in 10 high-dose-rate fractions or 45 Gy in 3.5–6 days as a low-dose-rate implant to 1–2 cm beyond the lumpectomy bed. The PROs and physician-reported outcomes of toxicity, cosmesis, and tx satisfaction at year-5 are reported here, defined as data submitted 54–78 months after tx.

Results.—Grade (G) 1–2 skin toxicity developed in 78% of the pts and G3 in 13% (no G4). The tx effects included skin dimpling/indentation

(37%), fibrosis (45%), telangiectasias (45%), skin catheter marks (54%), and symptomatic fat necrosis (15%). Breast asymmetry was reported in 73%. Rates of excellent-to-good cosmesis were similar between PROs (66%) and radiation oncologists (68%). The PROs of tx satisfaction at year-5 was 75%.

Conclusions.—RTOG 95-17 documents the year-5 skin toxicity and tx effects of mCathBrachy APBI, which are associated with PROs of good-to-excellent cosmesis and high tx satisfaction. This emphasizes the importance of PROs when assessing BrCa tx. National Surgical Adjuvant Breast and Bowel Project B39/RTOG 0413 will allow for definitive comparisons between APBI and whole breast radiation therapy.

► Stage I and II breast cancer patients in general have 2 options for local treatment of their disease. They can select modified radical mastectomy with some form of reconstruction or select conservative management with lumpectomy and radiation therapy. For many patients who do not live near a radiation facility, the organ preservation option is not feasible given the multiple weeks required for standard external beam irradiation. This same issue existed for our prostate cancer patients who wanted a nonsurgical approach until both low-dose rate brachytherapy and high-dose rate brachytherapy were perfected. Thus, this Radiation Therapy Oncology Group (RTOG) phase II trial was an important step toward understanding the possible radiation alternative of brachytherapy for our breast cancer patients.

Critical to this trial were the patient-reported outcomes because cosmesis (especially evaluated through the eyes of the patient) is one of the most important end points. Fortunately, the rate of excellent to good cosmesis at 5 years was similar for the radiation oncologists and the patients. Ultimately, however, to understand how this approach fares in terms of breast cancer control and cosmesis will only be understood via a phase III trial comparing this form of partial breast irradiation with standard whole breast irradiation. A trial looking at this question is ongoing within the National Surgical Adjuvant Breast and Bowel Project (B39) RTOG 0413. We anxiously await the results.

C. A. Lawton, MD

Comparative Effectiveness Study of Patient-Reported Outcomes After Proton Therapy or Intensity-Modulated Radiotherapy for Prostate Cancer

Hoppe BS, Michalski JM, Mendenhall NP, et al (Univ of Florida Proton Therapy Inst, Jacksonville; Washington Univ, St Louis, MO; et al)

Cancer 120:1076-1082, 2014

Background.—Data continue to emerge on the relative merits of different treatment modalities for prostate cancer. The objective of this study was to compare patient-reported quality-of-life (QOL) outcomes after proton therapy (PT) and intensity-modulated radiation therapy (IMRT) for prostate cancer.

Methods.—A comparison was performed of prospectively collected QOL data using the Expanded Prostate Cancer Index Composite (EPIC) questionnaire. QOL data were collected during the first 2 years after treatment for men who received PT and IMRT. PT was delivered to 1243 men at a single center at doses from 76 grays (Gy) to 82 Gy. IMRT was delivered to 204 men who were included in the Prostate Cancer Outcomes and Satisfaction with Treatment Quality Assessment (PROSTQA) study in doses from 75.6 Gy to 79.4 Gy. The Wilcoxon rank-sum test was used to compare EPIC outcomes by modality using baseline-adjusted scores at different time points. Individual questions were assessed by converting to binary outcomes and testing with generalized estimating equations.

Results.—No differences were observed in summary score changes for bowel, urinary incontinence, urinary irritative/obstructive, and sexual domains between the 2 cohorts. However, more men who received IMRT reported moderate/big problems with rectal urgency ($P = 0.02$) and frequent bowel movements ($P = 0.05$) than men who received PT.

Conclusions.—There were no differences in QOL summary scores between the IMRT and PT cohorts during early follow-up (up to 2-years). Response to individual questions suggests possible differences in specific bowel symptoms between the 2 cohorts. These outcomes highlight the need for further comparative studies of PT and IMRT.

▶ Given that health care costs in the United States are well beyond what we as a country can afford, we must find ways to better use our precious health care dollars. Diseases such as diabetes, heart disease, and cancer eat up the lion's share of these dollars and thus need to be the focus of study for improved valued as defined by quality/cost.

As oncologists it is the common cancers such as breast and prostate, given their sheer numbers, that can easily ratchet up our costs if we simply accept that new and expensive procedures are "better" than older ones without the science to prove these claims. This has been true for surgeons as well as radiation oncologists in the case of prostate cancer. The "robot" has been well marketed as better than the standard open radical prostatectomy despite clear data to support these claims. We must admit the same in radiation oncology with the explosion of intensity modulated radiation therapy (IMRT) and subsequently proton beam radiotherapy to treat localized prostate cancer.

Thus my hat is off to these authors for taking a serious scientific look at the toxicity end points of proton therapy versus IMRT for the treatment of localized prostate cancer. They found no clear differences between the 2 modalities at up to 2 years of follow-up and suggest the need for further scientific comparisons. In addition, they evaluated these end points with patient-reported outcomes, a known best way to assess the real experience of our patients. We look forward to more comparative effectiveness data before we conclude that more expensive proton therapy is worth the increased cost.

C. A. Lawton, MD

Impact of Dose to the Bladder Trigone on Long-Term Urinary Function After High-Dose Intensity Modulated Radiation Therapy for Localized Prostate Cancer

Ghadjar P, Zelefsky MJ, Spratt DE, et al (Memorial Sloan-Kettering Cancer Ctr, NY)

Int J Radiat Oncol Biol Phys 88:339-344, 2014

Purpose.—To determine the potential association between genitourinary (GU) toxicity and planning dose—volume parameters for GU pelvic structures after high-dose intensity modulated radiation therapy in localized prostate cancer patients.

Methods and Materials.—A total of 268 patients who underwent intensity modulated radiation therapy to a prescribed dose of 86.4 Gy in 48 fractions during June 2004-December 2008 were evaluated with the International Prostate Symptom Score (IPSS) questionnaire. Dose—volume histograms of the whole bladder, bladder wall, urethra, and bladder trigone were analyzed. The primary endpoint for GU toxicity was an IPSS sum increase ≥10 points over baseline. Univariate and multivariate analyses were done by the Kaplan-Meier method and Cox proportional hazard models, respectively.

Results.—Median follow-up was 5 years (range, 3-7.7 years). Thirty-nine patients experienced an IPSS sum increase ≥10 during follow-up; 84% remained event free at 5 years. After univariate analysis, lower baseline IPSS sum (P =.006), the V90 of the trigone (P =.006), and the maximal dose to the trigone (P =.003) were significantly associated with an IPSS sum increase ≥10. After multivariate analysis, lower baseline IPSS sum (P =.009) and increased maximal dose to the trigone (P =.005) remained significantly associated. Seventy-two patients had both a lower baseline IPSS sum and a higher maximal dose to the trigone and were defined as high risk, and 68 patients had both a higher baseline IPSS sum and a lower maximal dose to the trigone and were defined as low risk for development of an IPSS sum increase ≥10. Twenty-one of 72 high-risk patients (29%) and 5 of 68 low-risk patients (7%) experienced an IPSS sum increase ≥10 (P =.001; odds ratio 5.19).

Conclusions.—The application of hot spots to the bladder trigone was significantly associated with relevant changes in IPSS during follow-up. Reduction of radiation dose to the lower bladder and specifically the bladder trigone seems to be associated with a reduction in late GU toxicity.

▶ Significant improvements in our ability to design radiation treatment plans that are very conformal have been critical to allowing dose escalation for prostate cancer patients. Intensity modulated radiation therapy (IMRT) technology was a breakthrough in our ability to design such conformal treatment. Yet we all understood that this increase in conformality associated with IMRT came at a price in terms of increased heterogeneity. How much heterogeneity is tolerable and where those doses are placed has not been well studied. Thus the data presented here are the type of research that is needed to help all radiation oncologists design optimal conformal IMRT plans.

Given that low-dose rate brachytherapy for prostate cancer has resulted in some increase in International Prostate Symptom Score (IPSS) scores due to urinary radiation toxicity, it probably should not surprise us that increased IPSS scores can result in increased urinary toxicity from external beam irradiation as well. But just how much dose a bladder can tolerate and where that dose is placed has not been studied well.

Data from single institutions, such as that present in this article are important, and the message is clear that "hot spots" within the bladder trigone can result in increased IPSS scores for many patients. It will be important to look at these type of data in some of the cooperative group trials to see whether similar findings are detected. In the meantime, it behooves all radiation oncologists to be judicious in approving IMRT prostate plans with significant dose heterogeneity. Clearly the location of the "hot spots" is of concern.

C. A. Lawton, MD

Enzalutamide in Metastatic Prostate Cancer before Chemotherapy

Beer TM, for the PREVAIL Investigators (Oregon Health and Science Univ, Portland; et al)

N Engl J Med 371:424-433, 2014

Background.—Enzalutamide is an oral androgen-receptor inhibitor that prolongs survival in men with metastatic castration-resistant prostate cancer in whom the disease has progressed after chemotherapy. New treatment options are needed for patients with metastatic prostate cancer who have not received chemotherapy, in whom the disease has progressed despite androgen-deprivation therapy.

Methods.—In this double-blind, phase 3 study, we randomly assigned 1717 patients to receive either enzalutamide (at a dose of 160 mg) or placebo once daily. The coprimary end points were radiographic progression-free survival and overall survival.

Results.—The study was stopped after a planned interim analysis, conducted when 540 deaths had been reported, showed a benefit of the active treatment. The rate of radiographic progression-free survival at 12 months was 65% among patients treated with enzalutamide, as compared with 14% among patients receiving placebo (81% risk reduction; hazard ratio in the enzalutamide group, 0.19; 95% confidence interval [CI], 0.15 to 0.23; $P < 0.001$). A total of 626 patients (72%) in the enzalutamide group, as compared with 532 patients (63%) in the placebo group, were alive at the data-cutoff date (29% reduction in the risk of death; hazard ratio, 0.71; 95% CI, 0.60 to 0.84; $P < 0.001$). The benefit of enzalutamide was shown with respect to all secondary end points, including the time until the initiation of cytotoxic chemotherapy (hazard ratio, 0.35), the time until the first skeletal-related event (hazard ratio, 0.72), a complete or partial soft-tissue response (59% vs. 5%), the time until prostate-specific antigen (PSA) progression (hazard ratio, 0.17), and a rate of decline of at least 50% in PSA (78% vs. 3%) ($P < 0.001$ for all comparisons). Fatigue and hypertension were the most common clinically relevant adverse events associated with enzalutamide treatment.

Conclusions.—Enzalutamide significantly decreased the risk of radiographic progression and death and delayed the initiation of chemotherapy in men with metastatic prostate cancer. (Funded by Medivation and Astellas Pharma; PREVAIL ClinicalTrials.gov number, NCT01212991.)

▶ Prostate cancer continues to claim the lives of more than 30 000 men annually. Given these staggering numbers, it is critical that we continue to screen for this disease in an effort to find it when it is still curable. Yet prostate-specific antigen screening is not supported as a useful screening tool by Medicare and Medicaid (and thus is not paid for). So many patients now are found to have prostate cancer based on an abnormal digital rectal examination or painful bony metastasis.

Once the bony metastasis has developed, there is no cure for the disease, but there is still hope for successful treatment to prolong life. Androgen deprivation therapy is the first step to control metastatic prostate cancer, but this is only a temporary fix. Data published in this same journal in 2004 showed a survival benefit to the addition of docetaxel chemotherapy for these castrate-resistant patients. Yet chemotherapy comes with significant side effects of decreased white cell counts resulting in increased risk of infection, anemia, hair loss, and fatigue. So efforts to develop other noncytotoxic chemotherapy options are of merit.

Data from this trial in which patients with castrate-resistant prostate cancer were randomized to enzalutamide versus placebo before any cytotoxic chemotherapy is encouraging. Previously enzalutamide (an oral antiandrogen receptor inhibitor) was shown to increase survival in patients with metastatic castrate-resistant prostate cancer when given after cytotoxic chemotherapy. Based on these randomized results, we now know that enzalutamide, which has a much better toxicity profile compared with the side effects of chemotherapy, can be given before cytotoxic chemotherapy with the benefit in prostate cancer disease control still preserved.

C. A. Lawton, MD

Stereotactic Body Radiation Therapy Versus Intensity-Modulated Radiation Therapy for Prostate Cancer: Comparison of Toxicity

Yu JB, Cramer LD, Herrin J, et al (Yale School of Medicine, New Haven, CT; et al)

J Clin Oncol 32:1195-1201, 2014

Purpose.—Stereotactic body radiation therapy (SBRT) is a technically demanding prostate cancer treatment that may be less expensive than intensity-modulated radiation therapy (IMRT). Because SBRT may deliver a greater biologic dose of radiation than IMRT, toxicity could be increased. Studies comparing treatment cost to the Medicare program and toxicity are needed.

Methods.—We performed a retrospective study by using a national sample of Medicare beneficiaries age ≥66 years who received SBRT or IMRT as primary treatment for prostate cancer from 2008 to 2011. Each SBRT patient was matched to two IMRT patients with similar follow-up (6, 12, or 24 months). We calculated the cost of radiation therapy treatment to the Medicare program and toxicity as measured by Medicare claims; we used a random effects model to compare genitourinary (GU), GI, and other toxicity between matched patients.

Results.—The study sample consisted of 1,335 SBRT patients matched to 2,670 IMRT patients. The mean treatment cost was $13,645 for SBRT versus $21,023 for IMRT. In the 6 months after treatment initiation, 15.6% of SBRT versus 12.6% of IMRT patients experienced GU toxicity (odds ratio [OR], 1.29; 95% CI, 1.05 to 1.53; $P=.009$). At 24 months after treatment initiation, 43.9% of SBRT versus 36.3% of IMRT patients had GU toxicity (OR, 1.38; 95% CI, 1.12 to 1.63; $P=.001$). The increase in GU toxicity was due to claims indicative of urethritis, urinary incontinence, and/or obstruction.

Conclusion.—Although SBRT was associated with lower treatment costs, there appears to be a greater rate of GU toxicity for patients undergoing SBRT compared with IMRT, and prospective correlation with randomized trials is needed.

▶ Stereotactic body radiation therapy (SBRT) for localized prostate cancer has been advertised extensively by companies who sell equipment for such that it is quicker, cheaper, and equally effective from a cancer control and toxicity perspective. We clearly have limited data to address these claims and essentially no data comparing SBRT and standard intensity-modulated radiation therapy (IMRT) for this disease. But annually hundreds if not thousands of prostate cancer patients receive SBRT treatment assuming that we have these answers.

Given the precarious situation in which we find ourselves, we are stuck with the fact that until randomized trials are completed and reported we must look to retrospective data to try to address this SBRT versus IMRT comparison.

These authors are to be commended, as they performed an excellent analysis of cost and toxicity based on Medicare claims data in a retrospective matched comparison, weighted 2:1 IMRT versus SBRT. Their findings do support a cost savings for SBRT over IMRT ($13,645 vs $21,023). But this cost savings appears to come with a price in terms of genitourinary (GU) toxicity. The finding of increased GU toxicity at 6 months, 15.6% for SBRT versus 12.6% for IMRT, seems small enough that, despite the statistical difference, they could be tolerated. The real concern is the data at 24 months in which the delta is significantly larger, 43.9% for SBRT versus 36.3% for IMRT. These toxicities are concerning and include urethritis, urinary incontinence, or obstruction.

Until we have the randomized data that we need to address these significant toxicities, we simply must caution patients who wish to receive SBRT and treat them only on a multi-institutional registry or clinical randomized trial.

C. A. Lawton, MD

The Impact of Definitive Local Therapy for Lymph Node–Positive Prostate Cancer: A Population-Based Study

Rusthoven CG, Carlson JA, Waxweiler TV, et al (Univ of Colorado-Denver, Aurora)

Int J Radiat Oncol Biol Phys 88:1064-1073, 2014

Purpose.—To evaluate the survival outcomes for patients with lymph node–positive, nonmetastatic prostate cancer undergoing definitive local therapy (radical prostatectomy [RP], external beam radiation therapy [EBRT], or both) versus no local therapy (NLT) in the US population in the modern prostate specific antigen (PSA) era.

Methods and Materials.—The Surveillance, Epidemiology, and End Results database was queried for patients with T1-4N1M0 prostate cancer diagnosed from 1995 through 2005. To allow comparisons of equivalent datasets, patients were analyzed in separate clinical (cN+) and pathologically confirmed (pN+) lymph node–positive cohorts. Kaplan-Meier overall survival (OS) and prostate cancer-specific survival (PCSS) estimates were generated, with accompanying univariate log-rank and multivariate Cox proportional hazards comparisons.

Results.—A total of 796 cN+ and 2991 pN+ patients were evaluable. Among cN+ patients, 43% underwent EBRT and 57% had NLT. Outcomes for cN+ patients favored EBRT, with 10-year OS rates of 45% versus 29% ($P < .001$) and PCSS rates of 67% versus 53% ($P < .001$). Among pN+ patients, 78% underwent local therapy (RP 57%, EBRT 10%, or both 11%) and 22% had NLT. Outcomes for pN+ also favored local therapy, with 10-year OS rates of 65% versus 42% ($P < .001$) and PCSS rates of 78% versus 56% ($P < .001$). On multivariate analysis, local therapy in both the cN+ and pN+ cohorts remained independently associated with improved OS and PCSS (all $P < .001$). Local therapy was associated with favorable hazard ratios across subgroups, including patients aged ≥70 years and those with multiple positive lymph nodes. Among pN+ patients, no significant differences in survival were observed between RP versus EBRT and RP with or without adjuvant EBRT.

Conclusions.—In this large, population-based cohort, definitive local therapy was associated with significantly improved survival in patients with lymph node–positive prostate cancer.

▶ Annually in the United States more than 30 000 men die from prostate cancer. These numbers are still reflective of the prostate-specific antigen (PSA) screening era and earlier diagnosis. Now that our government does not support

PSA screening, the likelihood of patients presenting with more advanced disease will increase. Some of that advanced disease will present itself with clinically or pathologically involved regional lymph nodes, which are known to be a life-threatening feature of prostate cancer. Yet how to best treat patients with positive lymph nodes is a gray area indeed.

Many oncologists, including urologists and radiation oncologists, have considered positive lymph nodes consistent with systemic disease and, thus, feel that local therapy is not warranted. The studies trying to address the issue of treatment of the regional lymph nodes for clinical or microscopic involvement such as Radiation Therapy Oncology Group 94-13 have not provided clear answers. So a quandary remains.

In other adenocarcinomas, such as breast and rectal, the treatment with radiation for lymph node-positive disease impacts outcomes significantly so that there is no question that radiation to these affected lymph nodes is warranted. Thus, in the face of a lack of clear scientific data, this report is helpful. This review of the Surveillance, Epidemiology, and End Results database looking at lymph node-positive groups, clinically lymph node positive and pathologically lymph node positive, found a benefit to local therapy for both groups in terms of overall survival and prostate cancer-specific survival. These data are important to understand in detail and are important to communicate to our lymph node-positive patients who look to us for guidance as to the best treatment for their potentially fatal disease.

C. A. Lawton, MD

Declining use of brachytherapy for the treatment of prostate cancer

Mahmood U, Pugh T, Frank S, et al (Univ of Texas MD Anderson Cancer Ctr, Houston; et al)

Brachytherapy 13:157-162, 2014

Purpose.—To analyze the recent trends in the utilization of external beam radiation therapy (EBRT) and brachytherapy (BT) for the treatment of prostate cancer.

Methods and Materials.—Using the Surveillance, Epidemiology, and End Results (SEER) database, information was obtained for all patients diagnosed with localized prostate adenocarcinoma between 2004 and 2009 who were treated with radiation as local therapy. We evaluated the utilization of BT, EBRT, and combination BT + EBRT by the year of diagnosis and performed a multivariable analysis to determine the predictors of BT as treatment choice.

Results.—Between 2004 and 2009, EBRT monotherapy use increased from 55.8% to 62.0%, whereas all BT use correspondingly decreased from 44.2% to 38.0% (BT-only use decreased from 30.4% to 25.6%, whereas BT + EBRT use decreased from 13.8% to 12.3%). The decline of BT utilization differed by patient race, SEER registry, median county income, and National Comprehensive Cancer Network risk categorization (all $p < 0.001$), but not by patient age ($p = 0.763$) or marital status ($p = 0.193$). Multivariable analysis found that age, race, marital status, SEER registry, median county income, and National Comprehensive Cancer Network risk category were independent predictors of BT as treatment choice (all $p < 0.001$). Moreover, after controlling for all available patient and tumor characteristics, there was decreasing utilization of BT with increasing year of diagnosis (odds ratio for BT = 0.920, 95% confidence interval: 0.911–0.929, $p < 0.001$).

Conclusions.—Our analysis reveals decreasing utilization of BT for prostate cancer. This finding has significant implications in terms of national health care expenditure.

▶ Multiple treatment options exist for the hundreds of thousands of men in the United States who will have prostate cancer diagnosed this year to address their localized disease. If active surveillance is not their best option, successful and proven oncologic interventions include surgery and radiation therapy, including external beam, brachytherapy, or some combination. Each of these treatments comes with a cost in terms of expense in performing the procedure and loss of productivity of the patient as they recover from the intervention. In this era of trying to contain the burgeoning cost of health care, it is worth trying to understand each of these procedures and their outcomes in terms of cancer control and survival. Data presented here (obtained from Surveillance, Epidemiology, and End Results database) clearly show that the use of brachytherapy is declining, and the use of external beam radiation therapy is increasing. This change as the authors note is likely multifactorial, but it does not fall on deaf ears of the payers that this change occurred with the advent of intensity-modulated radiation therapy (IMRT), a clearly more costly yet not proven better treatment over brachytherapy.

Controlling the ever-increasing cost of health care is part of our job as oncologists; therefore, we need to be sure to apply new technology where it is needed and hopefully not where it is done solely due to increased reimbursement. If we as oncologists don't apply appropriate control on these expensive modalities someone else (like Centers for Medicare and Medicaid Services) will. This applies to the surgeons with their robot just as it does to the radiation oncologists with our IMRT, stereotactic body radiation therapy, and proton treatment.

C. A. Lawton, MD

Gleason 6 Prostate Cancer: Serious Malignancy or Toothless Lion?

Lepor H, Donin NM (Department of Urology, NYU Langone Medical Center, New York University School of Medicine, New York, New York)

Oncology (Williston Park) 28:16-22, 2014

Autopsy studies of men without known prostate cancer suggest that a substantial reservoir of prostate cancer that does not cause symptoms or death exists within the population. The majority of these cancers are

Gleason 6 tumors and are frequently detected by prostate-specific antigen-based prostate cancer screening. There is strong evidence from longitudinal cohort studies of men with both treated and untreated Gleason 6 prostate cancer to suggest that Gleason 6 disease, when not associated with higher-grade cancer, virtually never demonstrates the ability to metastasize and thus represents an indolent entity that does not require treatment. Whether Gleason 6 has a propensity to progress to higher-grade cancer is still under investigation. Because the term "cancer" has historically been used to represent a disease state that leads to progressive illness that is uniformly fatal without treatment, we believe Gleason 6 disease should not be labeled with this term. Our challenge now is to develop the technology to differentiate true Gleason 6 disease from the higher grades of dysplasia with which it can be associated.

▶ Expanding knowledge regarding prostate cancer like many of the common malignancies (breast, colon, and lung) has evolved significantly over the last several decades. Gleason scoring, first described in 1966, is a critical part of that evaluation in prostate cancer. Although important in its ability to define the more indolent from the more aggressive cancers, we are still struggling to understand the level of concern that both oncologists and patients should have regarding indolent cancers (today most often scored as Gleason score 6).

Prostate-specific antigen (PSA) screening, although controversial, is also critical in the understanding of this disease. The challenge here, of course, is the problem of potential over diagnosis and resultant treatment with mass screening. Yet all of this has to be balanced with the fact that over 30 000 men in the United States will die of prostate cancer this year. So what should oncologists and potential prostate cancer patients do?

The work outlined in this article is an excellent summary of the current understanding of Gleason Score 6 disease, PSA screening, and methods to sort out the best next steps for prostate cancer patients. Answers will come only with time and further research, but the push for better imaging such as multiparametric MRI to direct biopsies and better genetic understandings of patients with Gleason Score 6 disease are important directions for study. We desperately need these data as oncologists to be able to give our prostate cancer patients the answers they deserve to decrease overtreatment, and, just as importantly, avoid death from what can be a very aggressive malignancy.

C. A. Lawton, MD

AR-V7 and Resistance to Enzalutamide and Abiraterone in Prostate Cancer

Antonarakis ES, Lu C, Wang H, et al (Johns Hopkins Univ School of Medicine, Baltimore, MD)

N Engl J Med 371:1028-1038, 2014

Background.—The androgen-receptor isoform encoded by splice variant 7 lacks the ligand-binding domain, which is the target of enzalutamide and abiraterone, but remains constitutively active as a transcription factor. We hypothesized that detection of androgen-receptor splice variant 7 messenger RNA (AR-V7) in circulating tumor cells from men with advanced prostate cancer would be associated with resistance to enzalutamide and abiraterone.

Methods.—We used a quantitative reverse-transcriptase–polymerase-chain-reaction assay to evaluate AR-V7 in circulating tumor cells from prospectively enrolled patients with metastatic castration-resistant prostate cancer who were initiating treatment with either enzalutamide or abiraterone. We examined associations between AR-V7 status (positive vs. negative) and prostate-specific antigen (PSA) response rates (the primary end point), freedom from PSA progression (PSA progression–free survival), clinical or radiographic progression–free survival, and overall survival.

Results.—A total of 31 enzalutamide-treated patients and 31 abiraterone-treated patients were enrolled, of whom 39% and 19%, respectively, had detectable AR-V7 in circulating tumor cells. Among men receiving enzalutamide, AR-V7–positive patients had lower PSA response rates than AR-V7–negative patients (0% vs. 53%, $P = 0.004$) and shorter PSA progression–free survival (median, 1.4 months vs. 6.0 months; $P < 0.001$), clinical or radiographic progression–free survival (median, 2.1 months vs. 6.1 months; $P < 0.001$), and overall survival (median, 5.5 months vs. not reached; $P = 0.002$). Similarly, among men receiving abiraterone, AR-V7–positive patients had lower PSA response rates than AR-V7–negative patients (0% vs. 68%, $P = 0.004$) and shorter PSA progression–free survival (median, 1.3 months vs. not reached; $P < 0.001$), clinical or radiographic progression–free survival (median, 2.3 months vs. not reached; $P < 0.001$), and overall survival (median, 10.6 months vs. not reached, $P = 0.006$). The association between AR-V7 detection and therapeutic resistance was maintained after adjustment for expression of full-length androgen receptor messenger RNA.

Conclusions.—Detection of AR-V7 in circulating tumor cells from patients with castration-resistant prostate cancer may be associated with resistance to enzalutamide and abiraterone. These findings require large-scale prospective validation. (Funded by the Prostate Cancer Foundation and others.)

▶ There has been a plethora of advances in the medical management of metastatic prostate cancer in the past few years, such that patients have multiple options for second-line therapy and beyond for castrate-resistant disease. Yet what the next best step is after resistance to standard androgen-deprivation therapy has occurred is not known. With multiple options available, we need more research to develop the "best" second-line, third-line, and beyond treatment options for individual patients.

Clearly some of the new drugs developed for "castrate-resistant" prostate cancer have proven that many of these tumors are not truly androgen independent. Both enzalutamide and abiraterone, which have shown excellent results in this cohort of patients, modulate androgen receptors. Yet approximately 20% to 40% of castrate-resistant patients have no response (in terms of lowering prostate-specific antigen) to these agents. Understanding the biology behind this and other resistance to medical therapies is critical in selecting the next best options for these patients. Thus, the data presented here showing that detection of AR-V7 in circulating tumor cells may be associated with resistance to enzalutamide and abiraterone is the beginning of the type of data that we need to make the most appropriate choices for our castrate-resistant prostate cancer patients.

C. A. Lawton, MD

Radical Prostatectomy or Watchful Waiting in Early Prostate Cancer

Bill-Axelson A, Holmberg L, Garmo H, et al (Uppsala Univ Hosp, Sweden)
N Engl J Med 370:932-942, 2014

Background.—Radical prostatectomy reduces mortality among men with localized prostate cancer; however, important questions regarding long-term benefit remain.

Methods.—Between 1989 and 1999, we randomly assigned 695 men with early prostate cancer to watchful waiting or radical prostatectomy and followed them through the end of 2012. The primary end points in the Scandinavian Prostate Cancer Group Study Number 4 (SPCG-4) were death from any cause, death from prostate cancer, and the risk of metastases. Secondary end points included the initiation of androgen-deprivation therapy.

Results.—During 23.2 years of follow-up, 200 of 347 men in the surgery group and 247 of the 348 men in the watchful-waiting group died. Of the deaths, 63 in the surgery group and 99 in the watchful-waiting group were due to prostate cancer; the relative risk was 0.56 (95% confidence interval [CI], 0.41 to 0.77; $P = 0.001$), and the absolute difference was 11.0 percentage points (95% CI, 4.5 to 17.5). The number needed to treat to prevent one death was 8. One man died after surgery in the radical-prostatectomy group. Androgen-deprivation therapy was used in fewer patients who underwent prostatectomy (a difference of 25.0 percentage points; 95% CI, 17.7 to 32.3). The benefit of surgery with respect to death from prostate cancer was largest in men younger than 65 years of age (relative risk, 0.45) and in those with intermediate-risk prostate cancer (relative risk, 0.38). However, radical prostatectomy was associated with a reduced risk of metastases among older men (relative risk, 0.68; $P = 0.04$).

Conclusions.—Extended follow-up confirmed a substantial reduction in mortality after radical prostatectomy; the number needed to treat to prevent one death continued to decrease when the treatment was modified according to age at diagnosis and tumor risk. A large proportion of long-term survivors in the watchful-waiting group have not required any palliative treatment. (Funded by the Swedish Cancer Society and others.)

▶ Patients with localized prostate cancer have myriad treatment options to consider. Which option represents the best treatment for patients with localized early prostate cancer remains controversial. Certainly, most oncologists understand the low risk of death from prostate cancer for elderly men (greater than 75 years) with low-risk disease and, thus, the use of active surveillance for these patients as per the National Comprehensive Cancer Network guidelines is appropriate. But thousands of other younger men will have localized disease diagnosed for which both the patient and their treating oncologist wonder, what is the best approach? Consideration must be given to comorbidities and, thus, life expectancy, but also issue of the toxicity from progression of untreated disease.

This trial performed by the Scandinavian Prostate Cancer Group more than 20 years ago is critical to help us understand the potential benefit of treatment over observation for our localized prostate cancer patients. Inclusion criteria of age less than 75 years and life expectancy of greater than 10 years, no other cancers, T1 or T2 tumors, well-to-moderately well histology, prostate-specific antigen less than 50, and negative bone scan are also important as we try to assess which group of patients to apply these results.

In the end, we can learn a lot from these long-term results. Clearly, for the patients in this trial, there was a great benefit to treatment (in this trial the treatment was surgery, but certainly definitive radiation could be considered an equal alternative). Yet the magnitude of the benefit was greatest in the youngest patients (< 65 years) and those with intermediate-risk disease. So for these younger and less favorable patients, it is fairly clear that definitive treatment is helpful. What to do for more favorable and older patients still remains controversial. We await more data to help make the best treatment decisions for this group of patients.

C. A. Lawton, MD

24 Breast Cancer

Cognitive Impairment in Older Patients With Breast Cancer Before Systemic Therapy: Is There an Interaction Between Cancer and Comorbidity?

Mandelblatt JS, Stern RA, Luta G, et al (Georgetown Univ, Washington, DC; Boston Univ School of Medicine, MA; et al)
J Clin Oncol 32:1909-1918, 2014

Purpose.—To determine if older patients with breast cancer have cognitive impairment before systemic therapy.

Patients and Methods.—Participants were patients with newly diagnosed nonmetastatic breast cancer and matched friend or community controls age >60 years without prior systemic treatment, dementia, or neurologic disease. Participants completed surveys and a 55-minute battery of 17 neuropsychological tests. Biospecimens were obtained for *APOE* genotyping, and clinical data were abstracted. Neuropsychological test scores were standardized using control means and standard deviations (SDs) and grouped into five domain *z* scores. Cognitive impairment was defined as any domain *z* score two SDs below or ≥ two *z* scores 1.5 SDs below the control mean. Multivariable analyses evaluated pretreatment differences considering age, race, education, and site; comparisons between patient cases also controlled for surgery.

Results.—The 164 patient cases and 182 controls had similar neuropsychological domain scores. However, among patient cases, those with stage II to III cancers had lower executive function compared with those with stage 0 to I disease, after adjustment ($P = .05$). The odds of impairment were significantly higher among older, nonwhite, less educated women and those with greater comorbidity, after adjustment. Patient case or control status, anxiety, depression, fatigue, and surgery were not associated with impairment. However, there was an interaction between comorbidity and patient case or control status; comorbidity was strongly associated with impairment among patient cases (adjusted odds ratio, 8.77; 95% CI, 2.06 to 37.4; $P = .003$) but not among controls ($P = .97$). Only diabetes and cardiovascular disease were associated with impairment among patient cases.

Conclusion.—There were no overall differences between patients with breast cancer and controls before systemic treatment, but there may be pretreatment cognitive impairment within subgroups of patient cases with greater tumor or comorbidity burden.

▶ The message given to patients that they will require chemotherapy as part of their treatment strategy is a daunting one. Fear, anxiety, and depression can accompany that messaging, separate from the diagnosis of cancer itself. These symptoms are often the result of the perception that chemotherapy always makes one violently sick to your stomach, makes your hair fall out, and turns your brain into "mush," otherwise known as "chemo brain." Yet all oncologists are aware of the fact that many patients never have many of these symptoms. Nausea, much less vomiting, for example, is uncommon because of improved antiemetics.

Unfortunately, for breast cancer patients, the concern over "chemo brain" is real, as data have emerged showing its prevalence. Thus, ways to better understand who is most at risk is important so as to inform patients and help in prevention. These data evaluating cognition in older patients (> 60 years) who received chemotherapy for breast cancer and comparing them with age-matched controls is an excellent step in helping to understand this potential toxicity. Clearly these data shows some increased concern for cognitive changes in patients with increased tumor burden and comorbidities and are helpful to oncologists as they explain the risk of such changes to their breast cancer patients who need chemotherapy.

C. A. Lawton, MD

Society of Surgical Oncology–American Society for Radiation Oncology Consensus Guideline on Margins for Breast-Conserving Surgery With Whole-Breast Irradiation in Stages I and II Invasive Breast Cancer

Moran MS, Schnitt SJ, Giuliano AE, et al (Yale Univ, New Haven, CT; Harvard Med School, Boston, MA; Cedars Sinai Med Ctr, Los Angeles, CA; et al)

Int J Radiat Oncol Biol Phys 88:553-564, 2014

Purpose.—To convene a multidisciplinary panel of breast experts to examine the relationship between margin width and ipsilateral breast tumor recurrence (IBTR) and develop a guideline for defining adequate margins in the setting of breast conserving surgery and adjuvant radiation therapy.

Methods and Materials.—A multidisciplinary consensus panel used a meta-analysis of margin width and IBTR from a systematic review of 33 studies including 28,162 patients as the primary evidence base for consensus.

Results.—Positive margins (ink on invasive carcinoma or ductal carcinoma in situ) are associated with a 2-fold increase in the risk of IBTR compared with negative margins. This increased risk is not mitigated by favorable biology, endocrine therapy, or a radiation boost. More widely clear margins than no ink on tumor do not significantly decrease the rate of IBTR compared with no ink on tumor. There is no evidence that more widely clear margins reduce IBTR for young patients or for those with unfavorable biology, lobular cancers, or cancers with an extensive intraductal component.

Conclusions.—The use of no ink on tumor as the standard for an adequate margin in invasive cancer in the era of multidisciplinary therapy is associated with low rates of IBTR and has the potential to decrease re-excision rates, improve cosmetic outcomes, and decrease health care costs.

► For decades there has been a common belief that "in-breast" recurrence of breast cancer correlated with the width of the negative margin at the time of lumpectomy. This concept was so well engrained in many surgeons that women had to undergo multiple reexcisions to get to that "magic" margin width. This resulted in decreased cosmesis (the primary reason for breast conservation therapy), increased inconvenience, and increased cost. Therefore, this consensus guideline is critical for the best outcomes for our breast cancer patients treated with organ preservation. Essential to this guideline and its impact is the collaboration that occurred to develop it. It took both the breast surgeons and the breast radiation oncologists to recommend the best care for patients and thus this guideline (a joint effort of the Society of Surgical Oncology and the American Society for Radiation Oncology) represents the correct collaboration.

The authors are to be commended for addressing multiple aspects of this margin question including positive margins, negative margin width, and effect of systemic therapy, biological subtypes, and aspects of radiation therapy delivery, age, and lobular carcinoma in situ, in addition to invasive ductal carcinoma.

Guidelines like these can be helpful from a quality metric perspective going forward. It will be helpful to have more of these types of collaborative guidelines developed to ensure that all of our cancer patients are being treated with the best scientifically based care possible.

C. A. Lawton, MD

Uptake and Costs of Hypofractionated vs Conventional Whole Breast Irradiation After Breast Conserving Surgery in the United States, 2008–2013

Bekelman JE, Sylwestrzak G, Barron J, et al (Univ of Pennsylvania Perelman School of Medicine, Philadelphia; HealthCore, Wilmington, DE; et al)
JAMA 312:2542-2550, 2014

Importance.—Based on randomized evidence, expert guidelines in 2011 endorsed shorter, hypofractionated whole breast irradiation (WBI) for selected patients with early-stage breast cancer and permitted hypofractionated WBI for other patients.

Objectives.—To examine the uptake and costs of hypofractionated WBI among commercially insured patients in the United States.

Design, Setting, and Participants.—Retrospective, observational cohort study, using administrative claims data from 14 commercial health care plans covering 7.4% of US adult women in 2013, we classified patients with incident early-stage breast cancer treated with lumpectomy and WBI from 2008 and 2013 into 2 cohorts: (1) the hypofractionation-endorsed cohort (n = 8924) included patients aged 50 years or older without prior chemotherapy or axillary lymph node involvement and (2) the hypofractionation-permitted cohort (n = 6719) included patients younger than 50 years or those with prior chemotherapy or axillary lymph node involvement.

Exposures.—Hypofractionated WBI (3-5 weeks of treatment) vs conventional WBI (5-7 weeks of treatment).

Main Outcomes and Measures.—Use of hypofractionated and conventional WBI, total and radiotherapy-related health care expenditures, and patient out-of-pocket expenses. Patient and clinical characteristics included year of treatment, age, comorbid disease, prior chemotherapy, axillary lymph node involvement, intensity-modulated radiotherapy, practice setting, and other contextual variables.

Results.—Hypofractionated WBI increased from 10.6% (95% CI, 8.8%-12.5%) in 2008 to 34.5% (95% CI, 32.2%-36.8%) in 2013 in the hypofractionation-endorsed cohort and from 8.1% (95% CI, 6.0%-10.2%) in 2008 to 21.2% (95% CI, 18.9%-23.6%) in 2013 in the hypofractionation-permitted cohort. Adjusted mean total health care expenditures in the 1 year after diagnosis were $28 747 for hypofractionated and $31 641 for conventional WBI in the hypofractionation-endorsed cohort (difference, $2894; 95% CI, $1610-$4234; $P < .001$) and $64 273 for hypofractionated and $72 860 for conventional WBI in the hypofractionation-permitted cohort (difference, $8587; 95% CI, $5316-$12 017; $P < .001$). Adjusted mean total 1-year patient out-of-pocket expenses were not significantly different between hypofractionated vs conventional WBI in either cohort.

Conclusions and Relevance.—Hypofractionated WBI after breast conserving surgery increased among women with early-stage breast cancer in 14 US commercial health care plans between 2008 and 2013. However, only 34.5% of patients with hypofractionation-endorsed and 21.2% with hypofractionation-permitted early-stage breast cancer received hypofractionated WBI in 2013.

▶ Breast and prostate cancers represent the most common nonskin cancers for women and men, respectively, in the United States. Thus, changes in the management of either of these have far-reaching implications given the sheer number of cases.

Both of these glandular malignancies have the treatment option of organ preservation via the use of radiation therapy. Radiation therapy is standardly delivered at doses of 1.8 to 2.0 Gy/fraction, which results in multiple weeks of radiation therapy for patients, making it both inconvenient and expensive for patients and a cost concern for insurers. With the advent of hypofractionation and promising results in both prostate and breast cancer, we as oncologists are understanding that hypofractionation is an excellent option for many of these patients.

For the breast cancer patients in particular, multiple datasets have shown equivalence of the shorter hypofractionated schedules (approximately 3 vs the standard 5-6 weeks) in terms of control and toxicity to the standard fractionation schedules. Given these data, the authors of this article evaluated the adoption, or lack thereof, of hypofractionated regimens for intact breast cancer patients treated in the United States from 2008 to 2013. The authors found an increase in utilization of hypofractionation from 10.6% of hypofractionated endorsed patients to 34.5%. The conclusion of these authors that this adoption has been slow should be taken with some caution in that the long-term results of the breast cancer hypofractionation trials that are cited came out as recently as 2010 and 2011. It takes time for data like these to be processed by the practicing radiation oncologists. Thus, it will be fascinating to see similar analysis in the next few years to see if the adoption increases dramatically as one might expect. Clearly, increasing the utilization of hypofractionated regimens will result in increased convenience for the patients and decreased costs for the health care system.

C. A. Lawton, MD

Hypofractionation for Breast Cancer: Lessons Learned From Our Neighbors to the North and Across the Pond

Eblan MJ, Vanderwalde NA, Zeman EM, et al (Department of Radiation Oncology, UNC Lineberger Comprehensive Cancer Center, Chapel Hill, North Carolina)

Oncology (Williston Park) 28:536-546, 2014

Adjuvant whole breast irradiation was established within the standard of care for breast-conserving therapy in the early 1980s, following the results of major randomized trials comparing mastectomy vs breast-conserving surgery and radiation. Since that time, techniques and treatment strategies have evolved, but one major thread that carries forward is the need to balance cost, efficacy, complications, and convenience. Fortunately, data from randomized trials conducted in Canada and Great Britain provide a solid framework for the consideration of hypofractionated radiation in the treatment of breast cancer. In this review we discuss the rationale and underlying radiobiologic concepts for hypofractionation, and review the clinical trials and American Society for Radiation Oncology (ASTRO) guidelines supporting this approach. We also review the practical considerations for treatment planning, including dosimetric criteria and how to approach treatment of the node-positive patient. In the current era of healthcare reform and cost awareness, thoughtful utilization of hypofractionation may offer considerable savings to individual patients and the healthcare system–without compromising clinical outcomes or quality of life.

▶ The use of relatively small radiation fraction sizes used over a long period of time (many weeks) was predicated on the understanding that late-responding normal tissues, such as lung and spinal cord, have lower alpha/beta ratios and therefore increased sensitivity to dose per fraction compared with malignant cells. Most malignancies were thought to have high alpha/beta ratios and therefore less sensitivity to a change in fraction size. Data has emerged in many common tumors that suggest that this may not be correct. In prostate cancer, for example, we now understand that the alpha/beta is likely much lower than we previously thought. Like prostate cancer, breast cancer is now understood to have a lower alpha/beta than previously understood. Thus, the concept of larger fraction sizes over a shorter period of time is clinically reasonable.

These alpha/beta changes have been evaluated via clinical trials in breast cancer using hypofractionation. Prospective randomized data from both Canada and Great Britain with long follow-up have shown excellent results in terms of disease control and cosmesis to support the use of hypofractionation in selected patients. Although hypofractionation cannot be considered the standard radiation therapy for all breast cancer patients, many are appropriate and should be offered this more convenient and less costly option.

C. A. Lawton, MD

25 Myeloid Suppressor Cell Tumors

Autologous Transplantation and Maintenance Therapy in Multiple Myeloma

Palumbo A, Cavallo F, Gay F, et al (Univ of Turin, Italy; et al)

N Engl J Med 371:895-905, 2014

Background.—This open-label, randomized, phase 3 study compared melphalan at a dose of 200 mg per square meter of body-surface area plus autologous stem-cell transplantation with melphalan–prednisone–lenalidomide (MPR) and compared lenalidomide maintenance therapy with no maintenance therapy in patients with newly diagnosed multiple myeloma.

Methods.—We randomly assigned 273 patients 65 years of age or younger to high-dose melphalan plus stem-cell transplantation or MPR consolidation therapy after induction, and 251 patients to lenalidomide maintenance therapy or no maintenance therapy. The primary end point was progression-free survival.

Results.—The median follow-up period was 51.2 months. Both progression-free and overall survival were significantly longer with high-dose melphalan plus stem-cell transplantation than with MPR (median progression-free survival, 43.0 months vs. 22.4 months; hazard ratio for progression or death, 0.44; 95% confidence interval [CI], 0.32 to 0.61; $P < 0.001$; and 4-year overall survival, 81.6% vs. 65.3%; hazard ratio for death, 0.55; 95% CI, 0.32 to 0.93; $P = 0.02$). Median progression-free survival was significantly longer with lenalidomide maintenance than with no maintenance (41.9 months vs. 21.6 months; hazard ratio for progression or death, 0.47; 95% CI, 0.33 to 0.65; $P < 0.001$), but 3-year overall survival was not significantly prolonged (88.0% vs. 79.2%; hazard ratio for death, 0.64; 95% CI, 0.36 to 1.15; $P = 0.14$). Grade 3 or 4 neutropenia was significantly more frequent with high-dose melphalan than with MPR (94.3% vs. 51.5%), as were gastrointestinal adverse events (18.4% vs. 0%) and infections (16.3% vs. 0.8%); neutropenia and dermatologic toxic effects were more frequent with lenalidomide maintenance than with no maintenance (23.3% vs. 0% and 4.3% vs. 0%, respectively).

Conclusions.—Consolidation therapy with high-dose melphalan plus stem-cell transplantation, as compared with MPR, significantly prolonged progression-free and overall survival among patients with multiple myeloma who were 65 years of age or younger. Lenalidomide maintenance, as compared with no maintenance, significantly prolonged progression-free survival. (Funded by Celgene; ClinicalTrials.gov number, NCT00551928.)

▶ Multiple myeloma has essentially been a uniformly fatal disease until the advent of stem autologous transplant. Yet patients often live for many years after the diagnosis with the use of conventional chemotherapy without stem cell transplant. Thus, the push to employ stem cell autologous transplant sooner in the treatment course could cause some premature deaths and may not be warranted in many cases.

To try to address the above, this phase III randomized trial looked at newly diagnosed multiple myeloma patients older than 65 years of age and randomized them to high-dose melphalan and autologous stem cell transplant versus standard chemotherapy of melphalan, prednisone, and lenalidomide. In addition, they were subsequently randomized to maintenance lenalidomide versus no maintenance therapy. The results showing an overall benefit from the use of high-dose melphalan and stem cell transplant reinforces the need to perform this aggressive therapy upfront for these patients to achieve the best results.

The answer to the question regarding the need for maintenance lenalidomide was somewhat less clear in that it resulted in improvement in progression-free survival only. Given the follow-up of a median 51.2 months, perhaps longer follow-up will reveal an overall survival benefit for this maintenance treatment. We await further follow-up to support or negate this end point.

C. A. Lawton, MD

26 Cancer Screening

Final Trial Report of Sentinel-Node Biopsy versus Nodal Observation in Melanoma

Morton DL, for the MSLT Group (John Wayne Cancer Inst at Saint John's Health Ctr, Santa Monica, CA; et al)

N Engl J Med 370:599-609, 2014

Background.—Sentinel-node biopsy, a minimally invasive procedure for regional melanoma staging, was evaluated in a phase 3 trial.

Methods.—We evaluated outcomes in 2001 patients with primary cutaneous melanomas randomly assigned to undergo wide excision and nodal observation, with lymphadenectomy for nodal relapse (observation group), or wide excision and sentinel-node biopsy, with immediate lymphadenectomy for nodal metastases detected on biopsy (biopsy group).

Results.—No significant treatment-related difference in the 10-year melanoma-specific survival rate was seen in the overall study population (20.8% with and 79.2% without nodal metastases). Mean (±SE) 10-year disease-free survival rates were significantly improved in the biopsy group, as compared with the observation group, among patients with intermediate-thickness melanomas, defined as 1.20 to 3.50 mm (71.3 ± 1.8% vs. 64.7 ± 2.3%; hazard ratio for recurrence or metastasis, 0.76; $P = 0.01$), and those with thick melanomas, defined as >3.50 mm (50.7 ± 4.0% vs. 40.5 ± 4.7%; hazard ratio, 0.70; $P = 0.03$). Among patients with intermediate-thickness melanomas, the 10-year melanoma-specific survival rate was 62.1 ± 4.8% among those with metastasis versus 85.1 ± 1.5% for those without metastasis (hazard ratio for death from melanoma, 3.09; $P < 0.001$); among patients with thick melanomas, the respective rates were 48.0 ± 7.0% and 64.6 ± 4.9% (hazard ratio, 1.75; $P = 0.03$). Biopsy-based management improved the 10-year rate of distant disease–free survival (hazard ratio for distant metastasis, 0.62; $P = 0.02$) and the 10-year rate of melanoma-specific survival (hazard ratio for death from melanoma, 0.56; $P = 0.006$) for patients with intermediate-thickness melanomas and nodal metastases. Accelerated-failure-time latent-subgroup analysis was performed to account for the fact that nodal status was initially known only in the biopsy group, and a significant treatment benefit persisted.

Conclusions.—Biopsy-based staging of intermediate-thickness or thick primary melanomas provides important prognostic information and identifies patients with nodal metastases who may benefit from immediate complete lymphadenectomy. Biopsy-based management prolongs disease-free survival for all patients and prolongs distant disease—free survival and melanoma-specific survival for patients with nodal metastases from intermediate-thickness melanomas. (Funded by the National Cancer Institute, National Institutes of Health, and the Australia and New Zealand Melanoma Trials Group; ClinicalTrials.gov number, NCT00275496.)

▶ Common skin cancers related to sun exposure are on the rise and for the most part are easily addressed and not life-threatening. The less common skin cancer, melanoma, is also on a rise secondary to sun exposure and unfortunately can be a life-threatening disease pending depth of invasion and lymph node metastasis. Thus the most appropriate way to treat these potentially life-threatening cancers is critical to understand.

In 1994, the multicenter selective lymphadenectomy trial (MSLT-I) was started and randomized 2001 patients with primary cutaneous melanomas to wide excision and nodal observation versus wide excision and sentinel-node biopsy with immediate lymph node dissection for positive sentinel lymph nodes. The goal of this trial was 2-fold. First, the trial was attempting to evaluate the potential benefit of routine elective lymph node dissection (which some authors have fervently supported). Second, the trial was attempting to evaluate the potential toxicity improvement for patients who might be spared lymph node dissection.

The current report is the 10-year follow-up data showing the clear benefit of sentinel-node biopsy and subsequent lymph node dissection in patients with intermediate-thickness (1.20-3.50 mm) or thick (> 3.5 mm) primary melanomas. This type of long-term data from a phase III prospective randomized trial is exactly what is needed to support the need for lymph node dissection (a surgery with clear toxicities related to it especially in terms of lymphoderma). Understanding of the potential lack of benefit of such surgery for patients with more superficial melanomas is also critically needed, and we await such data.

C. A. Lawton, MD

Considerations for Observational Research Using Large Data Sets in Radiation Oncology

Jagsi R, Bekelman JE, Chen A, et al (Univ of Michigan, Ann Arbor; Univ of Pennsylvania Perelman School of Medicine, Philadelphia; Harvard Med School, Boston, MA; et al)

Int J Radiation Oncol Biol Phys 90:11-24, 2014

The radiation oncology community has witnessed growing interest in observational research conducted using large-scale data sources such as registries and claims-based data sets. With the growing emphasis on observational analyses in health care, the radiation oncology community must possess a sophisticated understanding of the methodological considerations of such studies in order to evaluate evidence appropriately to guide practice and policy. Because observational research has unique features that distinguish it from clinical trials and other forms of traditional radiation oncology research, the *International Journal of Radiation Oncology, Biology, Physics* assembled a panel of experts in health services research to provide a concise and well-referenced review, intended to be informative for the lay reader, as well as for scholars who wish to embark on such research without prior experience. This review begins by discussing the types of research questions relevant to radiation oncology that large-scale databases may help illuminate. It then describes major potential data sources for such endeavors, including information regarding access and insights regarding the strengths and limitations of each. Finally, it provides guidance regarding the analytical challenges that observational studies must confront, along with discussion of the techniques that have been developed to help minimize the impact of certain common analytical issues in observational analysis. Features characterizing a well-designed observational study include clearly defined research questions, careful selection of an appropriate data source, consultation with investigators with relevant methodological expertise, inclusion of sensitivity analyses, caution not to overinterpret small but significant differences, and recognition of limitations when trying to evaluate causality. This review concludes that carefully designed and executed studies using observational data that possess these qualities hold substantial promise for advancing our understanding of many unanswered questions of importance to the field of radiation oncology.

▶ As the desire for increased "value" for every aspect of medical care has occurred, we have to look closely at both quality and cost to address this value question. Cost is relatively straightforward in radiation oncology in terms of technology and personnel required to run such. Given that cost for radiation oncology are significant because our technology is quite advanced as are the personnel needed to run it well, our best option to improve value hinges on quality.

Quality improvement requires data. The reality is that the type of data we like to quote to address the role of radiation therapy in the treatment of malignancies comes from clinical trials. The gold standard of clinical trials of course is the phase III randomized trial. Yet the vast majority of the use of radiation therapy does not have that type of data to support it. Phase III randomized trials, although helpful, provide results that likely only apply to the population studied, not necessarily to the general population.

So we are challenged to find other data sources to help us best define quality radiation therapy. Registries or other large-scale databases can be a source of answers for us. When considering the large-scale datasets, we need to carefully determine the strengths and weaknesses of them. This article provides an excellent guide to the use of large datasets addressing the strengths and pitfalls of such. It provides a great resource to the practicing radiation oncologists on how to review results from large-scale databases that will significantly help determine the future of quality radiation therapy.

C. A. Lawton, MD

Chemoradiation Therapy Sequencing for Resected Pancreatic Adenocarcinoma in the National Cancer Data Base

Colbert LE, Hall WA, Nickleach D, et al (Emory Univ, Atlanta, GA; Biostatistics and Bioinformatics Shared Resource at Winship Cancer Inst, Atlanta, GA; et al)

Cancer 120:499-506, 2014

Background.—Pancreatic adenocarcinoma (PAC) has low overall survival (OS) rates and high recurrence rates following surgical resection. The role for preoperative radiation therapy (prRT) for PAC versus postoperative RT (poRT) remains uncertain. The authors used the National Cancer Data Base (NCDB) to report prRT outcomes for the largest multi-institutional patient cohort to date.

Methods.—NCDB data were obtained for all patients who underwent resection and external beam radiation (RT) for PAC from 1998 to 2002. Patients with metastatic (M1) disease, intraoperative RT, RT both before and after surgery, missing OS, or missing RT variables were excluded. Univariate (UV) and multivariate (MV) analysis were run using treatment characteristics, tumor characteristics, and patient demographics. The difference in patients' known characteristics was described by a chi-square test or analysis of variance.

Results.—A total of 5414 patients were identified. Of these, 277 received prRT and 5137 received poRT. Overall, 92.9% received chemotherapy and 7.1% received RT alone; 56% (2990 of 5307) of patients had stage III disease, according to American Joint Commission on Cancer (AJCC) staging manual, 5th edition. Median tumor size was 3 cm (range: 0-9.9 cm); 82% (199 of 244) of patients with prRT had negative surgical margins; 72% (3383 of 4699) of patients with poRT had negative margins. Forty-one percent (71 of 173) of patients with prRT were lymph node (LN)-positive; 65% (3159 of 4833) of patients with poRT were LN-positive. Median OS for patients with prRT was 18 months (95% CI = 18-19 months) and for patients with poRT, 19 months (95% CI = 17-22 months).

Conclusions.—Receipt of prRT was associated with lower stage, higher rates of negative margins, and lower rates of lymph node positivity at resection. However, there was no significant difference in median OS versus that of the poRT group.

► Pancreatic carcinoma is an aggressive, often fatal malignancy for which overall survival rates at 5 years are still less than 5%. So any potential therapeutic maneuver that might affect these terrible statistics is welcome. Preoperative radiation therapy and chemotherapy represents one such approach for which small, single-institution series have reported some potential improvement in terms of negative margins at the time of surgery and in some cases increased survival. Yet large datasets looking at preoperative vs postoperative chemoradiation do not exist. The reality is that not all questions like this one can be answered with level I data due to many issues, not the least of which is cost.

Large data sets such as the National Cancer Data Base represent registry-type "big data" to which we can look for some answers. This data bank reveals that preoperative radiation therapy was associated with lower stages at the time of surgery, higher rates of negative margins, and lower rates of positive lymph nodes. Yet overall survival was no different than in the postoperative radiation therapy group.

Although not answering all of our questions related to preoperative vs postop adjuvant treatment for resected pancreatic carcinoma, these data do give some clues as to potential benefit of preoperative radiation and the need for further study of systemic agents in addition to radiation and surgery. Going forward, registry data like this will be pivotal in guiding our therapies for this and many other malignancies when phase II and III data are not available.

C. A. Lawton, MD

Current Status and Recommendations for the Future of Research, Teaching, and Testing in the Biological Sciences of Radiation Oncology: Report of the American Society for Radiation Oncology Cancer Biology/ Radiation Biology Task Force, Executive Summary

Wallner PE, Anscher MS, Barker CA, et al (American Board of Radiology, Bethesda, MD; Virginia Commonwealth Univ, Richmond; Memorial Sloan-Kettering Cancer Ctr, NY; et al)

Int J Radiat Oncol Biol Phys 88:11-17, 2014

In early 2011, a dialogue was initiated within the Board of Directors (BOD) of the American Society for Radiation Oncology (ASTRO) regarding the future of the basic sciences of the specialty, primarily focused on the current state and potential future direction of basic research within radiation oncology. After consideration of the complexity of the issues involved and the precise nature of the undertaking, in August 2011, the BOD empanelled a Cancer Biology/Radiation Biology Task Force (TF). The TF was charged with developing an accurate snapshot of the current state of basic (preclinical) research in radiation oncology from the perspective of relevance to the modern clinical practice of radiation oncology as well as the education of our trainees and attending physicians in the biological sciences. The TF was further charged with making suggestions as to critical areas of biological basic research investigation that might be most likely to maintain and build further the scientific foundation and vitality of radiation oncology as an independent and vibrant medical specialty. It was not within the scope of service of the TF to consider the quality of ongoing research efforts within the broader radiation oncology space, to presume to consider their future potential, or to discourage in any way the investigators committed to areas of interest other than those targeted. The TF charge specifically precluded consideration of research issues related to technology, physics, or clinical investigations. This document represents an Executive Summary of the Task Force report.

▶ Appropriate use of radiation for cancer patients is based on radiation biology research. The 4 "Rs" of radiation biology (repair, reoxygenation, redistribution, and repopulation) remain as relevant today as they were when they first described decades ago. Our ability to advance our field depends not only on improvements in radiation therapy delivery, but more importantly on advances in the biological basis of radiation/cancer cell interactions and improvements in those interactions.

Understanding the need to support radiation biology research, the American Society of Radiation Oncology (ASTRO) Board of Directors convened a task force to address such in 2011. The group was charged with describing not only the current status of basic research in radiation oncology and education of trainees in such, but also with outlining critical areas for future research. The overarching goal of this task force was to describe the pathway for future investigations to support the vital role of radiation in eradicating cancer.

This article describes a critical road map for preclinical research in our field. This should be a blueprint for investigators and those supporting the investigators to help our cancer patients achieve their goal of being survivors with minimal toxicity.

C. A. Lawton, MD

National Trends in Prostate Cancer Screening Among Older American Men With Limited 9-Year Life Expectancies: Evidence of an Increased Need for Shared Decision Making

Drazer MW, Prasad SM, Huo D, et al (Univ of Chicago Med Ctr, IL; Med Univ of South Carolina, Charleston; et al)

Cancer 120:1491-1498, 2014

Background.—Prostate-specific antigen (PSA) screening for prostate cancer remains controversial. Most groups recommend informed decision making for men with 10 years of remaining life expectancy. The primary objective of this observational cohort study was to investigate the association between predicted 9-year mortality and prostate cancer screening among American men aged ≥65 years in 2005 and 2010. The second objective was to analyze the proportions of men who discussed screening with their physicians.

Methods.—Data were extracted from the 2005 and 2010 National Health Interview Surveys. Men aged ≥65 years without prostate cancer were divided into predicted 9-year mortality quartiles. The proportions of men confirming a screening PSA within the prior year were determined. Logistic regression was used to compare screening rates.

Results.—Screening rates for men aged ≥65 years were 48% in 2005 and 48% in 2010 ($P = .9$). Men ages 65 to 74 years who had <27% predicted 9-year mortality were most commonly screened, with 56% screened in 2010, compared with 34% of men aged ≥75 years with >75% predicted 9-year mortality. Approximately 55% of screened men aged ≥75 years who had ≥53% predicted 9-year mortality recalled discussing the advantages of screening, whereas 25% recalled discussing the disadvantages.

Conclusions.—Prostate cancer screening with PSA did not differ significantly between 2005 and 2010 for men aged ≥65 years based on predicted 9-year mortality. Approximately 33% of older men with a high likelihood of 9-year mortality were screened despite minimal clinical benefit. Twice as many men recalled discussing the potential advantages of screening compared with the disadvantages.

▶ Prostate-specific antigen (PSA) screening for prostate cancer is controversial. PSA screening unquestionably does increase the diagnosis of the disease, yet results of trials looking at the effect PSA screening on prostate cancer mortality are mixed. This finding has caused the United States Preventative Service Task Force to give PSA screening a grade D in 2012, which is a recommendation against PSA screening for prostate cancer. Both the American Urologic Association and American Society for Radiation Oncology have issued statements encouraging the appropriate use of PSA screening to help decrease the annual death rate from prostate cancer in the United States, which is a staggering 35 000-plus lives.

Given the above, it comes as no surprise that virtually everyone in the medical community can agree that routine PSA screening for men with limited life expectancy makes little sense. Thus, the data evaluating the use of PSA screening in patients older than 65 years are of particular interest. The fact that one-third of these men with relatively short life expectancy (high likelihood of 9-year mortality) were screened is very concerning. Equally distressing is the lack of discussion and PSA screening for many healthy younger men who could potentially benefit from such screening. There is, therefore, a serious need for education of both primary care clinicians and patients regarding the best use of PSA screening. At a minimum, it should begin with a discussion between the primary care physician and the patient on the potential risks verses benefits of PSA screening. This discussion will allow men to make more informed decisions with regard to this challenging screening question and sometimes lethal disease.

C. A. Lawton, MD

Proton Radiation Therapy for Head and Neck Cancer: A Review of the Clinical Experience to Date

Holliday EB, Frank SJ (Univ of Texas MD Anderson Cancer Ctr, Houston)

Int J Radiat Oncol Biol Phys 89:292-302, 2014

Proton beam radiation has been used for cancer treatment since the 1950s, but recent increasing interest in this form of therapy and the construction of hospital-based and clinic-based facilities for its delivery have greatly increased both the number of patients and the variety of tumors being treated with proton therapy. The mass of proton particles and their unique physical properties (ie, the Bragg peak) allow proton therapy to spare normal tissues distal to the tumor target from incidental irradiation. Initial observations show that proton therapy is particularly useful for treating tumors in challenging locations close to nontarget critical structures. Specifically, improvements in local control outcomes for patients with chordoma, chonodrosarcoma, and tumors in the sinonasal regions have been reported in series using proton. Improved local control and survival outcomes for patients with cancer of the head and neck region have also been seen with the advent of improvements in better imaging and multimodality therapy comprising surgery, radiation therapy, and chemotherapy. However, aggressive local therapy in the proximity of critical normal structures to tumors in the head and neck region may produce debilitating early and late toxic effects. Great interest has been expressed in evaluating whether proton therapy can improve outcomes, especially early and late toxicity, when used in the treatment of head and neck malignancies. This review summarizes the progress made to date in addressing this question.

▶ Proton radiation therapy in the treatment of cancer is certainly not a new technology. It has been available, albeit at limited locations, for clinical care for decades. Two facts are very clear with regard to protons today. First is that there is a plethora of facilities putting in proton-producing equipment. Second, the cost of these facilities and, thus, the cost of proton radiation therapy for patients and payers are high and considerably higher than standard photon beam irradiation. Thus, studying the most appropriate use of protons in all cancer types is laudable.

This review of the clinical experience to date using protons for head and neck cancer provides some insights and is an excellent compilation of the data available to date. I disagree with the authors' conclusions that proton versus photon comparisons cannot happen. Large registries can be and should be compiled to make these comparisons. These large registries are exactly what we need to prove whether the increased costs associated with proton therapy is justifiable. We are a nation going broke over technology improvements, many of which have not been "proven." We must stop this madness or there will be no health care dollars for any type of radiation therapy. Large registries can provide these essential comparative effectiveness data and therefore should be compiled.

C. A. Lawton, MD

Multitarget Stool DNA Testing for Colorectal-Cancer Screening

Imperiale TF, Ransohoff DF, Itzkowitz SH, et al (Indiana Univ School of Medicine, Indianapolis; Univ of North Carolina at Chapel Hill; Icahn School of Medicine at Mount Sinai, NY)
N Engl J Med 370:1287-1297, 2014

Background.—An accurate, noninvasive test could improve the effectiveness of colorectal-cancer screening.

Methods.—We compared a noninvasive, multitarget stool DNA test with a fecal immunochemical test (FIT) in persons at average risk for colorectal cancer. The DNA test includes quantitative molecular assays for *KRAS* mutations, aberrant *NDRG4* and *BMP3* methylation, and β-actin, plus a hemoglobin immunoassay. Results were generated with the use of a logistic-regression algorithm, with values of 183 or more considered to be positive. FIT values of more than 100 ng of hemoglobin per milliliter of buffer were considered to be positive. Tests were processed independently of colonoscopic findings.

Results.—Of the 9989 participants who could be evaluated, 65 (0.7%) had colorectal cancer and 757 (7.6%) had advanced precancerous lesions (advanced adenomas or sessile serrated polyps measuring ≥1 cm in the greatest dimension) on colonoscopy. The sensitivity for detecting colorectal cancer was 92.3% with DNA testing and 73.8% with FIT ($P = 0.002$). The sensitivity for detecting advanced precancerous lesions was 42.4% with DNA testing and 23.8% with FIT ($P < 0.001$). The rate of detection of polyps with high-grade dysplasia was 69.2% with DNA testing and 46.2% with FIT ($P = 0.004$); the rates of detection of serrated sessile polyps measuring 1 cm or more were 42.4% and 5.1%, respectively ($P < 0.001$). Specificities with DNA testing and FIT were 86.6% and 94.9%, respectively, among participants with nonadvanced or negative findings ($P < 0.001$) and 89.8% and 96.4%, respectively, among those with negative results on colonoscopy ($P < 0.001$). The numbers of persons who would need to be screened to detect one cancer were 154 with colonoscopy, 166 with DNA testing, and 208 with FIT.

Conclusions.—In asymptomatic persons at average risk for colorectal cancer, multitarget stool DNA testing detected significantly more cancers than did FIT but had more false positive results. (Funded by Exact Sciences; ClinicalTrials.gov number, NCT01397747.)

▶ Colorectal cancer kills on an average more than 50 000 men and women in the United States annually. It has been well documented that screening colonoscopy can reduce those deaths substantially. Yet most Americans do not get such screening for a variety of reasons. High on the list of reasons for Americans not getting a colonoscopy are cost and the invasive nature of the examination. Thus, development of noninvasive options is worth serious consideration.

One such noninvasive test is the fecal immunochemical test (FIT). Although this is clearly a much less-invasive potential screening option (one only needs a stool sample), it suffers from fairly low sensitivity for the detection of colorectal cancers. Advances have occurred in this area such that this current evaluation of the multitargeted stool DNA test is important and warranted.

Unfortunately, the results are mixed. Although the multitarget stool DNA test did substantially detect more cancers than the FIT, it also had more false-positive results. Clearly, these current noninvasive colorectal potential screening options are not ready for prime time and clearly not ready to take the place of screening colonoscopy. This work needs to continue so as to develop a less-invasive test to decrease the incidence and, thus, mortality of this often preventable and curable disease. Until such time as these lesser invasive screening options are proven, colonoscopy remains the standard.

C. A. Lawton, MD

Bevacizumab plus Radiotherapy–Temozolomide for Newly Diagnosed Glioblastoma

Chinot OL, Wick W, Mason W, et al (Centre Hospitaliere Universitaire Timone, Marseille; German Cancer Research Ctr, Heidelberg; Princess Margaret Hosp, Toronto, Canada; et al)
N Engl J Med 370:709-722, 2014

Background.—Standard therapy for newly diagnosed glioblastoma is radiotherapy plus temozolomide. In this phase 3 study, we evaluated the effect of the addition of bevacizumab to radiotherapy–temozolomide for the treatment of newly diagnosed glioblastoma.

Methods.—We randomly assigned patients with supratentorial glioblastoma to receive intravenous bevacizumab (10 mg per kilogram of body weight every 2 weeks) or placebo, plus radiotherapy (2 Gy 5 days a week; maximum, 60 Gy) and oral temozolomide (75 mg per square meter of body-surface area per day) for 6 weeks. After a 28-day treatment break, maintenance bevacizumab (10 mg per kilogram intravenously every 2 weeks) or placebo, plus temozolomide (150 to 200 mg per square meter per day for 5 days), was continued for six 4-week cycles, followed by bevacizumab monotherapy (15 mg per kilogram intravenously every 3 weeks) or placebo until the disease progressed or unacceptable toxic effects developed. The coprimary end points were investigator-assessed progression-free survival and overall survival.

Results.—A total of 458 patients were assigned to the bevacizumab group, and 463 patients to the placebo group. The median progression-free survival was longer in the bevacizumab group than in the placebo group (10.6 months vs. 6.2 months; stratified hazard ratio for progression or death, 0.64; 95% confidence interval [CI], 0.55 to 0.74; $P < 0.001$). The benefit with respect to progression-free survival was observed across subgroups. Overall survival did not differ significantly between groups (stratified hazard ratio for death, 0.88; 95% CI, 0.76 to 1.02; $P = 0.10$). The respective overall survival rates with bevacizumab and placebo were 72.4% and 66.3% at 1 year ($P = 0.049$) and 33.9% and 30.1% at 2 years ($P = 0.24$). Baseline health-related quality of life and performance status were maintained longer in the bevacizumab group, and the glucocorticoid requirement was lower. More patients in the bevacizumab group than in the placebo group had grade 3 or higher adverse events (66.8% vs. 51.3%) and grade 3 or higher adverse events often associated with bevacizumab (32.5% vs. 15.8%).

Conclusions.—The addition of bevacizumab to radiotherapy–temozolomide did not improve survival in patients with glioblastoma. Improved progression-free survival and maintenance of baseline quality of life and performance status were observed with bevacizumab; however, the rate of adverse events was higher with bevacizumab than with placebo. (Funded by F. Hoffmann–La Roche; ClinicalTrials.gov number, NCT00943826.)

▶ Although brain tumors in general result in less than half of cancer deaths annually compared with breast or prostate cancer, there are brain tumors like glioblastoma multiforme (GBM) that are almost uniformly lethal. These tumors in particular need to be studied in the hope of some breakthroughs. The use of temozolomide in addition to radiation was one such breakthrough for GBM patients. Although the survival improvement was only measured in months, it was still an important advance.

Because GMB tumors are very vascular and have been characterized with overexpression of vascular endothelial growth factor A (VEGF-A), testing the potential benefit of an anti-VEGF-A drug was important. Unfortunately, this phase III trial showed no survival benefit to the addition of Bevacizumab in the treatment of GBM. There was, however, improvement in progression-free survival of 4.4 months. Toxicity was an issue. Going forward, there may be a role for these types of drugs in helping GBM patients, assuming that the toxicities can be addressed.

This class of drugs and others need to be studied extensively to improve the lives of patients afflicted with this dreaded malignancy.

C. A. Lawton, MD

27 Gynecologic Cancers

The role of postoperative radiation therapy for endometrial cancer: Executive Summary of an American Society for Radiation Oncology evidence-based guideline

Klopp A, Smith BD, Alektiar K, et al (Univ of Texas MD Anderson Cancer Ctr, Houston; Memorial Sloan-Kettering Cancer Ctr, NY; et al)

Pract Radiat Oncol 4:137-144, 2014

Purpose.—To present evidence-based guidelines for adjuvant radiation in the treatment of endometrial cancer.

Methods and Materials.—Key clinical questions to be addressed in this evidence-based guideline on endometrial cancer were identified. A comprehensive literature review was performed to identify studies that included no adjuvant therapy, or pelvic radiation or vaginal brachytherapy with or without systemic chemotherapy. Outcomes included local control, survival rates, and overall assessment of quality of life.

Results.—Patients with grade 1 or 2 cancers with either no invasion or <50% myometrial invasion (MI), especially when no other high risk features are present, can be safely observed after hysterectomy. Vaginal cuff brachytherapy is as effective as pelvic radiation therapy at preventing vaginal recurrence for patients with grade 1 or 2 cancers with ≥50% MI or grade 3 tumors with ≥50% MI. Patients with grade 3 cancer with ≥50% MI or cervical stroma invasion may benefit from pelvic radiation to reduce the risk of pelvic recurrence. There is limited evidence for a benefit to vaginal cuff brachytherapy following pelvic radiation. Multimodality treatment is recommended for patients with positive nodes or involved uterine serosa, ovaries or fallopian tubes, vagina, bladder, or rectum.

Conclusions.—External beam and vaginal brachytherapy remain integral aspects of adjuvant therapy for endometrial cancer.

► Endometrial carcinoma is a common female cancer that usually presents in early stages. It is most often treated with upfront surgery, and postoperative treatment is dependent on stage, grade, and other factors.

Exactly when to apply postoperative radiation therapy, whether external beam or brachytherapy or both, remains somewhat controversial despite multiple trials trying to pinpoint the best use of each of these postoperative treatment modalities. Given the lack of clear and concise data for the use of postoperative radiation therapy in this disease, American Society for Radiation Oncology and the Society of Gynecologic Oncology convened this panel to systematically evaluate the science to date. This report, which is a summary of the entire guideline, provides an invaluable tool for practitioners as they try to provide the best data-driven care for their endometrial carcinoma patients. Its platform, which is question based, also provides some clear information for patients to digest as they try to understand which postoperative radiation options are the most appropriate for their cancer.

We definitely need more of these types of guidelines for many areas in which the use of radiation therapy definitively, preoperatively or postoperatively, is not clear.

C. A. Lawton, MD

Patterns of Radiation Therapy Practice for Patients Treated for Intact Cervical Cancer in 2005 to 2007: A Quality Research in Radiation Oncology Study

Eifel PJ, Ho A, Khalid N, et al (Univ of Texas MD Anderson Cancer Ctr, Houston; American College of Radiology Clinical Research Ctr, Philadelphia, PA; et al)

Int J Radiat Oncol Biol Phys 89:249-256, 2014

Purpose.—To assess practice patterns and compliance with clinical performance measures for radiation therapy (RT) for patients with intact carcinoma of the cervix.

Methods and Materials.—Trained research associates reviewed the records of 261 randomly selected patients who received RT for cervix carcinoma between 2005 and 2007 from 45 facilities randomly selected after stratification by practice type. National estimates of patient and treatment characteristics were calculated from survey data using SUDAAN statistical software.

Results.—From the survey data, we estimated that only 8% of US facilities treated on average more than 3 eligible patients per year. No small or medium nonacademic facilities in the survey treated more than 3 eligible patients per year. Approximately 65.5% of patients began treatment in a facility that treated 3 or fewer eligible patients per year. Although 87.5% of patients had brachytherapy as part of their treatment, the proportion treated with external beam RT only was about double that estimated from the 1996 to 1999 survey. The use of high-dose-rate brachytherapy sharply increased, particularly in small nonacademic facilities. Overall, patients treated in nonacademic facilities were more likely to have incomplete or protracted treatment; 43% of patients treated in small nonacademic facilities did not have treatment completed within 10 weeks. Also, patients treated in facilities that treated 3 or fewer eligible patients per year were significantly less likely to receive concurrent chemotherapy than were patients treated in other facilities.

Conclusion.—Survey results indicate a disturbingly high rate of noncompliance with established criteria for high-quality care of patients with cervical cancer. Noncompliance rates are particularly high in nonacademic facilities, especially those that treat relatively few patients with intact cervical cancer.

▶ "It takes a village" is a motto used to describe many aspects of life, including child rearing. The motto can be correlated with cancer care in that many cancers need to be treated via coordinated efforts with surgical, medical, and radiation oncology, not to mention primary care. When one is dealing with less common tumors like intact cervix cancer (given the decrease in numbers due to the Pap smear), it becomes even more difficult to have in-house expertise in each of these oncologic areas.

Understanding the need for expertise in surgical, medical, and radiation oncology for uncommon tumors like intact cervix cancer can lead to recommendations that such cases be referred to high-volume centers so that "the best and most up to date" care can be provided. The concern of not doing these referrals is that patients might receive lower quality care and resultant poor outcomes. This recommendation of patient referrals for uncommon tumors can be a challenge given the fiscal push in most centers not to send cases out.

The result of not referring these cases to a higher-volume center is seen in these data from the Quality Research in Radiation Oncology group. These data reinforce the need for patients with intact cervix cancer to be sent to facilities with significant volumes of such cases, as they found a concerning rate of noncompliance with established criteria for good cancer care for these patients, especially in nonacademic facilities who treat relatively few patients with intact cervix cancer.

C. A. Lawton, MD

28 Colorectal Cancer

Effect of PET Before Liver Resection on Surgical Management for Colorectal Adenocarcinoma Metastases: A Randomized Clinical Trial

Moulton C-A, Gu C-S, Law CH, et al (Univ Health Network, Toronto, Ontario, Canada; McMaster Univ, Hamilton, Ontario, Canada; Odette Cancer Centre, Toronto, Ontario, Canada; et al)

JAMA 311:1863-1869, 2014

Importance.—Patients with colorectal cancer with liver metastases undergo hepatic resection with curative intent. Positron emission tomography combined with computed tomography (PET-CT) could help avoid noncurative surgery by identifying patients with occult metastases.

Objectives.—To determine the effect of preoperative PET-CT vs no PET-CT (control) on the surgical management of patients with resectable metastases and to investigate the effect of PET-CT on survival and the association between the standardized uptake value (ratio of tissue radioactivity to injected radioactivity adjusted by weight) and survival.

Design, Setting, and Participants.—A randomized trial of patients older than 18 years with colorectal cancer treated by surgery, with resectable metastases based on CT scans of the chest, abdomen, and pelvis within the previous 30 days, and with a clear colonoscopy within the previous 18 months was conducted between 2005 and 2013, involving 21 surgeons at 9 hospitals in Ontario, Canada, with PET-CT scanners at 5 academic institutions.

Interventions.—Patients were randomized using a 2 to 1 ratio to PET-CT or control.

Main Outcomes and Measures.—The primary outcome was a change in surgical management defined as canceled hepatic surgery, more extensive hepatic surgery, or additional organ surgery based on the PET-CT. Survival was a secondary outcome.

Results.—Of the 263 patients who underwent PET-CT, 21 had a change in surgical management (8.0%; 95% CI, 5.0%-11.9%). Specifically, 7 patients (2.7%) did not undergo laparotomy, 4 (1.5%) had more extensive hepatic surgery, 9 (3.4%) had additional organ surgery (8 of whom had hepatic resection), and the abdominal cavity was opened in 1 patient but hepatic surgery was not performed and the cavity was closed. Liver resection was performed in 91% of patients in the PET-CT group and 92% of the control group. After a median follow-up of 36 months, the estimated mortality rate was 11.13 (95% CI, 8.95-13.68) events/1000 person-months for the PET-CT group and 12.71 (95% CI, 9.40-16.80) events/1000 person-months for the control group. Survival did not differ between the 2 groups (hazard ratio, 0.86 [95% CI, 0.60-1.21]; $P = .38$). The standardized uptake value was associated with survival (hazard ratio, 1.11 [90% CI, 1.07-1.15] per unit increase; $P < .001$). The C statistic for the model including the standardized uptake value was 0.62 (95% CI, 0.56-0.68) and without it was 0.50 (95% CI, 0.44-0.56). The difference in C statistics is 0.12 (95% CI, 0.04-0.21). The low C statistic suggests that the standard uptake value is not a strong predictor of overall survival.

Conclusions and Relevance.—Among patients with potentially resectable hepatic metastases of colorectal adenocarcinoma, the use of PET-CT compared with CT alone did not result in frequent change in surgical management. These findings raise questions about the value of PET-CT scans in this setting.

Trial Registration.—clinicaltrials.gov Identifier: NCT00265356.

▶ Positron emission tomography (PET) scanning for patients with many forms of cancer has been well studied and found to be exceedingly useful for many malignancies, most notably the lymphomas. Its role in many solid tumors is much less well understood, yet it is often performed, which increases costs for patients and payers. Identifying which patients are best served with this advanced technology is therefore important and worth careful study.

For patients with colorectal cancers and liver metastasis, PET scanning has been used and studied by some for more than a decade. But a large and systematic evaluation of PET-computed tomography (CT) versus CT alone (the standard) has not occurred. Patients with such liver metastasis from colorectal carcinoma often undergo "curative hepatic resection." Thus, knowing whether there are other occult lesions preoperatively via some sort of scanning is critical.

These data from Canada has evaluated the role of PET-CT for patients with hepatic metastases from colorectal cancer in a prospective randomized method, "the gold standard methodology." Their results showing no significant change in surgical management for patients receiving PET-CT versus CT alone puts the use of PET-CT into serious question for these patients. Given these data, hepatic surgeons need to think twice before order PET-CT over CT alone to decrease what could be wasteful spending of health care dollars.

C. A. Lawton, MD

PART FOUR

KIDNEY, WATER, AND ELECTROLYTES

RENEE GARRICK, MD

Introduction

Mediators and Modifiers of Kidney Disease

As the incidence of chronic kidney disease (CKD), has continued to rise its impact on individual morbidity and mortality and healthcare costs has become increasingly evident. To set the stage, we included the findings by McMahon and colleagues drawn from the data of the Framingham Offspring Study which suggest that risk factors associated with the ultimate development of CKD are identifiable more than 30 years prior to the diagnosis of CKD. This year's selections include several articles which highlight interventions which may help to mitigate the occurrence and progression of CKD. A high dietary fiber intake has been shown to reduce inflammation and improve mortality in patients with kidney disease. Studies this year demonstrated that high dietary fiber intake is directly associated with the estimated GFR(eGFR), and among patients with kidney disease was associated with reduced mortality and cancer risk. Previous work has suggested that diet can influence our acid-base balance, and that metabolic acidosis can hasten the progression of renal disease. This year data from the Multi-ethnic Study of Atherosclerosis demonstrated that even among patients with a normal baseline eGFR (>60 ml/min), and independent of albuminuria, a lower serum bicarbonate concentration was associated with a decline in kidney function. Along the same lines, Banerjee and colleagues observed that among patients with underlying CKD a high dietary acid load predicts the development of ESRD. In keeping with the same dietary theme, data collected over a 15 year period in the multi-ethnic, observational, Northern Manhattan study suggested that a Mediterranean-style diet was associated a greater preservation of eGFR. In addition to dietary changes, exercise is also an important part of a healthy lifestyle, and Chen and colleagues demonstrated that among patients with moderate to severe CKD, walking as little as 30 minutes a week slowed progression of CKD and reduced mortality. The final selection is a fascinating study from the basic science literature. Using a model of ureteral obstruction data from Mael-Ainin and associates suggest that periostin leads to renal injury via activation of the pro-fibrotic TGB-β pathway, and that inhibition of periostin expression can be renoprotective.

Hypertension and Kidney Disease

Among patients with CKD, the longitudinal control of blood pressure is believed to reduce the risk of disease progression. Data from Federally sponsored CRIC Study now suggests that time-updated systolic blood pressures of over 130 mm Hg readings are more strongly associated with renal disease progression than are independent, baseline office readings. These findings are clinically noteworthy and more data regarding the applicability to the practice setting will likely be forthcoming. Hypertension and proteinuria have been demonstrated to promote the progression of kidney disease, and the salt-sensitive, anti-proteinuria effect of inhibition of the renin-angiotensin system is well-established. A study by Hwang showed that among non-diabetic, hypertensive patients receiving angiotensin receptor blockade therapy, urinary albumin excretion was significantly reduced among those patients who received intensive dietary education, as compared to those without dietary counseling. Thus, supporting a role for appropriate, standardized patient education as a part of our treatment armamentarium. The next selection focuses on polycystic kidney disease which is the most common of the inherited renal lesions. The findings of the multi-centered NIDDK sponsored HALT trial demonstrated that combined ACE-ARB therapy did not improve outcomes, but a low blood pressure target (95/62 110/70 mm Hg), was reno-protective. The lower target was however associated with a higher incidence of dizziness and lightheadedness as compared to standard (120/82 to 130/80 mm Hg) targets. The final selection presents the clinically important results of the SYMPLICITY HTN-3 trial. Contrary to prior, smaller, non-blinded trials, the findings from this carefully conducted trial did not support the use of renal artery denervation as a treatment for resistant hypertension.

Diabetes and Kidney Disease

Studies this year continued to focus on mitigating the progression of diabetic kidney disease. Among patients with type I diabetes the development of macroalbuminuria (>300 mg/day), has long been considered a harbinger of irreversible, progressive kidney injury. Data from DCCT and EDIC groups demonstrated that through 10 years of follow-up among patients with macroalbuminuria about 50% had albumin excretion rates of less than 300 mg/day and preserved eGFR. Most, but not all, of these patients were receiving treatment with renin-angiotensin system inhibitors. In a separate study, the Joslin group evaluated the impact of glycemic control on the risk of progression to ESRD among type I diabetics with proteinuria. The data are gratifying, as they suggest that long-term, sustained improvement in glycemic control can slow progression of kidney injury and delay the onset of ESRD. The next two selections focus on kidney disease among individuals with type II diabetes. The first suggests that metformin use may be safe among patients with mild to moderate CKD (eGFR 30-60 ml/min/1.73 m^2), and the second demonstrates that among patients with eGFR between 15 and 59 ml/min treatment with pentoxifylline, along with renin-angiotensin system (RAS) inhibitors, significantly reduced albumin excretion and the decline in eGFR, as compared with treatment with RAS inhibitors alone.

Acute Kidney Injury

Well-defined studies have demonstrated that among non-pregnant, hospitalized patients without underlying kidney disease the incidence of AKI approaches 23%.[1] Other studies have shown that even with recovery from the acute kidney event, the long term risks of mortality and CKD remain increased. Thus, it is clearly important to correctly identify and follow these patients. The first election by Schetz and colleagues, stresses that when the serum creatinine is changing due to alterations in either creatinine production or excretion (I.e. is not in steady-state), renal function cannot be reliable judged by nomogram calculations (such as the estimated GFR), or by a 24 hour creatinine clearance. Thus, clinically, whenever possible, medications doses should be based on their actual serum levels, and follow-up measurements of GFR are necessary following clinical recovery. The next group of selections evaluates AKI and subsequent CKD in the setting of vascular surgery. A randomized study by Garg, demonstrated that off-pump CABG surgery was associated with a lower risk of AKI then was on-pump surgery, but the risk of long-term renal dysfunction after one year was similar (17.1 versus 15.2%). A study of almost 30,000 patients undergoing isolated CABG surgery, showed that postoperative AKI occurred in approximate 13% of patients and that even a small (0.3 mg/dl) increase in creatinine was associated with a 3-fold increase in the long-term risk of ESRD and others demonstrated that renal function progressively deteriorates for one year and beyond following endovascular repair of an abdominal aneurysm. As a group, these articles stress the long term risks of renal dysfunction, and he need for long-term renal follow up after and episode of even seemingly trivial AKI. Medications use often precipitates AKI and the next several selections focus on the risk of AKI associated with commonly used medications, such as gentamicin, vancomycin, and atypical antipsychotic agents, and the high risk of AKI associated with drugs of abuse. The final selections presents a fascinating analysis demonstrating that the high risk of AKI among African Americans may be related to socioeconomic disparities.

Selected Topics in Clinical Nephrology

The prevalence of CKD is approaching 15% of the US adult population, and the resources required to provide appropriate care are rapidly expanding. The selections this year focused on a number of topics that are of general importance to patients with underlying CKD. To begin, and Mendu and colleagues have effectively demonstrated that implementation of a chronic kidney disease "checklist" can help busy primary care providers monitor the clinical progress and outcome indicators of patients with CKD. The next several selections draw attention to clinical observations which are directly applicable to the care of our patients. For example, the data from the Chronic Renal Insufficiency Cohort (CRIC) study have demonstrated that after corrections for eGFR and proteinuria the presence and severity of retinopathy are not markers for the risk of CKD progression. Data from the prospective rheumatoid arthritis study cohort has suggested that the use of non-steroidal anti-inflammatory agents in patients with an eGFR of greater than 30 ml/min may be safer than previously believed. However, other previous data suggest that caution is warranted if patients are simultaneously using diuretics and renin-angiotensin system inhibitors.[2] Schrier and colleagues published and encyclopedic compendium regarding the factors that predict the progression of autosomal dominant polycystic kidney disease , and a retrospective cohort study of almost 1.2 million patients demonstrated that the risk of uroepithelial cancer, but not other cancer types, is increased in patients with an eGFR of <30. This will help physicians choose screening studies in a cost-effective manner. The next selection focuses on the appropriate initial use of radiation-sparing ultrasonography for the detection of nephrolithiasis. The results need to be carefully understood; if the initial ultrasound is negative and stone symptoms persist, additional more sensitive imaging (such as a stone-protocol CT) is required. Sodium polystyrene has received unfavorable publicity as a potassium lowering agent, so as a portent of things to come we included the phase 3 results of the HARMONIZE trial, which have demonstrated the efficacy and safety of sodium zirconium cyclosilicate to lower serum potassium among outpatients. We will stay tuned for further updates regarding its clinical application. The final entry focuses on the utility of antibody markers to help guide the therapy, and establish prognosis in patients with idiopathic membranous nephropathy, which in remains one of the most common causes of adult nephrotic syndrome. If the findings are supported by additional studies these markers may replace the current therapeutic approach.

Issues in Severe CKD and Dialysis

The renal community continues to focus on the morbidity and mortality of dialysis patients and those with severe chronic kidney failure. Cardiovascular disease and Infection are the two most common causes of death among the dialysis population. The large retrospective review by Sud and colleagues demonstrated that repetitive hospitalization for heart failure led to a step-wise increase in both the risk of ESRD, and the risk of death before ESRD. Perhaps increased after-hospital follow up care could alter this trend within this high-risk population. With regard to infectious illnesses, as compared to the general population, ESRD patients have an extremely high risk of methicillin resistant staphylococcal aureus (MRSA) infection. A large meta-analysis of almost 5600 dialysis patients identified that the risk of MRSA colonization is substantially greater among hemodialysis than peritoneal dialysis patients, and within 6-20 months about 20% of MRSA-colonized hemodialysis patients developed clinical infections. The potential sequelae of MRSA are well-known, and appropriate use of nasal mupirocin ointment in select patients may be beneficial. Cognitive function has shown to be impaired in both CKD and ESRD patients and this year studies in dialysis patients showed that reductions in both executive function and memory are associated with an increased risk of mortality. Other studies focusing on ESRD patients residing in skilled nursing facilities, demonstrated that over 40% of these patients either return to the ER or are readmitted within 30 days of hospital discharge. Taken together, these findings suggest that greater attention to home care support and transitional care may be beneficial among this population. The last selection reviews the quality of life and survival outcomes in elderly individuals who choose to forgo dialysis. This patient population is growing and it is important for us to become well-versed in patient centered care and shared decision making.

Renee Garrick, MD

References

1. Wang HE, Muntner P, Chertow GM, Warnock DG. Acute kidney injury and mortality in hospitalized patients. *Am J Nephrol.* 2012;35:349-355.
2. Lapi F, Azoulay L, Yin H, Nessim SJ, Suissa S. Concurrent use of diuretics, angiotensin-converting enzyme inhibitors, and angiotensin receptor blockers with non-steroidal anti-inflammatory drugs and the risk of acute kidney injury: nested case-control study. *BMJ.* 2013;346:e8525.

29 Mediators and Modifiers of Kidney Disease

Mid-Adulthood Risk Factor Profiles for CKD

McMahon GM, Preis SR, Hwang S-J, et al (Natl Heart, Lung, and Blood Inst's Framingham Heart Study and the Ctr for Population Studies, Framingham, MA; Boston Univ School of Public Health, MA; et al)

J Am Soc Nephrol 25:2633-2641, 2014

Early identification of CKD risk factors may allow risk factor modification and prevention of CKD progression. We investigated the hypothesis that risk factors are present ≥30 years before the diagnosis of CKD in a case-control study using data from the Framingham Offspring Study. Patients with incident CKD (eGFR ≤60 ml/min per 1.73 m^2) at examination cycles 6, 7, and 8 were age- and sex-matched 1:2 to patients without CKD at baseline (examination 5). CKD risk factors were measured at each examination cycle. Logistic regression models, adjusted for age, sex, and time period, were constructed to compare risk factor profiles at each time point between cases and controls. During follow-up, 441 new cases of CKD were identified and matched to 882 controls (mean age 69.2 years, 52.4% women). Those who ultimately developed CKD were more likely to have hypertension (odds ratio [OR], 1.76; 95% confidence interval [CI], 1.23 to 2.51), obesity (OR, 1.71; 95% CI, 1.14 to 2.59), and higher triglyceride levels (OR, 1.43; 95% CI, 1.12 to 1.83) 30 years before CKD diagnosis, and were more likely to have hypertension (OR, 1.38; 95% CI, 1.07 to 1.79), higher triglyceride levels (OR, 1.35; 95% CI, 1.11 to 1.64), lower HDLc (OR, 0.89; 95% CI, 0.81 to 0.97), and diabetes (OR, 2.90; 95% CI, 1.59 to 5.29) 20 years before CKD diagnosis. These findings demonstrate that risk factors for CKD are identifiable ≥30 years before diagnosis and suggest the importance of early risk factor identification in patients at risk for CKD.

▶ Chronic kidney disease (CKD) is largely asymptomatic, and most studies evaluating risk factors for occurrence or progression span a limited number of years. The data presented here are drawn from the Framingham Study Offspring Cohort, which began enrollment in 1971, and represent a unique opportunity to evaluate the long-term impact of a variety of risk factors believed to be associated with the ultimate development of CKD. A prospective, nested case-control model was used, and participants were eligible for inclusion into the study if they were free of kidney disease at baseline. Estimated glomerular filtration rate was calculated using the CKD-epi equation,[1] and data were available on all of the risk factors tracked in the Framingham study, including hypertension (defined as ≥140/90), diabetes, body mass index, lipid profiles, the presence of albuminuria, and smoking history. Limitations of the Framingham database include the lack of longitudinal information on other potential CKD risk factors such as dietary habits and activity levels, and it primarily enrolled individuals of European ancestry, so the results may not be easily generalized. However, the cohort is well defined, and data are quite interesting. As shown in Figure 4 in the original article, the presence of risk factors (diabetes, hypertension, smoking, and obesity) portend the development of CKD by as many as 30 years before its clinical occurrence. As the authors point out, CKD should be considered "a life course disease." Although it's not yet known with certainty whether it is possible to mitigate the progression of CKD, appropriate screening and therapeutic interventions for patients at greatest risk do seem clinically prudent.

R. Garrick, MD

Reference

1. Levey AS, Stevens LA, Schmid CH, et al. CKD-EPI (chronic kidney disease epidemiology collaboration): a new equation to estimate glomerular filtration rate. *Ann Intern Med.* 2009;150:604-612.

Low Serum Bicarbonate and Kidney Function Decline: The Multi-Ethnic Study of Atherosclerosis (MESA)

Driver TH, Shlipak MG, Katz R, et al (Univ of California, San Francisco; Univ of Washington, Seattle; et al)

Am J Kidney Dis 64:534-541, 2014

Background.—Among populations with established chronic kidney disease (CKD), metabolic acidosis is associated with more rapid progression of kidney disease. The association of serum bicarbonate concentrations with early declines in kidney function is less clear.

Study Design.—Retrospective cohort study.

Setting & Participants.—5,810 participants in the Multi-Ethnic Study of Atherosclerosis (MESA) with a baseline estimated glomerular filtration rate (eGFR) >60 mL/min/1.73 m^2 using the CKD-EPI (CKD Epidemiology Collaboration) creatinin–cystatin C equation.

Predictors.—Serum bicarbonate concentrations.

Outcomes.—Rapid kidney function decline (eGFR decline >5% per year) and incident reduced eGFR (eGFR <60 mL/min/1.73 m^2 with minimum rate of eGFR loss of 1 mL/min/1.73 m^2 per year).

Results.—Average bicarbonate concentration was 23.2 ± 1.8 mEq/L. 1,730 (33%) participants had rapid kidney function decline, and 487 had incident reduced eGFR during follow-up. Each 1-SD lower baseline bicarbonate concentration was associated with 12% higher adjusted odds of rapid kidney function decline (95% CI, 6%-20%) and higher risk of incident reduced eGFR (adjusted incidence rate ratio, 1.11; 95% CI, 1.03-1.20) in models adjusting for demographics, baseline eGFR, albuminuria, and CKD risk factors. The OR for the associations of bicarbonate level <21 mEq/L relative to 23-24 mEq/L was 1.35 (95% CI, 1.05-1.73) for rapid kidney function decline, and the incidence rate ratio was 1.16 (95% CI, 0.83-1.62) for incident reduced eGFR.

Limitations.—Cause of metabolic acidosis cannot be determined in this study.

Conclusions.—Lower serum bicarbonate concentrations are associated independently with rapid kidney function decline independent of eGFR or albuminuria in community-living persons with baseline eGFR >60 mL/min/1.73 m^2. If confirmed, our findings suggest that metabolic acidosis may indicate either early kidney disease that is not captured by eGFR or albuminuria or may have a causal role in the development of eGFR <60 mL/min/1.73 m^2 (Fig 2).

▶ Bicarbonate (CO_2) levels are used to assess the acid—base status of patients. A low level can be a sign of either metabolic acidosis or respiratory alkalosis. In the absence of clear pulmonary disease, however, low CO_2 in the setting of renal disease is nearly always due to metabolic acidosis. The significance of this acidosis is a subject of much interest. Studies have linked low CO_2 to many clinical parameters including increased incidence of functional

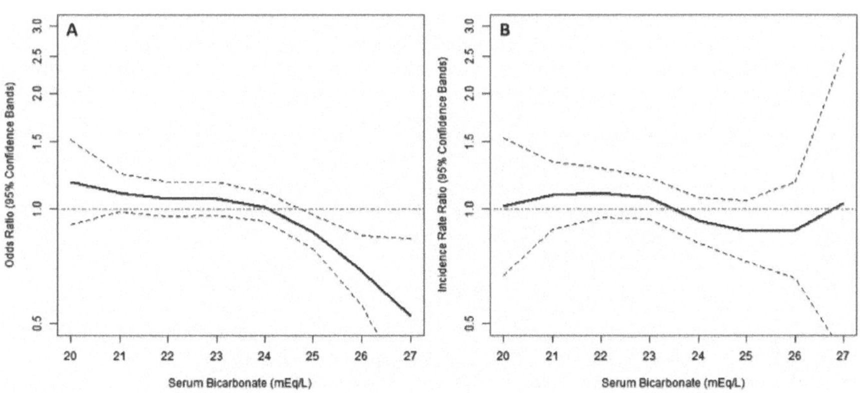

FIGURE 2.—(A) Adjusted association of serum bicarbonate level with risk of (A) rapid kidney function decline and (B) incident reduced estimated glomerular filtration rate (eGFR) in MESA (Multi-Ethnic Study of Atherosclerosis). Spline analysis adjusted for age, race, sex, education, diabetes mellitus, hypertension, smoking, body mass index, high-density lipoprotein cholesterol level, eGFR, diuretic use, and albuminuria. Solid line represents the point estimate and dotted lines represent 95% confidence interval. (Reprinted from American Journal of Kidney Diseases. Driver TH, Shlipak MG, Katz R, et al. Low serum bicarbonate and kidney function decline: the multi-ethnic study of atherosclerosis (MESA). *Am J Kidney Dis.* 2014;64:534-541, Copyright 2014, with permission from the National Kidney Foundation, Inc.)

limitation,[1] worsening bone disease,[2] and even progression of established chronic kidney disease.[3] This study by Driver et al used the The Multi-Ethnic Study of Atherosclerosis study cohort to examine the effect of low CO_2 on the incidence of kidney disease in subjects with initially normal kidney function. They evaluated 5810 participants with baseline estimated glomerular filtration rate (eGFR) >60 mL/min. In this cohort, the distribution of CO_2 levels was normal with a mean of 23 $\pm$ 1.8 mEq/L. In follow-up examination it was noted that those with lower serum CO_2 had higher odds of rapid kidney function decline and incident reduced GFR (Fig 2). Each 1.8 lower baseline CO_2 concentration was associated with 10% higher odds of renal functional decline. Levels under 21 mmol/L demonstrated 35% higher odds of renal decline compared with the reference CO_2 of 23 to 24 mmol/L (odds ratio 1.15 vs 1.00). CO_2 levels of 25 to 27 mmol/L demonstrated the lowest odds ratio of renal functional decline at 0.84. The presence or absence of microalbuminuria did not affect these odds significantly. There are several plausible explanations for the potential relationship between CO_2 levels and progression of renal disease, including the activation of complement by generated ammonium or that lower CO_2 is a marker for tubular dysfunction rather than being an independent cause for renal damage.

This study is significant because it suggests that CO_2, an inexpensive and widely available test, may be an earlier marker for renal risk than even eGFR or increased urinary albumin excretion assessment. It also suggests, as do some small studies,[4] that CO_2 supplementation may retard the progression of CKD. These are diagnostic and therapeutic avenues that are ripe for well-designed investigations.

M. Klein, MD

References

1. Yenchek R, Ix JH, Rifkin DE, et al. Association of serum CO_2 with incident functional limitation in older adults. *Clin J Am Soc Nephrol.* 2014;9:2111-2116.
2. Lemann J Jr, Adams ND, Wilz DR, Brenes LG. Acid and mineral balances and bone in familial proximal renal tubular acidosis. *Kidney Int.* 2000;58:1267-1277.
3. Shah SN, Abramowitz M, Hostetter TH, Melamed ML. Serum CO_2 levels and the progression of kidney disease: a cohort study. *Am J Kidney Dis.* 2009;54:270-277.
4. de Brito-Ashurst I, Varagunam M, Raftery MJ, Yaqoob MM. CO_2 supplementation slows progression of CKD and improves nutritional status. *J Am Soc Nephrol.* 2009;20:2075-2084.

High Dietary Acid Load Predicts ESRD among Adults with CKD

Banerjee T, for the Centers for Disease Control and Prevention Chronic Kidney Disease Surveillance Team (Univ of California, San Francisco; et al)
J Am Soc Nephrol 26:1-8, 2015

Small clinical trials have shown that a reduction in dietary acid load (DAL) improves kidney injury and slows kidney function decline;

however, the relationship between DAL and risk of ESRD in a population-based cohort with CKD remains unexamined. We examined the association between DAL, quantified by net acid excretion (NAEes), and progression to ESRD in a nationally representative sample of adults in the United States. Among 1486 adults with CKD age ≥20 years enrolled in the National Health and Nutrition Examination Survey III, DAL was determined by 24-h dietary recall questionnaire. The development of ESRD was ascertained over a median 14.2 years of follow-up through linkage with the Medicare ESRD Registry. We used the Fine–Gray competing risks method to estimate the association of high, medium, and low DAL with ESRD after adjusting for demographics, nutritional factors, clinical factors, and kidney function/damage markers and accounting for intervening mortality events. In total, 311 (20.9%) participants developed ESRD. Higher levels of DAL were associated with increased risk of ESRD; relative hazards (95% confidence interval) were 3.04 (1.58 to 5.86) for the highest tertile and 1.81 (0.89 to 3.68) for the middle tertile compared with the lowest tertile in the fully adjusted model. The risk of ESRD associated with DAL tertiles increased as eGFR decreased (P trend=0.001). Among participants with albuminuria, high DAL was strongly associated with ESRD risk (P trend=0.03). In conclusion, high DAL in persons with CKD is independently associated with increased risk of ESRD in a nationally representative population.

▶ As the incidence of CKD has increased, search for modifiable risk factors has similarly become more intense. This study, drawn from the 1988–94 National Health and Nutrition Examination Survey (NHANES III), analyzed the dietary acid load (DAL) of almost 1500 patients followed for a median span of approximately 14 years. The statistical analysis was adjusted for multiple factors including hypertension and diabetes, and results were stratified based on estimated glomerular filtration rate (≥45 and ≤45 mL/min/1.73 m^2) and by the presence of absence of albuminuria (≥ or ≤30 mg/g creatinine). The median value for DAL was 47.24 mEq. Patients who consumed a low-acid diet were 3 times less likely to progress to dialysis than were those who consumed a high dietary acid load. A graded association between tertiles of DAL and progression to ESRD was most pronounced in patients with more advanced CKD, and among patients with albuminuria, a high DAL was significantly associated with the risk of end-stage renal disease ($P < .001$).

The findings are in keeping with prior small studies that showed a favorable association between both alkali supplements and diets rich in vegetable and the rate of disease progression.[1-4] The concept is attractive in its simplicity. The investigators note that the typical Western diet is rich in foods that are net-acidifying (meat fish and grains), in contrast to net alkalizing foods such as fruits, vegetables, and legumes. The physiology behind these observations has yet to be definitively determined. One suggested mechanism is tubular toxicity caused by increased ammonium excretion that occurs as a result of the increased net acid load. Other suggested mechanisms include activation of the renin-angiotensin or complement systems. The study is well done, statistically valid, and is the first longitudinal demonstration that modification of DAL may alter the rate of progression of renal disease. Confirmation of these observational findings will require multicenter observational studies, but it would seem reasonable to incorporate these findings into our clinical armamentarium while awaiting the results of such studies.

R. Garrick, MD

References

1. Goraya N, Simoni J, Jo C-H, Wesson DE. A comparison of treating metabolic acidosis in CKD stage 4 hypertensive kidney disease with fruits and vegetables or sodium bicarbonate. *Clin J Am Soc Nephrol.* 2013;8:371-381.
2. de Brito-Ashurst I, Varagunam M, Raftery MJ, et al. Bicarbonate supplementation slows progression of CKD and improves nutritional status. *J Am Soc Nephrol.* 2009;20:2075-2084.
3. Wesson DE, Simoni J. Acid retention during kidney failure induces endothelin and aldosterone production which lead to progressive GFR decline, a situation ameliorated by alkali diet. *Kidney Int.* 2010;78:1128-1135.
4. Wesson DE, Simoni J, Broglio K, et al. Acid retention accompanies reduced GFR in humans and increases plasma levels of endothelin and aldosterone. *Am J Physiol Renal Physiol.* 2011;300:F830-F883.

The Association between a Mediterranean-Style Diet and Kidney Function in the Northern Manhattan Study Cohort

Khatri M, Moon YP, Scarmeas N, et al (Columbia Univ, NY; et al)
Clin J Am Soc Nephrol 9:1868-1875, 2014

Background and Objectives.—Various dietary strategies have been investigated to slow kidney function decline. However, it is unknown whether a Mediterranean diet, which has been associated with improved cardiovascular risk, is associated with change in kidney function.

Design, Setting, Participants, & Measurements.—This study used the Northern Manhattan Study, a prospective, multiethnic, observational cohort of participants who were stroke free at baseline. Data were collected between 1993 and 2008. Serum creatinine measurements were taken a mean 6.9 years apart. A baseline dietary questionnaire was extrapolated into a previously used 9-point scoring system (MeDi). The primary outcome was incident eGFR <60 ml/min per 1.73 m^2 using the Modification of Diet in Renal Disease formula. A secondary outcome was the upper quartile of annualized eGFR decline (≥2.5 ml/min per 1.73 m^2 per year). Conditional logistic regression models adjusted for demographics and baseline vascular risk factors.

Results.—Mean baseline age was 64 years, with 59% women and 65% Hispanics ($N = 900$); mean baseline eGFR was 83.1 ml/min per 1.73 m^2. Incident eGFR <60 ml/min per 1.73 m^2 developed in 14%. In adjusted models, every 1-point increase in the MeDi score, indicating increasing adherence to a Mediterranean diet, was associated with decreased odds of incident eGFR <60 ml/min per 1.73 m^2 (odds ratio, 0.83; 95% confidence interval, 0.71 to 0.96) and decreased odds of being in the upper quartile of eGFR decline (odds ratio, 0.88; 95% confidence interval, 0.79 to 0.98).

Conclusions.—A Mediterranean diet was associated with a reduced, incidence of eGFR <60 ml/min per 1.73 m^2 and upper quartile of eGFR decline in a multiethnic cohort.

► Previous studies have suggested that high-fiber, low-acid, and low-protein diets may help slow the progression of chronic kidney injury.[1-3] The data from the observational, prospective, multiethnic Northern Manhattan Study extends the list of potentially beneficial diets to include the Mediterranean diet. These findings are even more interesting when evaluated in the context of the data by Gutierrez and colleagues, which demonstrated that among patients with stage 3 to 5 chronic kidney disease (CKD), consumption of a so-called Southern diet (fried food, organ meats, sweetened drinks), was associated with a 50% increase in risk of death.[4] In the current study, individuals with a score of 5 or higher (indicating good adherence to Mediterranean diet), were 50% less likely to develop CKD and were about 40% less likely to have a rapid decline in kidney function. Moreover, every 1-point increase in compliance with the Mediterranean diet decreased the risk of CKD by 17%.

Of interest, the impact of adherence to Mediterranean diet on the progression of kidney disease was more marked among nondiabetics than among diabetics. Theoretically, the biological efficacy of a Mediterranean diet may be linked to improved endothelial cell function with a reduction in intrarenal inflammatory mediators, and transglomerular pressure. This might explain why the effects were less marked in diabetics, many of whom were already on angiotensin-converting enzyme inhibitor or angiotensin receptor blocker therapy, because the impact (delta change) would likely be less among those patients.

Limitations of the study include that the use of dietary histories reduces the ability to know whether the diets fully mimicked a well-defined Mediterranean diet, as well as its observational design, which limit the ability to control for additional, independent factors that may have affected disease progression. Randomized, controlled trials will be needed to fully assess the impact of diet on the progression of renal injury. In the meantime, these findings, and those of Gutiérrez and colleagues[4] are clinically valuable, and among patients with renal injury, appropriate dietary modifications should be encouraged.

R. Garrick, MD

References

1. Banerjee T, Crews DC, Wesson DE, et al. High dietary acid load predicts ESRD among adults with CKD. *J Am Soc Nephrol.* 2015;26:1-8.
2. Hong Xu H, Xiaoyan Huang X, Riserus U, et al. Dietary fiber, kidney function, inflammation, and mortality risk. *Clin J Am Soc Nephrol.* 2014;9:2104-2110.
3. Klahr S, Levey AS, Beck GJ, et al. Modification of diet in renal disease study group: the effects of dietary protein restriction and blood-pressure control on the progression of chronic renal disease. *N Engl J Med.* 1994;330:877-884.

4. Gutiérrez OM, Muntner P, Rizk DV, et al. Dietary patterns and risk of death and progression to ESRD in individuals with CKD: a cohort study. *Am J Kidney Dis.* 2014;64:204-213.

Association of Walking with Survival and RRT Among Patients with CKD Stages 3–5

Chen I-R, Wang S-M, Liang C-C, et al (China Med Univ Hosp, Taichung, Taiwan; et al)
Clin J Am Soc Nephrol 9:1183-1189, 2014

Background and Objectives.—Patients with CKD can benefit from an increase in physical activity. Walking is one of the most common exercises in patients with CKD; however, the association of walking with outcomes in patients with CKD is not clear. This study investigated the association of walking with overall mortality and RRT in patients with CKD stages 3–5.

Design, Setting, Participants, & Measurements.—All patients with CKD stages 3–5 in the CKD program of China Medical University Hospital from June 2003 to May 2013 were enrolled. The risks of overall mortality and RRT were analyzed using competing-risks regressions.

Results.—A total of 6363 patients (average age, 70 years) during a median of 1.3 (range = 0.6–2.5) years of follow-up were analyzed. There were 1341 (21.1%) patients who reported walking as their most common form of exercise. The incidence density rate of overall mortality was 2.7 per 100 person-years for walking patients and 5.4 for nonwalking ones. The incidence density rate of RRT was 22 per 100 person-years for walking patients and 32.9 for nonwalking ones. Walking, independent of patients' age, renal function, and comorbidity, was linked to lower overall mortality and lower RRT risk in the multivariate competing-risks regression. The adjusted subdistribution hazard ratio (SHR) of walking was 0.67 (95% confidence interval [95% CI], 0.53 to 0.84; $P < 0.001$) for overall mortality and 0.79 (95% CI, 0.73 to 0.85; $P < 0.001$) for the risk of RRT. The SHRs of overall mortality were 0.83, 0.72, 0.42, and 0.41 for patients walking 1–2, 3–4, 5–6, and ≥7 times per week, and the SHRs of RRT were 0.81, 0.73, 0.57, and 0.56, respectively.

Conclusions.—Walking is the most popular form of exercise in patients with CKD and is associated with lower risks of overall mortality and RRT. The benefit of walking is independent of patients' age, renal function, and comorbidity.

▶ These types of data are uplifting. Walking for as little as 30 minutes once a week was shown to reduce mortality and the rate of progression to dialysis among patients with stage 3 to 5 CKD (Figure 1 in the original article). Moreover, the effects of walking were graded, so walking 1 to 2, 3 to 4, 5 to 6, and 7 or more times per week had progressive reductions in the risk for death of 17%, 28%, 58%, and 59%, respectively. Similarly, increased frequency of walking reduced the risk of progression to end-stage renal disease by 19%, 27%, 43%, and 44%. The data were adjusted for erythropoietin use, body mass index, renal function, and comorbid conditions (diabetes, chronic glomerulonephritis, hypertension, coronary artery disease, stroke, or cancer within the past 5 years). A related article[1] suggests that exercise may have antiinflammatory effects in chronic kidney disease (CKD) as demonstrated by changes in neutrophil degranulation, activation of T lymphocytes (CD69 expression) and monocytes (CD86 and human leukocyte antigen—DR expression), and plasma infiammatory markers (interleukin [IL]-6, IL-10, soluble tumor necrosis factor receptors). In that study,[1] both acute exercise and 6 months of regular walking exercise induced a systemic antiinflammatory environment. These findings provide compelling evidence that walking is safe, may have positive effects on immune function, and has the potential both to improve mortality and to slow the progression of CKD. There are few other things that are of such potential benefit and still free.

A. Kapoor, MD

Reference

1. Viana JL, Kaosmadakis GC, Watson EL, et al. Evidence for anti-inflammatory effects of exercise in CKD. *J Am Soc Nephrol.* 2014;25:2121-2130.

Inhibition of Periostin Expression Protects against the Development of Renal Inflammation and Fibrosis

Mael-Ainin M, Abed A, Conway SJ, et al (Tenon Hosp, Paris, France; Indiana Univ School of Medicine, Indianapolis; et al)
J Am Soc Nephrol 25:1724-1736, 2014

Increased renal expression of periostin, a protein normally involved in embryonic and dental development, correlates with the decline of renal function in experimental models and patient biopsies. Because periostin has been reported to induce cell differentiation, we investigated whether it is also involved in the development of renal disease and whether blocking its abnormal expression improves renal function and/ or structure. After unilateral ureteral obstruction in wild-type mice, we observed a progressive increase in the expression and synthesis of periostin in the obstructed kidney that associated with the progression of renal lesions. In contrast, mice lacking the periostin gene showed less injury-induced interstitial fibrosis and inflammation and were protected against structural alterations. This protection was associated with a preservation of the renal epithelial phenotype. *In vitro*, administration of TGF-β to renal epithelial cells increased the expression of periostin several-fold, leading to subsequent loss of the epithelial phenotype. Furthermore, treatment of these cells with periostin increased the expression of collagen I and stimulated the phosphorylation of FAK, p38, and ERK 42/44. In vivo delivery of antisense oligonucleotides to inhibit periostin expression protected animals from L-NAME–induced renal injury. These data strongly suggest that periostin mediates renal disease in response to TGF-β and that blocking periostin may be a promising therapeutic strategy against the development of CKD.

▶ Chronic kidney disease (CKD) is progressive and incurable. Once initiated, the cellular alterations leading to end organ failure invariably progress. Effective therapies to mitigate disease progression are clearly needed. The biopsy of end-stage disease reveals accumulation of extracellular matrix and scarring fibrosis. Periostin (also known as osteoblast-specific factor-2), is an extracellular protein that is normally expressed during early development. It is present in low levels in healthy adults; however, its expression increases following tissue injury. Periostin expression has been demonstrated in a variety of inflammatory conditions including hypertension-mediated left ventricular hypertrophy and rheumatoid arthritis, among others. This elegant research study used a model of unilateral ureteral obstruction and is the first to demonstrate that stimulation (via administration of tumor growth factor [TGF]-beta) and inhibition (via antisense oligonucleotides) of periostin synthesis and expression correlates with renal injury. Activation of the TGF-beta pathway is believed to be a pivotal event in the progression of renal fibrosis. In fact, the beneficial effects of angiotensin receptor inhibition and blockade are, in part, believed to be mediated via inhibition of TGF expression.

The results suggest that rather than simply serving as a biomarker for the presence of renal injury, periostin may be a modifiable mediator of renal injury. We chose to include this study because it is so novel, and as the research unfolds, it may open doors to new treatments for CKD.

R. Garrick, MD

30 Hypertension and Kidney Disease

Time-Updated Systolic Blood Pressure and the Progression of Chronic Kidney Disease: A Cohort Study

Anderson AH, for the Chronic Renal Insufficiency Cohort Study Investigators (Univ of Pennsylvania Perelman School of Medicine, Philadelphia; et al)

Ann Intern Med 162:258-265, 2015

Background.—Previous reports of the longitudinal association between achieved blood pressure (BP) and end-stage renal disease (ESRD) among patients with chronic kidney disease (CKD) have not incorporated time-updated BP with appropriate covariate adjustment.

Objective.—To assess the association between baseline and time-updated systolic blood pressure (SBP) with CKD progression.

Design.—Observational, prospective cohort study. (ClinicalTrials.gov: NCT00304148)

Setting.—7 U.S. clinical centers.

Patients.—Patients in the Chronic Renal Insufficiency Cohort Study ($n = 3708$) followed for a median of 5.7 years (25th to 75th percentile, 4.6 to 6.7 years).

Measurements.—The mean of 3 seated SBP measurements made up the visit-specific SBP. Time-updated SBP was the mean of that and all previous visits. Outcomes were ESRD and the composite end point of ESRD or halving of the estimated glomerular filtration rate. Analyses investigating baseline and time-updated SBP used Cox proportional hazards models and marginal structural models, respectively.

Results.—Systolic blood pressure was 130 mm Hg or greater at all visits in 19.2% of patients. The hazard ratio for ESRD among patients with SBP of 130 to 139 mm Hg, compared with SBP less than 120 mm Hg, was 1.46 (95% CI, 1.13 to 1.88) using only baseline data and 2.37 (CI, 1.48 to 3.80) using time-updated data. Among patients with SBP of 140 mm Hg or greater, corresponding hazard ratios were 1.46 (CI, 1.18 to 1.88) and 3.37 (CI, 2.26 to 5.03) for models using only baseline data and those using time-updated data, respectively.

Limitation.—Blood pressure was measured once annually, and the cohort was not a random sample.

Conclusion.—Time-updated SBP greater than 130 mm Hg was more strongly associated with CKD progression than analyses based on baseline SBP.

▶ Both observational studies and clinical trials have provided strong evidence linking progression of chronic kidney disease (CKD) to blood pressure control.[1-5] However, in patients with CKD, the optimal blood pressure target remains elusive. Thus, recent recommendations suggest that the target blood pressure for individuals with CKD and diabetes are a systolic blood pressure less than 140/90, rather than less than 130/80, as previously described. The current study sought to evaluate the whether CKD progression is better predicted by time-updated blood pressure readings compared with 1-time measurements. The data were drawn from the well-defined Chronic Renal Insufficiency Cohort Study. Approximately 3700 patients were enrolled in this multicenter trial over a 5-year period. The annual sitting blood pressure for each visit was based on the average of 3 seated readings. The time-updated systolic blood pressure was the average of that blood pressure and all previous blood pressure readings. Patients were followed for a median of 5.7 years, the analysis was adjusted for time-updated covariates, and the end points were progression to end-stage renal disease, or a 50% in the estimated glomerular filtration rate. Time-updated values were better able to predict progression of renal disease, and progression was most marked in individuals with blood pressure readings greater than 130/80. The data suggest that timed-average readings offer insight into the longitudinal impact hypertension on the progression of renal disease. The data from this cohort also suggest that regardless of the presence of diabetes or hypertension, a time-updated blood pressure greater than 130/80 is associated with increased risk of progression of CKD. The study does have limitations; for example, the findings are based on readings from annual visits, and the data may be confounded by unknown variables (such as exact types of and compliance with, blood pressure medications). The findings are not intended to definitively define the target blood pressure for a individual patient. However, these observations are clinically relevant, applicable to practice settings, and again demonstrate the need for randomized, prospective trials to help bring clarity to current practice guidelines.

R. Garrick, MD

References

1. Eknoyan G, Lameire N. KDIGO 2012 clinical practice guideline for the evaluation and management of chronic kidney disease. *Kidney Int Suppl.* 2013;3:1-150.
2. US Renal Data System. *2013 USRDS Annual Data Report: Atlas of Chronic Kidney Disease and End-Stage Renal Disease in the United States.* Bethesda, MD: National Institute of Diabetes and Digestive and Kidney Diseases; 2013.
3. Lv J, Ehteshami P, Sarnak MJ, et al. Effects of intensive blood pressure lowering on the progression of chronic kidney disease: a systematic review and meta-analysis. *CMAJ.* 2013;185:949-957.

4. Bangalore S, Kumar S, Lobach I, Messerli FH. Blood pressure targets in subjects with type 2 diabetes mellitus/impaired fasting glucose: observations from traditional and Bayesian random-effects meta-analyses of randomized trials. *Circulation.* 2011;123:2799-2810.
5. Chobanian AV, Bakris GL, Black HR, et al; National heart, lung, and blood institute joint national committee on prevention, detection, evaluation, and treatment of high blood pressure. The seventh report of the joint national committee on prevention, detection, evaluation, and treatment of high blood pressure: the JNC 7 report. *JAMA.* 2003;289:2560-2572.

Effects of Intensive Low-Salt Diet Education on Albuminuria among Nondiabetic Patients with Hypertension Treated with Olmesartan: A Single-Blinded Randomized, Controlled Trial

Hwang JH, Chin HJ, Kim S, et al (Chung-Ang Univ Hosp, Seoul, South Korea; Univ Bundang Hosp, Seong-Nam, South Korea; et al)
Clin J Am Soc Nephrol 9:2059-2069, 2014

Background and Objectives.—The antiproteinuric effect of a renin-angiotensin-aldosterone system blockade can be magnified by dietary salt restriction. This study sought to determine the effect of intensive low-salt diet education on BP and urine albumin excretion in nondiabetic patients with hypertension and albuminuria.

Design, Setting, Participants, & Measurements.—This study was conducted between March of 2012 and March of 2013 as an open-label, randomized, controlled trial. After a run-in period of 8 weeks, all patients received the angiotensin II receptor blocker olmesartan (40 mg daily). Patients were then divided into two groups. One group was treated for another 8 weeks with angiotensin II receptor blocker plus conventional low-salt diet education, and the other group was treated for 8 weeks with angiotensin II receptor blocker plus intensive low-salt diet education. The final analyses was performed with 245 completed patients.

Results.—The amount of daily albuminuria was significantly decreased from 0 (566.0 [25.0–5398.6] mg/d) to 8 weeks (282.5 [16.1–4898.5] mg/d; $P < 0.001$). From 8 to 16 weeks, the 24-hour urinary sodium excretion was decreased by 36.0 ± 5.9 mmol/d in the intensive education group and 8.8 ± 4.9 mmol/d in the conventional education group (interaction $P < 0.001$). Patients who completed intensive low-salt diet education exhibited greater decreases in urinary albumin excretion than the control group (change in albuminuria from 8 to 16 weeks, −154.0 versus 0.4 mg/d; $P = 0.01$). Urinary albumin excretion tended to decrease as the 24-hour urinary sodium excretion amount decreased ($R = 0.32$; 95% confidence interval, 0.20 to 0.43; $P < 0.001$).

Conclusions.—The 24-hour urinary albumin excretion was decreased more in patients in the intensive low-salt diet education group than

patients in the conventional education group. Weekly intensive education on a low-salt diet would be a suitable method for clinical practice.

▶ Albuminuria is a known risk factor in individuals with and without diabetes for cardiovascular disease, end-stage renal disease (ESRD), hospitalization, and all-cause mortality.[1] Lowering of albuminuria with the help of renin-angiotensin-aldosterone system (RAAS) blockade not only prevent the progression to ESRD but also reduces cardiovascular events.[2] In this trial, the authors tried to investigate the efficacy of low-salt diet education on albuminuria in patients already on angiotensin receptor blockers.

This is an open-label, case-control, randomized, and controlled clinical trial done in South Korea. The study population consisted of nondiabetics with relatively controlled hypertension. Eight weeks before the initiation, all RAAS antagonist and diuretics were discontinued for a run-in and blood pressure was controlled on alternate medications. On week 0, olmesartan 40 mg daily was started in all the patients. At week 8, patients were randomized 1:1 in conventional education versus intensive education regarding a low-salt diet. Patients with intensive education received a close monitoring and 30-minute weekly phone feedback by a dietary consultant. The primary end point was change in albuminuria by week 16. There was a significant reduction of albuminuria in intensive group (from 278 to 178 mg/d) compared with the conventional group (from 258 to 231 mg/d) without any significant change in the blood pressure or serum creatinine. Subgroup analysis showed that sodium reduction (achieved in only 60% of intensive group arm) of 25% or more was associated with significant reduction in albuminuria regardless of randomization.

Overall, this is an interesting and well-performed study offering additional proof that, independent from blood pressure, lowering dietary sodium lowers albuminuria. The authors also demonstrated that compliance was sustained through education and follow-up (weekly, in this case) dietary counseling. Limitations, which may impede generalization of the findings, are that the patient population was relatively healthy and homogenous, with good blood pressure control, and at initiation, patients were consuming a relatively low-salt diet, compared with the typical US population. For clinical practice, the findings support the use of a low-salt diet, and dietary education as important adjuvant measures in this high-risk population.

R. Garrick, MD

References

1. Gerstein HC, Mann JF, Yi Q, et al; HOPE Study Investigators. Albuminuria and risk of cardiovascular events, death, and heart failure in diabetic and nondiabetic individuals. *JAMA*. 2001;286:421-426.
2. Balamuthusamy S, Srinivasan L, Verma M, et al. Renin angiotensin system blockade and cardiovascular outcomes in patients with chronic kidney disease and proteinuria: a meta-analysis. *Am Heart J*. 2008;155:791-805.

A Controlled Trial of Renal Denervation for Resistant Hypertension

Bhatt DL, for the SYMPLICITY HTN-3 Investigators (Brigham and Women's Hosp, Boston, MA; et al)

N Engl J Med 370:1393-1401, 2014

Background.—Prior unblinded studies have suggested that catheter-based renal-artery denervation reduces blood pressure in patients with resistant hypertension.

Methods.—We designed a prospective, single-blind, randomized, sham-controlled trial. Patients with severe resistant hypertension were randomly assigned in a 2:1 ratio to undergo renal denervation or a sham procedure. Before randomization, patients were receiving a stable antihypertensive regimen involving maximally tolerated doses of at least three drugs, including a diuretic. The primary efficacy end point was the change in office systolic blood pressure at 6 months; a secondary efficacy end point was the change in mean 24-hour ambulatory systolic blood pressure. The primary safety end point was a composite of death, end-stage renal disease, embolic events resulting in end-organ damage, renovascular complications, or hypertensive crisis at 1 month or new renal-artery stenosis of more than 70% at 6 months.

Results.—A total of 535 patients underwent randomization. The mean (±SD) change in systolic blood pressure at 6 months was −14.13 ± 23.93 mm Hg in the denervation group as compared with −11.74 ± 25.94 mm Hg in the sham-procedure group ($P < 0.001$ for both comparisons of the change from baseline), for a difference of −2.39 mm Hg (95% confidence interval [CI], −6.89 to 2.12; $P = 0.26$ for superiority with a margin of 5 mm Hg). The change in 24-hour ambulatory systolic blood pressure was −6.75 ± 15.11 mm Hg in the denervation group and −4.79 ± 17.25 mm Hg in the sham-procedure group, for a difference of −1.96 mm Hg (95% CI, −4.97 to 1.06; $P = 0.98$ for superiority with a margin of 2 mm Hg). There were no significant differences in safety between the two groups.

Conclusions.—This blinded trial did not show a significant reduction of systolic blood pressure in patients with resistant hypertension 6 months after renal-artery denervation as compared with a sham control.

▶ Resistant hypertension, defined as a persistent blood pressure (B/P) greater than 140/90 despite the optimal use of 3 antihypertensive medications, occurs in about 10% of all the hypertensive patients and is a major cause of morbidity and mortality in this population.[1] More than 50 years ago, the role of the renal sympathetic innervations in resistant hypertension became apparent. Thus, surgical interventions, including total or partial sympathectomy and even nephrectomies, were performed in the hope of achieving B/P control.[2,3] Recently, nonrandomized and randomized unblinded trials[4,5] have suggested that catheter-based radiofrequency ablation of renal sympathetic enervation is a potentially effective treatment for resistant hypertension.

To negate the limitations of previous suboptimal studies and in response to the US Food and Drug Administration's request, the investigators of SYMPLICITY III designed this prospective, single-blind, randomized trial, which included a sham-controlled model. The study enrolled 535 patients with 2:1 random assignment into catheter ablation versus a renal angiography sham procedure. The primary efficacy end point was a reduction in BP with a superiority margin of 5 mm Hg based on office blood pressure readings. The secondary end point was the change in ambulatory B/P 6 months after the procedure.

The results (Figures 1 and 2 in the original article) have reverberated across the medical community. Both the sham and denervation groups had impressive drops in blood pressure by 14.3 vs 11.74 mm Hg. This was the problem, as the denervation failed to show a benefit over control group. So why are these results different from previous ones? Unlike other studies, this was a sham-controlled, blinded trial, which is an effective way to study a new medical device. The findings again demonstrate the important need for randomized controlled trials and stress that the placebo effect is real and impressive. The results demonstrate that renal denervation is relatively safe procedure, but its antihypertensive efficacy is questionable. Whether additional data will establish a place for renal denervation remains to be seen, but in the meantime, the results teach us that medication compliance and close monitoring, together, can achieve impressive B/P control.

S. Chugh, MD

References

1. Sarafidis PA, Georgianos P, Bakris GL. Resistant hypertension—its identification and epidemiology. *Nat Rev Nephrol.* 2013;9:51-58.
2. Vertes V, Cangiano JL, Berman LB, Gould A. Hypertension in end-stage renal disease. *N Engl J Med.* 1969;280:978-981.
3. Grimson KS, Orgain ES, Anderson B, Broome RA, Longino FH. Results of treatment of patients with hypertension by total thoracic and partial to total lumbar sympathectomy, splanchnicectomy and celiac ganglionectomy. *Ann Surg.* 1949; 129:850-871.
4. Krum H, Schlaich M, Whitbourn R, et al. Catheter-based renal sympathetic denervation for resistant hypertension: a multicentre safety and proof-of-principle cohort study. *Lancet.* 2009;373:1275-1281.
5. Symplicity HTN-2 Investigators. Renal sympathetic denervation in patients with treatment-resistant hypertension (the SYMPLICITY HTN-2 trial): a randomised controlled trial. *Lancet.* 2010;376:1903-1909.

Blood Pressure in Early Autosomal Dominant Polycystic Kidney Disease

Schrier RW, for the HALT-PKD Trial Investigators (Univ of Colorado, Denver; et al)

N Engl J Med 371:2255-2266, 2014

Background.—Hypertension is common in autosomal dominant polycystic kidney disease (ADPKD) and is associated with increased total kidney volume, activation of the renin–angiotensin–aldosterone system, and progression of kidney disease.

Methods.—In this double-blind, placebo-controlled trial, we randomly assigned 558 hypertensive participants with ADPKD (15 to 49 years of age, with an estimated glomerular filtration rate [GFR] >60 ml per minute per 1.73 m^2 of body-surface area) to either a standard blood-pressure target (120/70 to 130/80 mm Hg) or a low blood-pressure target (95/60 to 110/75 mm Hg) and to either an angiotensin-converting–enzyme inhibitor (lisinopril) plus an angiotensin-receptor blocker (telmisartan) or lisinopril plus placebo. The primary outcome was the annual percentage change in the total kidney volume.

Results.—The annual percentage increase in total kidney volume was significantly lower in the low-blood-pressure group than in the standard-blood-pressure group (5.6% vs. 6.6%, $P = 0.006$), without significant differences between the lisinopril–telmisartan group and the lisinopril–placebo group. The rate of change in estimated GFR was similar in the two medication groups, with a negative slope difference in the short term in the low-blood-pressure group as compared with the standard-blood-pressure group ($P < 0.001$) and a marginally positive slope difference in the long term ($P = 0.05$). The left-ventricular-mass index decreased more in the low-blood-pressure group than in the standard-blood-pressure group (−1.17 vs. −0.57 g per square meter per year, $P < 0.001$); urinary albumin excretion was reduced by 3.77% with the low-pressure target and increased by 2.43% with the standard target ($P < 0.001$). Dizziness and light-headedness were more common in the low-blood-pressure group than in the standard-blood-pressure group (80.7% vs. 69.4%, $P = 0.002$).

Conclusions.—In early ADPKD, the combination of lisinopril and telmisartan did not significantly alter the rate of increase in total kidney volume. As compared with standard blood-pressure control, rigorous blood-pressure control was associated with a slower increase in total kidney volume, no overall change in the estimated GFR, a greater decline in the left-ventricular-mass index, and greater reduction in urinary albumin excretion.

▶ Hypertension occurs early in autosomal dominant polycystic kidney disease (ADPKD) and is strongly associated with cardiovascular morbidity and progression to end-stage renal disease in this patient population.[1] Renin release and activation of the renin-angiotensin-aldosterone system (RAAS) from enlarging cysts is believed to be central to the incident hypertension.[2] RAAS activation has also been shown in animal studies to have an important role in promoting mitogenesis and renal mass growth, but this has not been fully evaluated in clinical trials.[3] With this understanding, two fundamental questions arise in the management of these patients. First, what are the preferred medications and the optimal blood pressure target, and second, does dual angiotensin-converting enzyme inhibitor (ACE-I)/angiotensin II receptor blocker (ARB) blockade offer additive reno-protection to slow cyst growth and chronic kidney disease progression?

With these questions in mind, the investigators performed this multicenter, double-blind, placebo-controlled trial comparing low blood pressure target (95/60 to 110/75 mm Hg) to standard blood pressure target (120/70 to 130/80 mm Hg) and the effect of ARB (telmisartan)/ACE-I (lisinopril) combination versus monotherapy with an ACE-I (lisinopril). The primary endpoint was the percentage change in the total kidney volume over time. The secondary outcomes were the rate of change in estimated glomerular filtration rate (eGFR), albuminuria, and left ventricular mass index over time of follow-up (8 years).

Kidney size increased less and eGFR was stable in the low blood pressure group compared with those with standard blood pressure targets. In the other arm, patients with ACE-I/ARB combination therapy had similar increase in kidney size compared with monotherapy with no significant change in the eGFR between groups. In secondary endpoints, only the group with low blood pressure showed a decrease in left ventricular mass index (−1.17 vs −0.57 g per square meter per year, $P < .001$) and also urinary albumin excretion (−3.77% vs +2.43%). The favorable outcomes in low blood pressure group, however, were associated with more frequent episodes of dizziness and lightheadedness (80.7% vs 69.4%, $P = .002$).

In summary, this trial demonstrated that combination therapy with ACE-I and ARB offered no greater renal protection than did therapy with ACE-I alone. These findings are reminiscent of those in type II diabetics[4] and provide further evidence that use of combination ACE-I/ARB therapy is typically not superior to monotherapy with regard to progression of renal injury. The optimal blood pressure control in these patients still unsettled. This trial did show that achieving a lower target blood pressure was associated with a smaller increase in renal mass, left ventricular mass index, and urinary albumin excretion, but the long-term outcome is not yet known, and side effects were more frequent among the low blood pressure group. The HALT study was well designed and well executed and will certainly inform our decision making with regard to combination therapy. In addition, the findings suggest that, when clinically tolerated, lower blood pressure targets may be preferable for patients with ADPKD.

S. Chugh, MD

References

1. Schrier RW. Hypertension and autosomal dominant polycystic kidney disease. *Am J Kidney Dis.* 2011;57:811-813.
2. Chapman AB, Johnson A, Gabow PA, Schrier RW. The renin-angiotensin-aldosterone system and autosomal dominant polycystic kidney disease. *N Engl J Med.* 1990;323:1091-1096.
3. Thomas W, Dooley R, Harvey BJ. Aldosterone as a renal growth factor. *Steroids.* 2010;75:550-554.

4. Mann JF, Schmieder RE, McQueen M, et al. Renal outcomes with telmisartan, ramipril, or both, in people at high vascular risk (the ONTARGET study): a multicentre, randomised, double-blind, controlled trial. *Lancet*. 2008;372:547.

31 Diabetes and Kidney Disease

Renal Outcomes in Patients with Type 1 Diabetes and Macroalbuminuria

de Boer IH, for the Diabetes Control and Complications Trial/Epidemiology of Diabetes Interventions and Complications (DCCT/EDIC) Research Group (Univ of Washington, Seattle; et al)

J Am Soc Nephrol 25:2342-2350, 2014

Macroalbuminuria, defined as urine albumin excretion rate (AER) ≥300 mg/d, has long been considered a stage of irreversible kidney damage that leads reliably to GFR loss. We examined the long-term renal outcomes of persons with type 1 diabetes who developed incident macroalbuminuria during the Diabetes Control and Complications Trial (DCCT)/Epidemiology of Diabetes Interventions and Complications (EDIC) study. One hundred fifty-nine participants developed incident macroalbuminuria and were subsequently followed for a median duration of 9 years (maximum of 25 years). At the time of macroalbuminuria diagnosis, mean (SD) age was 37 (9) years, mean (SD) duration of diabetes was 17 (5) years, median AER was 524 mg/d, and mean (SD) eGFR was 108 (20) ml/min per 1.73 m^2. Ten years after macroalbuminuria diagnosis, the cumulative incidence of a sustained reduction in AER to <300 mg/d was 52%, mostly but not entirely under treatment with renin-angiotensin system inhibitors. The cumulative incidence of impaired GFR (sustained eGFR <60 ml/min per 1.73 m^2) 10 years after macroalbuminuria diagnosis was 32%, including 16% who developed ESRD. Lower hemoglobin A1c and BP and regression to AER <300 mg/d were associated with reduced risk of developing impaired GFR. In conclusion, people with type 1 diabetes who develop macroalbuminuria are at high risk of progressive kidney disease. However, through at least 10 years of follow-up, AER could often be controlled, and GFR frequently remained in the normal range.

▶ Urine albumin excretion (UAE) > 300 mg/day, called macroalbuminuria (MA), has been predictably linked to declining renal function and underlying kidney damage in diabetics. The Diabetes Control and Complications Trial/ Epidemiology of Diabetes Interventions and Complications trials were designed to study the differential effects of intensive vs conventional therapies in type I diabetes mellitus.[1,2] After 25 years of follow-up, the incidence of MA in the intensive vs conventional therapies were 6% and 17%, respectively. Prior evaluation of this cohort demonstrated a 50-fold increased risk of impaired glomerular filtration rate (GFR) in those patients who developed MA.

De Boer et al used the data collected from this important trial to examine incident MA and its long-term renal outcomes up to 25 years later. A total of 159 participants ultimately developed MA with median UAE 524 mg/24 hr and mean GFR over 100 mL/min. In 61 patients, the MA actually regressed, thereby reducing the 10-year sustained MA prevalence to only 52%. In 14 (13%) of these subjects, the levels actually resolved to below the level of microalbuminuria (30 mg/day). All but 2 of these "regressors" maintained estimated GFR (eGFR) > 60 mL/min for the complete duration of follow-up. Those who regressed to levels < 300 mg/day enjoyed an 89% reduction in developing sustained renal impairment. Renin-angiotensin-aldosterone system inhibition (RI) was used in all but 4 incident patients during this trial. In fact, the use of RI increased from 31% to 88% during the posttrial observation period.

The investigators found that after a median of 9 years of follow-up, the mean eGFR declined by 5.4 mL/min annually. They determined the cumulative incidence of impaired GFR and end-stage renal disease after 15 years of sustained MA were 42% and 15%, respectively. Not surprisingly, lower hemoglobin A1c, lower blood pressure, and lower rates of MA at diagnosis were associated with a decreased risk of impaired renal function. The incidence of nephrotic range proteinuria (> 3000 mg/day) was 25%, occurring after 15 years of sustained MA in 85% of the macroalbuminuric subjects.

This analysis demonstrates well that MA contributes substantially to the risk of progression of renal disease in type I diabetes. Nevertheless, the majority of patients with incident MA maintained eGFR > 60 mL/min through the end of the follow-up, and more than half regressed to micro or normal albuminuria.

An interesting editorial that accompanies this article[3] cautioned against crediting the use of RI for the observed high rate of regression as possibly misleading because of problems with study design. The editorial cogently warned against using posttrial observational studies to infer benefits or risks of interventions that did not have a proper control group in the posttrial period. Such extension trials are prone to both "selection" and "indication" bias due to the lack of such a control group. They cite as an example the fact that more RI (88%) was used in the sustained MA group compared with the regressed or normoalbuminuric group (67%). This, they note, could have resulted in misattributing effects of RI use when the actual differences could be due to variations in the urine protein levels themselves. They conclude that De Boers' study, although important and timely, should properly be used as a starting point for properly controlled trials in this field.

M. Klein, MD

References

1. The Diabetes Control and Complications Trial Research Group. The effect of intensive treatment of diabetes on the development and progression of long-term complications in insulin-dependent diabetes mellitus. *N Engl J Med.* 1993;329: 977-986.
2. (DCCT/EDIC) Study Research Group. Intensive diabetes treatment and cardiovascular disease in patients with type 1 diabetes. The diabetes control and

complications trial/epidemiology of diabetes interventions and complications. *N Engl J Med.* 2005;353:2643-2653.
3. Lambers Heerspink HJ, de Zeeuw D. Are post-trial observational studies useful? *J Am Soc Nephrol.* 2014;25:2148-2150.

Improved Glycemic Control and Risk of ESRD in Patients with Type 1 Diabetes and Proteinuria

Skupien J, Warram JH, Smiles A, et al (Brigham and Women Hosp, Boston, MA; et al)

J Am Soc Nephrol 25:2916-2925, 2014

Most patients with type 1 diabetes (T1D) and proteinuria have poor glycemic control and a high risk of ESRD. We investigated whether long-term improvement of glycemic control reduces risk of ESRD in a prospective 7- to 15-year follow-up observation of 349 patients with CKD stages 1–3 enrolled in the Joslin Proteinuria Cohort of adults with T1D. All patients developed proteinuria between 1990 and 2004 and were followed until 2011 to ascertain onset of ESRD and deaths unrelated to ESRD. Furthermore, we analyzed data from 279 patients with ≥3 years of clinic follow-up available to assess the level of glycemic control after enrollment. Average HbA_{1c} during the 5 years before study enrollment (prebaseline) was compared with HbA_{1c} (postbaseline) averaged during the first half of follow-up (median, 5.1 years).Median prebaseline HbA_{1c} was 9.3%, decreasing to 8.7% postbaseline. Cumulative risk of ESRD after 15 years was significantly lower for patients whose HbA_{1c} decreased than for those whose HbA_{1c} increased or remained poor (29% versus 42%; $P < 0.001$). The difference between these groups was not visible at 5 years of follow-up but became visible at 10 and 15 years of follow-up. In multivariate Cox regression analysis of ESRD risk, the hazard ratio corresponding to a 1–percentage point improvement in postbaseline HbA_{1c} was 0.76 (95% confidence interval, 0.63 to 0.91; $P = 0.003$). In conclusion, results of this study suggest that long-term sustained improvement in HbA_{1c} decelerates eGFR loss and delays the onset of ESRD in patients with T1D and proteinuria.

▶ These data shed light on a long-standing complicated question: does tight glycemic control alter the rate of progression to end-stage renal disease (ESRD) in type I diabetics? The question can only be answered through long-term follow-up because the time course of progression in type I diabetes is quite variable. These investigators prospectively followed (for 7-15 years), approximately 350 adult type I diabetics, with CKD stage 1 through 3, who were enrolled in the Joslin proteinuria cohort. Patients had been following in the Joslin clinic for a median of 19 years and in the majority of patients, proteinuria had been present for less than 3 years. The cohort was enrolled between 1991 and 2004 and followed through 2011. Preenrollment hemoglobin A_{1c}

(HbA_{1c}) measurements and serial follow-up data were analyzed, and the difference between pre-and post baseline HbA_{1c} was used to assess the exposure to ambient glucose.

The cohorts medium glomerular filtration rate was 85 mL/min/1.73 m^2, and the majority of patients' blood pressure was close to therapeutic target (median 130/78 mm Hg), and about 70% of the patients were on treatment with either an angiotensin-converting enzyme inhibitor or angiotensin receptor blocker. The relatively low use of RAS altering agents reflects the fact that the cohort began in 1991. At the time of enrollment, most patients had poor glycemic control (prebaseline median HgA_{1c} 9.3%). Figure 3 in the original article demonstrates acumen of risk of ESRD according to pre-and postbaseline HgA_{1c}. Approximately 10% of patients had a rapid deterioration or renal function. Among the others, improved glycemic control, especially among those with the poorest initial control, was associated with a reduction in the rate of decline in renal function.

This is the first long-term cohort follow-up of type I diabetics has become available. Weaknesses of the study are the absence of randomization and the fact that the HgA_{1c} levels were not the same degree of frequency and were obtained in unevenly spaced time intervals across the study in all patients. Nonetheless, the findings give us reason to be optimistic regarding progression of renal disease in type I diabetes mellitus. The degree of glycemic control required to slow the progression of renal disease was clinically quite achievable. The finding fact that renal outcomes and progression to ESRD might be improved in this very high-risk population with type I diabetes mellitus and proteinuria is certainly noteworthy.

R. Garrick, MD

Metformin in Patients With Type 2 Diabetes and Kidney Disease: A Systematic Review

Inzucchi SE, Lipska KJ, Mayo H, et al (Yale Univ School of Medicine, New Haven, CT; Univ of Texas Southwestern Med Ctr, Dallas; et al)
JAMA 312:2668-2675, 2014

Importance.—Metformin is widely viewed as the best initial pharmacological option to lower glucose concentrations in patients with type 2 diabetes mellitus. However, the drug is contraindicated in many individuals with impaired kidney function because of concerns of lactic acidosis.

Objective.—To assess the risk of lactic acidosis associated with metformin use in individuals with impaired kidney function.

Evidence Acquisition.—In July 2014, we searched the MEDLINE and Cochrane databases for English-language articles pertaining to metformin, kidney disease, and lactic acidosis in humans between 1950 and June 2014.We excluded reviews, letters, editorials, case reports, small case series, and manuscripts that did not directly pertain to the topic area or that met other exclusion criteria. Of an original 818 articles, 65 were included in this review, including pharmacokinetic/metabolic studies, large case series, retrospective studies, meta-analyses, and a clinical trial.

Results.—Although metformin is renally cleared, drug levels generally remain within the therapeutic range and lactate concentrations are not substantially increased when used in patients with mild to moderate chronic kidney disease (estimated glomerular filtration rates, 30-60 mL/min per 1.73 m^2). The overall incidence of lactic acidosis in metformin users varies across studies from approximately 3 per 100 000 person-years to 10 per 100 000 person-years and is generally indistinguishable from the background rate in the overall population with diabetes. Data suggesting an increased risk of lactic acidosis in metformin-treated patients with chronic kidney disease are limited, and no randomized controlled trials have been conducted to test the safety of metformin in patients with significantly impaired kidney function. Population-based studies demonstrate that metformin may be prescribed counter to prevailing guidelines suggesting a renal risk in up to 1 in 4 patients with type 2 diabetes mellitus—use which, in most reports, has not been associated with increased rates of lactic acidosis. Observational studies suggest a potential benefit from metformin on macrovascular outcomes, even in patients with prevalent renal contraindications for its use.

Conclusions and Relevance.—Available evidence supports cautious expansion of metformin use in patients with mild to moderate chronic kidney disease, as defined by estimated glomerular filtration rate, with appropriate dosage reductions and careful follow-up of kidney function.

▶ Metformin has been the mainstay of therapy in type 2 diabetes mellitus (DMII) since the mid-1990s. Concern about lactic acidosis seen with other biguanides such as phenformin was assuaged by limited US Food and Drug Administration approval of metformin to patients with normal renal function, thereby minimizing the risk for cumulative toxicity. Consequently, the current labeling recommends against the use in chronic kidney disease (CKD) stages 3 or lower. Nevertheless, as many as 25% of patients with DMII, are using metformin counter to these recommendations because it has been both effective and well tolerated.

This review by Inzucchi et al systematically evaluated more than 800 relevant studies in an attempt to determine the actual safety of prescribing this effective drug in patients with significant renal dysfunction.

They noted that despite decreased drug clearance in mild to moderate CKD, the levels remained in a safe range. They described a study in CKD with estimated glomerular filtration rate (eGFR) < 30 cc/min where the median trough level of measured metformin was only 8.88 mcmol/L.[1] This is well below the upper therapeutic range of 20 mcmol/L. One trial studying 97 metformin users found no association between plasma lactate levels and renal status between 3 discreet groups of eGFR levels.[2] These findings were replicated in at least 4 other reviewed trials. Apparently, the differing metabolic and pharmacokinetic properties of metformin and phenformin, although both biguanides, result in differing therapeutic and adverse effects.

Other studies were reviewed comprising more than 100 000 metformin users establishing the incidence of lactic acidosis at between 3 to 10 per 100 000 person-years of therapy. Interestingly, patients on sulfourea drugs had, in 1 study, an incidence of 4.8 per 100 000 person years. So the lactic acidosis incidence may be not much different from the background levels.

Much data demonstrate the efficacy of metformin use with mortality rates of 6.3% of users vs 9.8% of nonusers. This benefit persisted statistically even when GFR was under 30 cc/min. Cardiovascular mortality benefits with metformin monotherapy exceeded the benefits seen with other agents. Patients using metformin with moderate renal failure (eGFR 45-60) had lower risks of acidosis and/or infection than using other single agents.[3] Only 1 study demonstrated an elevated hazard ratio 6.37 versus HR 4.06 in users and nonusers, respectively. But the authors felt this study had many limitations including poor documentary evidence of lactic acidosis and of renal function.

This is an important article because the authors conclude that the benefits of using metformin outweigh the small risks of lactic acidosis in patients with clearances between 30 and 60 cc/min. They point to the already routine use of this drug in patients with mild to moderate CKD without convincing evidence of increased harm. Therefore, the authors recommend a change in the prescribing guidelines to permit metformin use in stage 3 CKD.

M. Klein, MD

References

1. Frid A, Sterner GN, Löndahl M, et al. Novel assay of metformin levels in patients with type 2 diabetes and varying levels of renal function: clinical recommendations. *Diabetes Care*. 2010;33:1291-1293.
2. Lim VC, Sum CF, Chan ES, Yeoh LY, Lee YM, Lim SC. Lactate levels in Asian patients with type 2 diabetes mellitus on metformin and its association with dose of metformin and renal function. *Int J Clin Pract*. 2007;61:829-833.
3. Ekström N, Schiöler L, Svensson AM, et al. Effectiveness and safety of metformin in 51 675 patients with type 2 diabetes and different levels of renal function: a cohort study from the Swedish National Diabetes Register. *BMJ Open*. 2012;2. e001076.

Effect of Pentoxifylline on Renal Function and Urinary Albumin Excretion in Patients with Diabetic Kidney Disease: The PREDIAN Trial

Navarro-González JF, Mora-Fernández C, Muros de Fuentes M, et al (Univ Hosp Nuestra Señora de Candelaria, Santa Cruz de Tenerife, Spain)
J Am Soc Nephrol 26:220-229, 2015

Diabetic kidney disease (DKD) is the leading cause of ESRD. We conducted an open-label, prospective, randomized trial to determine whether pentoxifylline (PTF), which reduces albuminuria, in addition to renin-angiotensin system (RAS) blockade, can slow progression of renal disease in patients with type 2 diabetes and stages 3–4 CKD. Participants were assigned to receive PTF (1200 mg/d) ($n = 82$) or to a control group ($n = 87$) for 2 years. All patients received similar doses of RAS inhibitors. At study end, eGFR had decreased by a mean ± SEM of 2.1 ± 0.4 ml/min per 1.73 m^2 in the PTF group compared with 6.5 ± 0.4 ml/min per 1.73 m^2 in the control group, with a between-group difference of 4.3 ml/min per 1.73 m^2 (95% confidence interval [95% CI], 3.1 to 5.5 ml/min per 1.73 m^2; $P < 0.001$) in favor of PTF. The proportion of patients with a rate of eGFR decline greater than the median rate of decline (0.16 ml/min per 1.73 m^2 per month) was lower in the PTF group than in the control group (33.3% versus 68.2%; $P < 0.001$). Percentage change in urinary albumin excretion was 5.7% (95% CI, −0.3% to 11.1%) in the control group and −14.9% (95% CI, −20.4% to −9.4%) in the PTF group ($P = 0.001$). Urine TNF-α decreased from a median 16 ng/g (interquartile range, 11–20.1 ng/g) to 14.3 ng/g (interquartile range, 9.2–18.4 ng/g) in the PTF group ($P < 0.01$), with no changes in the control group. In this population, addition of PTF to RAS inhibitors resulted in a smaller decrease in eGFR and a greater reduction of residual albuminuria.

▶ These data are noteworthy. Pentoxifylline is a nonspecific phosphodiesterase inhibitor and an antiinflammatory agent that is used in patients with claudication and alcoholic hepatitis. Although they have not yet been replicated in other centers, the safety and long history of pentoxifylline use makes these findings quite interesting and worthy of additional study. In this single-center randomized controlled trial, type II diabetics with proteinuria (urine albumin > 30 mg/day and estimated glomerular filtration (eGFR) rate 15 to 59 mL/min/1.73 m^2), receiving an angiotensin-converting enzyme (ACE) inhibitor or angiotensin receptor blocker (ARB) were randomly assigned to pentoxifylline (600 mg twice daily) or no therapy. At 2 years, compared with the control group, pentoxifylline use was associated with a smaller decline in eGFR and significant reduction in protein excretion.

Diabetes is the most common cause of ESRD in United States.[1] Several strategies have been described to delay the progression of kidney disease in diabetic nephropathy. These include adequate glycemic control, which targets Hb1c levels <7%[2]; blood pressure control with target less than 140/90[3]; and use of ACE inhibitor or ARB therapy for reduction of proteinuria. Although proteinuria itself is a surrogate marker, several trials have demonstrated that a reduction in protein spillage is associated with a slowing of the rate of progression of renal disease.[4-7] In the ONTARGET trial, combination ACE inhibitor and ARB therapy was shown to be superior to monotherapy for reducing proteinuria but was associated with worse renal outcomes. This finding dampened our enthusiasm for combined ACE inhibitor/ARB therapy.[8] Other strategies used to reduce proteinuria include medications such as spironolactone, eplerenone, verapamil, and diltiazem and nonpharmacological maneuvers such as weight loss and a low-salt diet.

The mechanism of action of pentoxifylline is uncertain, but it may be linked to its antiinflammatory activity as evidenced by reduced urinary excretion of tumor necrosis factor-alfa in the treatment group.

Larger randomized trials will be required before it becomes accepted as standard antiproteinuric therapy in type II diabetes. However, these early data suggest that pentoxifylline may be a viable adjuvant treatment option for patients with type II diabetes. Its efficacy in patients who are unable to tolerate ACE inhibitor or ARB therapy will also be of interest.

R. Lamba, MD

References

1. American Diabetes Association. Position statement: diabetic nephropathy. *Diabetes Care*. 1999;22:S66-S69.
2. DCCT/EDIC Research Group, de Boer IH, Sun W, Cleary PA, et al. Intensive diabetes therapy and glomerular filtration rate in type 1 diabetes. *N Engl J Med*. 2011;365:2366.
3. James PA, Oparil S, Carter BL, et al. 2014 evidence-based guideline for the management of high blood pressure in adults: report from the panel members appointed to the eighth joint national committee (JNC 8). *JAMA*. 2014;311:507.
4. Patel A, ADVANCE Collaborative Group, MacMahon S, et al. Effects of a fixed combination of perindopril and indapamide on macrovascular and microvascular outcomes in patients with type 2 diabetes mellitus (the ADVANCE trial): a randomised controlled trial. *Lancet*. 2007;370:829.
5. Barnett AH, Bain SC, Bouter P, et al. Angiotensin-receptor blockade versus converting-enzyme inhibition in type 2 diabetes and nephropathy. *N Engl J Med*. 1952;2004:351.
6. Pohl MA, Blumenthal S, Cordonnier DJ, et al. Independent and additive impact of blood pressure control and angiotensin II receptor blockade on renal outcomes in the irbesartan diabetic nephropathy trial: clinical implications and limitations. *J Am Soc Nephrol*. 2005;16:3027.
7. Brenner BM, Cooper ME, de Zeeuw D, et al. Effects of losartan on renal and cardiovascular outcomes in patients with type 2 diabetes and nephropathy. *N Engl J Med*. 2001;345:861.
8. Mann JF, Schmieder RE, McQueen M, et al. Renal outcomes with telmisartan, ramipril, or both, in people at high vascular risk (the ONTARGET study): a multicentre, randomised, double-blind, controlled trial. *Lancet*. 2008;372:547.

32 Acute Kidney Injury

The impact of using estimated GFR versus creatinine clearance on the evaluation of recovery from acute kidney injury in the ICU
Schetz M, Garrick R, Van den Berghe G (KU Leuven Univ, Belgium)
Intensive Care Med 40:1709-1717, 2014

Purpose.—To quantify the error in evaluating recovery from acute kidney injury (AKI) with estimated GFR (eGFR) in relation to ICU stay.

Methods.—Secondary analysis performed on the database of the EPaNIC trial. In a cohort of patients who developed AKI during ICU stay we compared eGFR with measured creatinine clearance (Clcr) at ICU discharge. Recovery of kidney function was assessed by comparison with baseline eGFR and the accuracy of eGFR to detect "potential CKD status" defined by Clcr was quantified. The same analysis was performed in subgroups with different ICU stay. Multivariate regression was performed to determine independent predictors of the eGFR−Clcr difference.

Results.—A total of 757 patients were included. The bias (limits of agreement (LOA)) between eGFR and Clcr at ICU discharge related to ICU stay, increasing from +1.3 (−37.4/+40) ml/min/1.73 m^2 in patients with short stay to +34.7 (−54.4/+123.8) ml/min/1.73 m^2 in patients with ICU stay of more than 14 days. This resulted in a significantly different incidence of complete recovery with the two evaluation methods and reduced sensitivity to detect "potential CKD status" with eGFR in patients with prolonged ICU stay. Independent predictors of the bias included creatinine excretion on the last day in ICU, baseline eGFR, ICU stay, gender, and age.

Conclusion.—Compared to Clcr, discharge eGFR results in overestimation of renal recovery in patients with prolonged ICU stay and in reduced accuracy of "CKD staging". Since age, gender and race do not change during ICU stay the same conclusion can be drawn with regard to plasma creatinine.

▶ Serum creatinine must be in steady state (ie, it cannot be changing quickly over time) to be used in nomograms or formulas for the calculation of the estimated glomerular filtration rate (eGFR). If serum creatinine is not in steady state, the actual glomerular filtration rate can be grossly overestimated. This article is a post hoc analysis of a cohort from the ePaNIC trial conducted in

Belgium,[1] which evaluated the nutritional care of intensive care unit (ICU) patients. The authors looked at the estimation of renal function based on either the Modification of Diet in Renal Disease—calculated eGFR[2] or a measured 24-hour urine creatinine clearance in the cohort of patients who developed stage 1 through 3 acute kidney injury (AKI). They made 2 key, clinically relevant observations.

First, the degree of discrepancy between eGFR and creatinine clearance in individuals with AKI worsens as the length of stay in the ICU increases. For those in the ICU between 8 and 14 days, the discrepancy was 10 mL/min/1.73 m^2. For patients with ICU stays of more than 2 weeks, the eGFR overestimated the creatinine clearance (measured by 24-hr urine) by 25 mL/min/1.73 m^2.

The second observation is that even for individuals who did not developed AKI, the loss of muscle mass that occurs during illness[3] lowers urinary creatinine excretion, and so the 24-hour urine creatinine collection may also overestimate the actual GFR, as measured by a gold standard such as Inulin or iothalamate.

These findings certainly should help inform our decisions with regard to the care of the critically ill. For patients with AKI and changing creatinine levels, the results warn us that using the eGFR may substantially overestimate actual renal function and give a false sense of security with regard to the extent of renal recovery and the need for long-term outpatient CKD follow-up.

With regard to all patients, the results caution us that endogenous markers such as creatinine and cystatin C also have limitations, especially in the ICU setting.[4,5] Best advice, be mindful of these limitations: adjust dosages based on serum drug levels whenever possible, and err on the side of caution when evaluating recovery and the need for long-term follow-up in patients who have had an episode of AKI.

R. Garrick, MD

References

1. Casaer MP, Mesotten D, Hermans G, et al. Early versus late parenteral nutrition in critically ill adults. *N Engl J Med.* 2011;365:506-517.
2. Levey AS, Bosch JP, Lewis JB, Greene T, Rogers N, Roth D. A more accurate method to estimate glomerular filtration rate from serum creatinine: a new prediction equation. Modification of Diet in Renal Disease Study Group. *Ann Intern Med.* 1999;130:461-470.
3. Baxmann AC, Ahmed MS, Marques NC, et al. Influence of muscle mass and physical activity on serum and urinary creatinine and serum cystatin C. *Clin J Am Soc Nephrol.* 2008;3:348-354.
4. Prowle JR, Kolic I, Purdell-Lewis J, Taylor R, Pearse RM, Kirwan CJ. Serum creatinine changes associated with critical illness and detection of persistent renal dysfunction after AKI. *Clin J Am Soc Nephrol.* 2014;9:1015-1023.
5. Kirwan CJ, Philips BJ, Macphee IA. Estimated glomerular filtration rate correlates poorly with four-hour creatinine clearance in critically ill patients with acute kidney injury. *Crit Care Res Pract.* 2013;2013:406075.

Kidney Function After Off-Pump or On-Pump Coronary Artery Bypass Graft Surgery: A Randomized Clinical Trial

Garg AX, for the CORONARY Investigators (Western Univ, London, Ontario, Canada)

JAMA 311:2191-2198, 2014

Importance.—Most acute kidney injury observed in the hospital is defined by sudden mild or moderate increases in the serum creatinine concentration, which may persist for several days. Such acute kidney injury is associated with lower long-term kidney function. However, it has not been demonstrated that an intervention that reduces the risk of such acute kidney injury better preserves long-term kidney function.

Objectives.—To characterize the risk of acute kidney injury with an intervention in a randomized clinical trial and to determine if there is a difference between the 2 treatment groups in kidney function 1 year later.

Design, Setting, and Participants.—The Coronary Artery Bypass Grafting Surgery Off- or On-pump Revascularisation Study (CORONARY) enrolled 4752 patients undergoing first isolated coronary artery bypass graft (CABG) surgery at 79 sites in 19 countries. Patients were randomized to receive CABG surgery either with a beating-heart technique (off-pump) or with cardiopulmonary bypass (on-pump). From January 2010 to November 2011, 2932 patients (from 63 sites in 16 countries) from CORONARY were enrolled into a kidney function substudy to record serum creatinine concentrations during the postoperative period and at 1 year. The last 1-year serum creatinine concentration was recorded on January 18, 2013.

Main Outcomes and Measures.—Acute kidney injury within 30 days of surgery (≥50% increase in serum creatinine concentration from prerandomization concentration) and loss of kidney function at 1 year (≥20% loss in estimated glomerular filtration rate from prerandomization level).

Results.—Off-pump (n = 1472) vs on-pump (n = 1460) CABG surgery reduced the risk of acute kidney injury (17.5% vs 20.8%, respectively; relative risk, 0.83 [95% CI, 0.72-0.97], *P* = .01); however, there was no significant difference between the 2 groups in the loss of kidney function at 1 year (17.1% vs 15.3%, respectively; relative risk, 1.10 [95% CI, 0.95-1.29], *P* = .23). Results were consistent with multiple alternate continuous and categorical definitions of acute kidney injury or kidney function loss, and in the subgroup with baseline chronic kidney disease.

Conclusions and Relevance.—Use of off-pump compared with on-pump CABG surgery reduced the risk of postoperative acute kidney injury, without evidence of better preserved kidney function with off-pump CABG surgery at 1 year. In this setting, an intervention that reduced the risk of mild to moderate acute kidney injury did not alter longer-term kidney function.

Trial Registration.—clinicaltrials.gov Identifier: NCT00463294.

► Acute kidney injury (AKI) has been reported in up to 5% to 7% of hospitalized patients.[1,2] It is routinely associated with mortality of up to 40% to 50%, and this can be even higher in intensive care unit patients.[3] It leads to long-term renal and extra-renal morbidities and is an underrecognized cause of chronic kidney disease (CKD), with 19% to 31% progressing to CKDIII/IV and 12.5% progressing further to dialysis.[4] There is no cure for AKI, and hence all efforts need to be focused on its prevention.

Decreased perfusion and inflammation are some of the factors that play a role in the development of AKI after on-pump cardiac surgery.[5] Off-pump coronary artery bypass grafting (CABG), developed as an alternate to on-pump CABG procedures, do not involve cannulation or clamping of the aorta, the heart is not chemically arrested, and the pulsatility of blood flow is maintained. This is presumed to improve hemodynamic stability, avoid inflammation, and prevent microthrombi.[6,7] A meta-analysis published in 2010 noted that there was a lower incidence of AKI in Off-pump CABG, but it did not affect the need for dialysis.[8] The current study by Garg et al evaluated whether off-pump CABG preserved long-term kidney function. The results demonstrate that off-pump (n = 1472) versus on-pump (n = 1460) CABG surgery reduced the risk of acute kidney injury (17.5% vs 20.8%, respectively; relative risk, 0.83 [95% confidence interval [CI], 0.72-0.97], $P = .01$); however, there was no significant difference between the 2 groups in the loss of kidney function at 1 year (17.1% vs 15.3%, respectively; relative risk, 1.10 [95% CI, 0.95-1.29], $P = .23$).

This study confirms that off-pump CABG can prevent postoperative AKI, which, in itself, is a significant benefit. The failure to show a benefit on renal function at 1 year may, in part, reflect the inherent insensitivity of using the serum creatinine as the marker of kidney function, and longer follow-up may be needed to demonstrate a separation between these groups. The Coronary Trial remains the largest trial to look at the prevention of AKI in patients undergoing CABG. The addition of novel biomarkers or longer follow-up may ultimately give guidance as to the best surgical approach for these patients.

R. Morey, MD

References

1. Hou SH, Bushinsky DA, Wish JB, Cohen JJ, Harrington JT. Hospital-acquired renal insufficiency: a prospective study. *Am J Med.* 1983;74:243-248.
2. Shusterman N, Strom BL, Murray TG, Morrison G, West SL, Maislin G. Risk factors and outcome of hospital-acquired acute renal failure. Clinical epidemiologic study. *Am J Med.* 1987;83:65-71.
3. Uchino S, Kellum JA, Bellomo R, et al. Acute renal failure in critically ill patients: a multinational, multicenter study. *JAMA.* 2005;17:813-818.
4. Goldberg R, Dennen P. Long-term outcomes of acute kidney injury. *Adv Chronic Kidney Dis.* 2008;15:297-307.
5. Thiele RH, Isbell JM, Rosner MH. AKI associated with cardiac surgery. *Clin J Am Soc Nephrol.* 2015;10:500-514.
6. Shekar PS. On-pump and off-pump coronary artery bypass grafting. *Circulation.* 2006;113:e51-e52.
7. Sellke FW, DiMaio JM, Caplan LR, et al; American Heart Association. Comparing on-pump and off-pump coronary artery bypass grafting: numerous studies but few conclusions: a scientific statement from the American Heart Association council on cardiovascular surgery and anesthesia in collaboration with the interdisciplinary working group on quality of care and outcomes research. *Circulation.* 2005;31:2858-2864.

8. Seabra VF, Alobaidi S, Balk EM, Poon AH, Jaber BL. Off-pump coronary artery bypass surgery and acute kidney injury: a meta-analysis of randomized controlled trials. *Clin J Am Soc Nephrol.* 2010;5:1734-1744.

Acute Kidney Injury After Coronary Artery Bypass Grafting and Long-Term Risk of End-Stage Renal Disease

Rydén L, Sartipy U, Evans M, et al (Karolinska Univ Hosp, Stockholm, Sweden; et al)

Circulation 130:2005-2011, 2014

Background.—Acute kidney injury (AKI) is a common complication after coronary artery bypass grafting (CABG) and is associated with adverse outcomes. However, the relationship between AKI after CABG and the long-term risk of end-stage renal disease (ESRD) is unknown.

Methods and Results.—This study included 29 330 patients who underwent primary isolated CABG in Sweden between 2000 and 2008. AKI was classified according to the Acute Kidney Injury Network (AKIN) classification: stage 1, >0.3 mg/dL (>26 μmol/L) or 50% to 100% increase; stage 2, 100% to 200% increase; and stage 3, >200% increase from the preoperative to postoperative serum creatinine level. Cox proportional hazards regression analysis was used to calculate hazard ratios with 95% confidence intervals for ESRD in AKIN stage 1 and stage 2 to 3. Postoperative AKI occurred in 13% of patients. During a mean follow-up of 4.3 ± 2.4 years, 123 patients (0.4%) developed ESRD, including 50 (1.6%) in AKIN stage 1, 29 (5.2%) in AKIN stage 2 to 3, and 44 (0.2%) without AKI after CABG. After multivariable adjustment, the hazard ratio for ESRD was 2.92 (95% confidence interval, 1.87–4.55) for AKIN stage 1 and 3.81 (95% confidence interval, 2.14–6.79) for AKIN stage 2 to 3.

Conclusions.—This nationwide study of patients who underwent CABG found that a small increase in the postoperative serum creatinine level was associated with an almost 3-fold increase in the long-term risk of ESRD after adjustment for a number of confounders, including preoperative renal function (Fig 2).

► Acute kidney injury (AKI) is a common complication after cardiopulmonary bypass (CPB). Severity can range from a small transient increase in creatinine to a severe loss of function with oliguria and the need for renal replacement therapy. Various cohorts have noted that these episodes of AKI are correlated with poor outcomes. In the past, it was assumed that transient reversible changes in creatinine were of little significance if baseline creatinine was restored before discharge. However, data are accumulating suggesting that the true risks of in-hospital AKI are much higher than previously thought. One recent study found that readmission rates, a major Medicare quality indicator, were significantly higher in those who experienced an episode of AKI compared with those who did not (11% vs 15% $P < .001$).[1] A recent meta-analysis found that an episode of AKI after CPB is associated with a doubling of early mortality rate.[2] Another found that the long-term risk of stage 4 or 5 CKD development

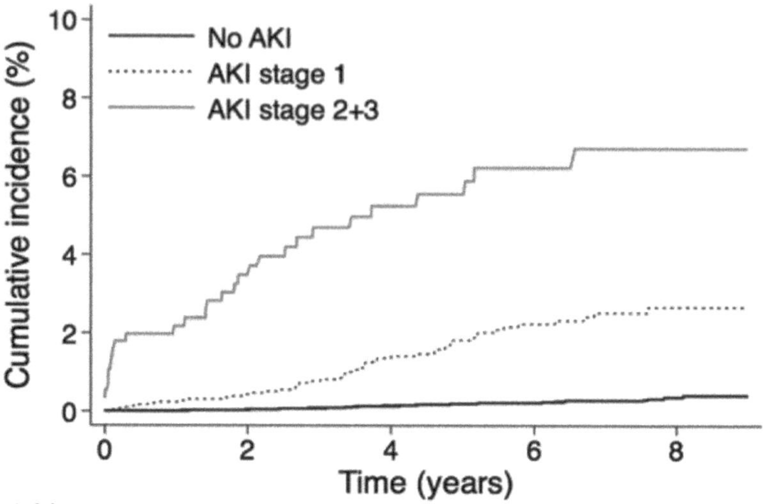

Number at risk

No AKI	25609	20105	13755	7326	1371
AKI stage 1	3159	2399	1723	925	214
AKI stage 2+3	562	383	269	149	28

FIGURE 2.—Cumulative incidence of end-stage renal disease according to the Acute Kidney Injury Network (AKIN) classification of acute kidney injury (AKI) in 29 330 patients who underwent primary isolated coronary artery bypass grafting in Sweden between 2000 and 2008. (Reprinted from Rydén L, Sartipy U, Evans M, et al. Acute kidney injury after coronary artery bypass grafting and long-term risk of end-stage renal disease. *Circulation*. 2014;130:2005-2011, with permission from American Heart Association, Inc.)

increased 29-fold after an episode of AKI, which required dialysis.[3] This study by Ryden et al evaluated data from more than 29 000 patients who underwent coronary artery bypass grafting (CABG), culled from the SWEDEHEART registry. They found the postoperative incidence of AKI using the Acute Kidney Injury Network staging to be as high as 13%, with most classified as stage 1 AKI. They also determined that after a median of 4.3 years, 0.4% of the studied patients had subsequent end-stage renal disease (ESRD) requiring renal replacement therapy (hemodialysis and peritoneal dialysis, transplant). This risk was higher in those with higher stages of post-CABG AKI (Fig 2). They found that the incidence of death or ESRD increased progressively with each stage of AKI experienced (14%: no AKI; 27%: stage 1; 38%: stages 2 or 3). Even with very small postoperative increases in creatinine of 0.3 mg/dL there was a 3-fold increase in the risk of ESRD during the follow-up period.

This study is important because it suggests strongly that even mild AKI in the postoperative setting can have profound effects on the future morbidity. Of course, causation could not be determined by this retrospective analysis. The authors recognized the possibility that the occurrence of AKI could simply be a marker of underlying renal disease that results in late ESRD, but the data are compelling enough to warrant more caution to minimize the risk of AKI whenever possible.

R. Garrick, MD

References

1. Koulouridis I, Price LL, Madias NE, Jaber BL. Hospital-acquired acute kidney injury and hospital readmission: a cohort study. *Am J Kidney Dis.* 2015;65: 275-282.
2. Pickering JW, James MT, Palmer SC. Acute kidney injury and prognosis after cardiopulmonary bypass: a meta-analysis of cohort studies. *Am J Kidney Dis.* 2015; 65:283-293.
3. Lo LJ, Go AS, Chertow GM, et al. Dialysis-requiring acute renal failure increases the risk of progressive chronic kidney disease. *Kidney Int.* 2009;76:893-899.

A systematic review and meta-analysis indicates underreporting of renal dysfunction following endovascular aneurysm repair

Karthikesalingam A, Bahia SS, Patel SR, et al (St George's Hosp NHS Trust, London, UK; et al)
Kidney Int 87:442-451, 2015

Deterioration in renal function has been described after endovascular repair of abdominal aortic aneurysms (EVRs). The etiology is multifactorial and represents an important therapeutic target. A need exists to quantitatively summarize incidence and severity of renal dysfunction after EVR to allow better-informed attempts to preserve renal function and improve life expectancy. Here a systematic search was performed using Medline and Embase for renal function after EVR applying PRISMA statements. Univariate and multivariate random-effects meta-analyses were performed to estimate pooled postoperative changes in serum creatinine and creatinine clearance at four time points after EVR. Clinically relevant deterioration in renal function was also estimated at 1 year or more after EVR. Pooled probability of clinically relevant deterioration in renal function at 1 year or more was 18% (95% confidence interval of 14–23%, I^2 of 82.5%). Serum creatinine increased after EVR by 0.05 mg/dl at 30 days/1 month, 0.09 mg/dl at 1 month to 1 year, and 0.11 mg/dl at 1 year or more (all significant). Creatinine clearance decreased after EVR by 5.65 ml/min at 1 month–1 year and by 6.58 ml/min at 1 year or more (both significant). Thus, renal dysfunction after EVR is common and merits attention.

▶ This study is of interest because typically once a patient has cleared the initial perioperative period, clinicians, and likely patients too, tend to believe that they are "out of the woods." However, this large retrospective, multivariant meta-analysis of approximately 1900 patients calls attention to the fact that renal function deteriorates during, and perhaps beyond, the first postoperative year after endovascular repair (EVR) of abdominal aortic aneurysms (AAA). The greatest deterioration in renal function occurred 1 year after EVR in 18% of patients with a mean decline of estimated glomerular filtration rate of 6.58 mL/min during that time frame. The ability to evaluate long-term renal survival was limited because few of the studies had information regarding progression to dialysis. Obviously, a perfectly matched control group is not possible in a retrospective review. However, the authors did seek to evaluate the annual change in renal function within a community cohort of nearly 10 000 patients aged over 66. Within this cohort, among nondiabetics and those with normal baseline renal function, there was little or no deterioration in renal function over 1 year.[1]

These patients require long-term surveillance for recurrence of their AAA (which often entails the use of radio iodine), and it has been postulated that contrast-induced nephropathy may be a major contributing factor to the observed decline in kidney function. Thus, alternative surveillance strategies such as serial Doppler ultrasounds and noncontrast scans deserve serious consideration.[2,3] The current data clearly highlight the need for long-term renal surveillance in all patients following AAA repair.

M. Brogan, MD

References

1. Hemmelgarn BR, Zhang J, Manns BJ, et al. Progression of kidney dysfunction in the community-dwelling elderly. *Kidney Int.* 2006;69:2155-2161.
2. Karthikesalingam A, Al-Jundi W, Jackson D, et al. Systematic review and meta-analysis of duplex ultrasonography, contrast-enhanced ultrasonography or computed tomography for surveillance after endovascular aneurysm repair. *Br J Surg.* 2012;99:1514-1523.
3. Holt PJ, Karthikesalingam A, Patterson BO, et al. Aortic rupture and sac expansion after endovascular repair of abdominal aortic aneurysm. *Br J Surg.* 2012; 99:1657-1664.

Risk of AKI with Gentamicin as Surgical Prophylaxis

Bell S, Davey P, Nathwani D, et al (Natl Health Service Tayside, Dundee, UK; Univ of Dundee, UK; Scottish Medicines Consortium, Glasgow, UK; et al)
J Am Soc Nephrol 25:2625-2632, 2014

In 2009, the Scottish government issued a target to reduce *Clostridium difficile* infection by 30% in 2 years. Consequently, Scottish hospitals changed from cephalosporins to gentamicin for surgical antibiotic prophylaxis. This study examined rates of postoperative AKI before and after this policy change. The study population comprised 12,482 adults undergoing surgery (orthopedic, urology, vascular, gastrointestinal, and gynecology) with antibiotic prophylaxis between October 1, 2006, and September 30, 2010 in the Tayside region of Scotland. Postoperative AKI was defined by the Kidney Disease Improving Global Outcomes criteria. The study design was an interrupted time series with segmented regression analysis. In orthopedic patients, change in policy from cefuroxime to flucloxacillin (two doses of 1 g) and single-dose gentamicin (4 mg/kg) was associated with a 94% increase in AKI ($P = 0.04$; 95% confidence interval, 93.8% to 94.3%). Most patients who developed AKI after prophylactic gentamicin had stage 1 AKI, but some patients developed persistent stage 2 or stage 3 AKI. The antibiotic policy change was not associated with a significant increase in AKI in the other groups. Regardless of antibiotic regimen, however, rates of AKI were high (24%) after vascular surgery, and increased steadily after gastrointestinal surgery. Rates could only be ascertained in 52% of urology patients and 47% of gynecology patients because of a lack of creatinine testing. These results suggest that gentamicin should be avoided in orthopedic patients in the perioperative period. Our findings also raise concerns about the increasing prevalence of postoperative AKI and failures to consistently measure postoperative renal function.

▶ The study reminds us of the need to be vigilant regarding unintended consequences. Thus, in 2009, in an attempt to reduce the incidence of *Clostridium difficile* infection, the Scottish government changed perioperative antibiotic prophylaxis from cephalosporins to gentamicin. The change in antibiotic use mostly focused on orthopedic surgery cases, and subsequently among these patients, a small study suggested the change may have inadvertently increased the rate of postoperative acute kidney injury (AKI).[1,2] The current large population study extended those earlier observations. Using interrupted time series analyses the authors demonstrated that in patients undergoing orthopedic surgery, the change in treatment regimen resulted in a significant increase in postoperative AKI (defined by the Kidney Disease: Improving Global Outcomes criteria). A second somewhat unexpected finding was a very high incidence of postoperative AKI in patients undergoing vascular procedures regardless of the antibiotic regimen used. This finding may reflect high baseline comorbidity potentially related to underlying generalized vascular. A third finding was that perioperative creatinine testing in Scotland is not standardized, a finding that is likely true in other countries as well. Taken together the findings are quite interesting. Although the majority of patients had mild AKI (increase in creatinine of $\geq$0.3 mg/dL or an increase in baseline creatinine of 150%-200%), more significant persistent degrees of AKI did occur. After adjustment for age, gender, and use of other nephrotoxic drugs, only the change in policy was significantly associated with an increase in AKI. A strength of this study was its use of interrupted time analyses, which allows nonrandomized trials to control for trends existing before and after points of intervention. In addition, the study was population-based and therefore effectively mirrors the routine environment of clinical care. The findings caution clinicians to be selective and cautious when using gentamicin in the perioperative setting and also highlight the need to monitor renal function perioperatively, especially in high-risk patients such as those undergoing vascular surgery.

R. Lamba, MD

References

1. Challagundla SR, Knox D, Hawkins A, et al. Renal impairment after high-dose flucloxacillin and single-dose gentamicin prophylaxis in patients undergoing elective hip and knee replacement. *Nephrol Dial Transplant.* 2013;28:612-619.

2. Chertow GM, Burdick E, Honour M, Bonventre JV, Bates DW. Acute kidney injury, mortality, length of stay, and costs in hospitalized patients. *J Am Soc Nephrol.* 2005;16:3365-3370.

Vancomycin-Associated Nephrotoxicity in the Critically Ill: A Retrospective Multivariate Regression Analysis

Hanrahan TP, Harlow G, Hutchinson J, et al (The Univ of Queensland, Brisbane, Australia; Univ Hosp Birmingham, UK; et al)
Crit Care Med 42:2527-2536, 2014

Objectives.—To evaluate the influence of vancomycin dose, serum trough concentration, and dosing strategy on the evolution of acute kidney injury in critically ill patients.

Design.—Retrospective, single-center, observational study.

Setting.—University Hospital ICU, Birmingham, UK.

Patients.—All critically ill patients receiving vancomycin from December 1, 2004, to August 31, 2009.

Intervention.—None.

Measurements and Main Results.—The prevalence of new onset nephrotoxicity was reported using Risk, Injury, Failure, Loss, End-stage renal disease criteria, and independent factors predictive of nephrotoxicity were identified using logistic regression analysis. Complete data were available for 1,430 patients. Concomitant vasoactive therapy (odds ratio = 1.633; $p < 0.001$), median serum vancomycin (odds ratio = 1.112; $p < 0.001$), and duration of therapy (odds ratio = 1.041; $p \leq 0.001$) were significant positive predictors of nephrotoxicity. Intermittent infusion was associated with a significantly greater risk of nephrotoxicity than continuous infusion (odds ratio = 8.204; $p \leq 0.001$).

Conclusions.—In a large dataset, higher serum vancomycin concentrations and greater duration of therapy are independently associated with increased odds of nephrotoxicity. Furthermore, continuous infusion is associated with a decreased likelihood of nephrotoxicity compared with intermittent infusion. This large dataset supports the use of continuous infusion of vancomycin in critically ill patients.

▶ The conundrum surrounding vancomycin use continues. Methicillin-resistant *Staphylococcus aureus* (MRSA) infections are extremely common among critically ill intensive care unit (ICU) patients. Infections with MRSA have a much higher risk of morbidity and mortality then do methicillin sensitive Staphylococcal illnesses.[1] Vancomycin remains the common agent of choice for the treatment of MRSA. Vancomycin trough levels under 10 mL/L have been associated with the development of vancomycin resistance, and this has prompted the maintenance of higher trough levels, which, in turn, may increase the risk of nephrotoxicity.[2-5] The current large retrospective cohort study was drawn from a single tertiary care center and evaluated the nephrotoxic risks of various vancomycin serum concentrations and dosing regimens (intermittent or continuous infusion) in critically ill patients. Complete treatment data were available on approximately 65% of the ICU patients who receive vancomycin (1430 patients). The estimated glomerular filtration rate (eGFR) was calculated using the Modification of Diet in Renal Disease (MDRD)[6] formula, and the primary endpoint of new onset nephrotoxicity was defined per the RIFLE acute kidney injury classification system.[7] Disease severity was assessed by the sequential organ failure assessment (SOFA) score.

Within the cohort, 1% of the patients develop nephrotoxicity. The rate of nephrotoxicity was highest in the intermittent infusion group compared with patients who received continuous dosing regimens, although interestingly the SOFA scores were highest in the continuous group. Of note, a survival advantage was not detected with continuous therapy. Thus, as suggested by the SOFA scores, confounding, unmeasured, variables may have been present. The median vancomycin serum concentration (18.9 vs 14.2 mg/L), duration of vancomycin treatment (8.1 vs 4 days), and simultaneous use of vasoactive therapy were all predictors of nephrotoxicity. Of greater clinical utility than the median serum concentration was the finding that the threshold for nephrotoxicity was 23.7 mg/L (sensitivity 0 .65; specificity 0.74; area under the curve = .727).

The findings of this retrospective cohort analysis agree with those of a previous meta-analyses that suggested continuous infusion was associated with less nephrotoxicity than intermittent dosing regimens.[8] In addition, the data confirm that vancomycin is indeed nephrotoxic especially given over a long period of time with higher trough levels in critically ill patients. Obviously this study carries with it all of the problems of a retrospective cohort analysis and the inability to establish either causality or to correct for all possible confounding variables. Nonetheless while awaiting concurrent head-to-head trials of various treatment regimens, these new and useful data can help guide clinical care.

R. Garrick, MD

References

1. Hanberger H, Walther S, Leone M, et al; EPIC II Group of Investigators. Increased mortality associated with methicillin-resistant *Staphylococcus aureus* (MRSA) infection in the intensive care unit: results from the EPIC II study. *Int J Antimicrob Agents.* 2011;38:331-335.
2. van Duijn PJ, Dautzenberg MJ, Oostdijk EA. Recent trends in antibiotic resistance in European ICUs. *Curr Opin Crit Care.* 2011;17:658-665.
3. Howden BP, Ward PB, Charles PG, et al. Treatment outcomes for serious infections caused by methicillin-resistant *Staphylococcus aureus* with reduced vancomycin susceptibility. *Clin Infect Dis.* 2004;38:521-528.
4. Wong-Beringer A, Joo J, Tse E, et al. Vancomycin-associated nephrotoxicity: A critical appraisal of risk with high-dose therapy. *Int J Antimicrob Agents.* 2011;37:95-101.
5. Rybak M, Lomaestro B, Rotschafer JC, et al. Therapeutic monitoring of vancomycin in adult patients: a consensus review of the American society of health-system pharmacists, the infectious diseases society of America, and the society of infectious diseases pharmacists. *Am J Health Syst Pharm.* 2009;66:82-98.
6. Levey AS, Bosch JP, Lewis JB, et al. A more accurate method to estimate glomerular filtration rate from serum creatinine: a new prediction equation. Modification of diet in renal disease study group. *Ann Intern Med.* 1999;130:461-470.

7. Bellomo R, Ronco C, Kellum JA, et al; Acute Dialysis Quality Initiative Workgroup. Acute renal failure—definition, outcome measures, animal models, fluid therapy and information technology needs: the second international consensus conference of the acute dialysis quality initiative (ADQI) group. *Crit Care.* 2004;8:R204-R212.
8. Cataldo MA, Tacconelli E, Grilli E, et al. Continuous versus intermittent infusion of vancomycin for the treatment of gram-positive infections: systematic review and meta-analysis. *J Antimicrob Chemother.* 2012;67:17-24.

Atypical Antipsychotic Drugs and the Risk for Acute Kidney Injury and Other Adverse Outcomes in Older Adults: A Population-Based Cohort Study

Hwang YJ, Dixon SN, Reiss JP, et al (London Health Sciences Centre, Ontario, Canada; et al)
Ann Intern Med 161:242-248, 2014

Background.—Several adverse outcomes attributed to atypical antipsychotic drugs, specifically quetiapine, risperidone, and olanzapine, are known to cause acute kidney injury (AKI). Such outcomes include hypotension, acute urinary retention, and the neuroleptic malignant syndrome or rhabdomyolysis.

Objective.—To investigate the risk for AKI and other adverse outcomes associated with use of atypical antipsychotic drugs versus nonuse.

Design.—Population-based cohort study.

Setting.—Ontario, Canada, from 2003 to 2012.

Patients.—Adults aged 65 years or older who received a new outpatient prescription for an oral atypical antipsychotic drug ($n = 97\,777$) matched 1:1 with those who did not receive such a prescription.

Measurements.—The primary outcome was hospitalization with AKI (assessed by using a hospital diagnosis code and, in a subpopulation, serum creatinine levels) within 90 days of prescription for atypical antipsychotic drugs.

Results.—Atypical antipsychotic drug use versus nonuse was associated with a higher risk for hospitalization with AKI (relative risk [RR], 1.73 [95% CI, 1.55 to 1.92]). This association was consistent when AKI was assessed in a subpopulation for which information on serum creatinine levels was available (5.46% vs. 3.34%; RR, 1.70 [CI, 1.22 to 2.38]; absolute risk increase, 2.12% [CI, 0.80% to 3.43%]). Drug use was also associated with hypotension (RR, 1.91 [CI, 1.60 to 2.28]), acute urinary retention (RR, 1.98 [CI, 1.63 to 2.40]), and all-cause mortality (RR, 2.39 [CI, 2.28 to 2.50]).

Limitation.—Only older adults were included in the study.

Conclusion.—Atypical antipsychotic drug use is associated with an increased risk for AKI and other adverse outcomes that may explain the observed association with AKI. The findings support current safety concerns about the use of these drugs in older adults.

▶ Atypical antipsychotic drugs are commonly prescribed for the management of behavioral symptoms associated with dementia. This population-based cohort study matched otherwise similar groups of drug recipients and nonrecipients among adult outpatients aged ≥65 using a previously validated database. The investigators sought to identify and quantify whether the use of these drugs is associated with the occurrence of acute kidney injury that is severe enough to require hospitalization.

Patient characteristics, drug use, covariant information, and outcome data were drawn from multiple Ontario and Canadian data sources. Data analysis included a carefully derived propensity score based on a logistic regression model with 91 selected variables.

The results are compelling. Drug recipients (risperidone, quetiapine, olanzapine, in decreasing order of prescribing frequency) were older (mean age 80.7 yr), more likely to dwell in long-term care facilities (~24%), and were more frequently diagnosed with dementia, psychiatric illnesses, Parkinson disease, and cardiovascular diseases. The relative risk for hospitalization for acute kidney injury (AKI) within 90 days of the initiation of medication was significantly increased, as was all-cause mortality (6.8% in recipients vs 3.1% in nonrecipients). Within 90 days of initial use, these agents were also associated with an increased risk of acute urinary retention, pneumonia, ventricular arrhythmia, and acute myocardial infarction. The risks of rhabdomyolysis and malignant neuroleptic syndrome were not significantly increased.

This study is the first population-based study to systematically evaluate the risks of AKI associated with the use of antipsychotic medications. Although observational in nature and at risk for confounding by unmeasured health characteristics (such as AKI risk from dementia-related deficiencies in fluid intake), the cohorts were carefully defined and matched, and the temporal association between medication initiation and hospitalization was carefully tracked. Millions of doses of atypical antipsychotic drugs are consumed annually. The risk-benefit of these agents in the elderly should be considered and patients carefully monitored for avoidable adverse events.

R. Garrick, MD

Nephrotoxic Effects of Common and Emerging Drugs of Abuse

Pendergraft WF III, Herlitz LC, Thornley-Brown D, et al (Univ of North Carolina at Chapel Hill; Columbia Univ Med Ctr, NY; Univ of Alabama at Birmingham; et al)

Clin J Am Soc Nephrol 9:1996-2005, 2014

The kidneys can be injured in diverse ways by many drugs, both legal and illegal. Novel associations and descriptions of nephrotoxic effects of common and emerging drugs of abuse have appeared over the past several years. Anabolic androgenic steroids, illicitly used by athletes and others for decades to increase muscle mass and decrease body fat, are emerging as podocyte toxins given recent descriptions of severe forms of FSGS in long-term abusers. Synthetic cannabinoids, a new group of compounds with marijuana-like effects, recently became popular as recreational drugs and have been associated with an atypical form of AKI. 3,4-

Methylenedioxymethamphetamine, commonly known as ecstasy, is a widely used synthetic recreational drug with mood-enhancing properties and a constellation of toxicities that can result in death. These toxic effects include hyperthermia, hypotonic hyponatremia due to its arginine vasopressin secretagogue–like effects, rhabdomyolysis, and cardiovascular collapse. Cocaine, a serotonin-norepinephrine-dopamine reuptake inhibitor that serves as an illegal stimulant, appetite suppressant, and anesthetic, also causes vasoconstriction and rhabdomyolysis. Recent adulteration of much of the world's supply of cocaine with levamisole, an antihelminthic agent with attributes similar to but distinct from those of cocaine, appears to have spawned a new type of ANCA-associated systemic vasculitis. This review discusses the nephrotoxic effects of these common and emerging drugs of abuse, of which both community and health care providers should become aware given their widespread abuse. Future investigation into pathogenetic mechanisms associated with these drugs is critical and may provide a window into ways to lessen and even prevent the nephrotoxic effects of these drugs of abuse and perhaps allow a deeper understanding of the nephrotoxicities themselves.

▶ Many over-the-counter preparations (including nutraceuticals), prescription medications, and elicit agents have hemodynamic or other systemic side effects and may have secondary renal toxicities. Some are directly nephrotoxic. Often, more than 1 compound is ingested, and therefore the specificity of the renal lesion is not always clear-cut. Many of these agents are widely abused. For example, anabolic steroids can cause focal glomerular sclerosis and proteinuria, which may reach nephrotic range level.[1] Synthetic marijuana ("spice" and "K2") is available over-the-counter and is frequently abused by high school students.[2] Its use has been associated with acute tubular necrosis, which may require dialysis. Its toxicity may be related either to direct renal cellular effects medicated through renal cannabinoid receptors or to gastrointestinal fluid losses and associated hemodynamic instability. Ecstasy, which can promote profound hyponatremia, has led to several deaths. Its toxicity is believed to be mediated through increased release of both serotonin and arginine vasopressin. Almost 40% of college students admit to trying and using ecstasy.[3] Other commonly used and abused compounds reviewed include cocaine and levamisole-adulterated cocaine, which has been linked to an antineutrophil cytoplasmic antibody–associated vasculitis and necrotizing glomerulonephritis. Sadly, given their widespread availability, it is necessary for clinicians to be aware of the clinical and renal pathophysiologic effects of these agents.

R. Garrick, MD

References

1. Kanayama G, Hudson JI, Pope HG Jr. Illicit anabolic-androgenic steroid use. *Horm Behav.* 2010;58:111-121.
2. Johnston LD, O'Malley PM, Bachman JG, Schulenberg JE. *Monitoring the Future National Survey Results on Drug Use, 1975-2012, Volume I: Secondary School*

Students. Ann Arbor, MI: Institute for Social Research, University of Michigan; 2013.

3. Peroutka SJ. Incidence of recreational use of 3,4-methylenedimethoxymethamphetamine (MDMA, "ecstasy") on an undergraduate campus. *N Engl J Med*. 1987;317:1542-1543.

Explaining the Racial Difference in AKI Incidence

Grams ME, Matsushita K, Sang Y, et al (Johns Hopkins Univ School of Medicine, Baltimore, MD; Johns Hopkins Univ Bloomberg School of Public Health, Baltimore, MD)

J Am Soc Nephrol 25:1834-1841, 2014

African Americans face higher risk of AKI than Caucasians. The extent to which this increased risk is because of differences in clinical, socioeconomic, or genetic risk factors is unknown. We evaluated 10,588 African-American and Caucasian participants in the Atherosclerosis Risk in Communities study, a community-based prospective cohort of middle-aged individuals. Participants were followed from baseline study visit (1996–1999) to first hospitalization for AKI (defined by billing code), ESRD, death, or December 31, 2010. African-American participants were slightly younger (61.7 versus 63.1 years, $P < 0.001$), were more often women (64.5% versus 53.2%, $P < 0.001$), and had higher baseline eGFR compared with Caucasians. Annual family income, education level, and prevalence of health insurance were lower among African Americans than Caucasians. The unadjusted incidence of hospitalized AKI was 7.4 cases per 1000 person-years among African Americans and 5.8 cases per 1000 person-years among Caucasians ($P = 0.002$). The elevated risk of AKI among African Americans persisted after adjustment for demographics, cardiovascular risk factors, kidney markers, and time-varying number of hospitalizations (adjusted hazard ratio, 1.20; 95% confidence interval [95% CI], 1.01 to 1.43; $P = 0.04$); however, accounting for differences in income and/or insurance by race attenuated the association ($P > 0.05$). High-risk *APOL1* variants did not associate with AKI among African Americans (demographic-adjusted hazard ratio, 1.07; 95% CI, 0.69 to 1.65; $P = 0.77$). In summary, the higher risk of AKI among African Americans may be related to disparities in socioeconomic status.

▶ The incidence of acute kidney injury (AKI), chronic kidney disease (CKD), and end-stage renal disease (ESRD), are greater in African Americans than Caucasians. At the same time, the incidence of hypertension, diabetes, and poverty are also greater within the African American population. Grams and colleagues used the well-described community-based prospective cohort from the atherosclerosis risk in communities (ARIC) study to evaluate whether these risk factors, or genetic alterations such as the presence of high-risk *APOL1*, contribute to the observed racial differences in the incidence of AKI. The results are startling. Over a follow-up period of approximately 13 years, the unadjusted incidence of AKI among African Americans appeared to be approximately 30% higher than that seen among Caucasians. This disparity persisted even after adjustment for a number of demographic and cardiovascular factors such as age, hypertension, and diabetes. However, when the data were adjusted based on socioeconomic differences the racial disparity noted in the incidence of AKI disappeared almost entirely. Thus, after carefully accounting for multiple potential confounding variables the data from this well-defined cohort suggest that the increased risk of AKI among African Americans is substantially influenced by differences in socioeconomic class, rather than just by underlying genetic variables or prevalent comorbidities. Additional analysis suggested that the presence of health insurance and access to care were both influenced by socioeconomic status.

The ARIC cohort is well defined, has been carefully followed longitudinally, and its data have been extensively validated. The findings of this study are unique. These data are bit of a game changer. They suggest that AKI and possibly CKD and ESRD are not more common among African Americans simply because of the higher prevalence of diabetes, hypertension, and other related comorbidities but, rather, are strongly influenced by poverty and access to care. These data should be considered as new systems of health care delivery are being developed and implemented.

R. Garrick, MD

33 Selected Topics in Clinical Nephrology

Implementation of a CKD Checklist for Primary Care Providers

Mendu ML, Schneider LI, Aizer AA, et al (Brigham and Women's Hosp, Boston, MA; Harvard Radiation Oncology Program, Boston, MA; et al)

Clin J Am Soc Nephrol 9:1526-1535, 2014

Background and Objectives.—CKD is associated with significant morbidity, mortality, and financial burden. Practice guidelines outlining CKD management exist, but there is limited application of these guidelines. Interventions to improve CKD guideline adherence have been limited. This study evaluated a new CKD checklist (a tool outlining management guidelines for CKD) to determine whether implementation in an academic primary care clinic improved adherence to guidelines.

Design, Setting, Participants, & Measurements.—During a 1-year period (August 2012–August 2013), a prospective study was conducted among 13 primary care providers (PCPs), four of whom were assigned to use a CKD checklist incorporated into the electronic medical record during visits with patients with CKD stages 1–4. All providers received education regarding CKD guidelines. The intervention and control groups consisted of 105 and 263 patients, respectively. Adherence to CKD management guidelines was measured.

Results.—A random-effects logistic regression analysis was performed to account for intra-group correlation by PCP assignment and adjusted for age and CKD stage. CKD care improved among patients whose PCPs were assigned to the checklist intervention compared with controls. Patients in the CKD checklist group were more likely than controls to have appropriate annual laboratory testing for albuminuria (odds ratio [OR], 7.9; 95% confidence interval [95% CI], 3.6 to 17.2), phosphate (OR, 3.5; 95% CI, 1.5 to 8.3), and parathyroid hormone (OR, 8.1; 95% CI, 4.8 to 13.7) ($P < 0.001$ in all cases). Patients in the CKD checklist group had higher rates of achieving a hemoglobin A1c target<7% (OR, 2.7; 95% CI, 1.4 to 5.1), use of an angiotensin-converting enzyme inhibitor or angiotensin-receptor blocker (OR, 2.1; 95% CI, 1.0 to 4.2), documentation of avoidance of nonsteroidal anti-inflammatory drugs (OR, 41.7; 95% CI, 17.8 to 100.0), and vaccination for annual influenza (OR, 2.1; 95% CI, 1.1 to 4.0) and pneumococcus (OR, 4.7; 95% CI, 2.6 to 8.6) ($P < 0.001$ in all cases).

Conclusions.—Implementation of a CKD checklist significantly improved adherence to CKD management guidelines and delivery of CKD care.

▶ At least 13% of the population is classified as having kidney disease.[1] Reducing the incidence and progression of chronic kidney disease (CKD) is an appropriate public health goal. It is generally understood that the scientific roadmap for accomplishing this goal has not yet been definitively determined. However, there is evidence to suggest that individualized care that is both evidence-based and standardized can improve compliance with best practice guidelines and can improve outcomes.[2,3] Mendu and colleagues prospectively utilized a standardized, electronic checklist to help guide CKD care being provided over a one year period by 13 primary care practitioners. The checklist was based on widely accepted practice guidelines promulgated by nephrology specialty societies and the National Institutes of Health.[4-6] Although the results are not perfect, they are gratifying and do support the hypothesis that standardized checklists can improve compliance with practice-based guidelines and may thereby favorably influence outcomes. In fact, of the 105 patients in the checklist group, 80 had been seen by the same primary care physician in the previous year, yet during the year of the checklist intervention, the compliance with implementing practice guidelines increased. The authors were unable to show improvement in blood pressure control, but that is not entirely surprising because other factors such as patient education and dietary modifications were not parts of the checklist tool. In addition, provider education was limited to a single 30-minute session, and although this may have improved the practitioners' willingness to participate, more detailed education may improve these results. For practice guidelines to be widely accepted and implemented, they will need to be seamlessly embedded into the clinical workflow. Moreover, to sustain their use, it will be necessary to demonstrate that compliance with standardized practice guidelines improves health outcomes. Both of these are worthwhile goals.

R. Garrick, MD

References

1. US Renal Data System Annual Report 2104, Vol. 1. http://www.usrds.org/2014/download/V1_Ch_i_Intro_14.pdf. Accessed April 18, 2015.
2. Gawande A. The checklist: If something so simple can transform intensive care, what else can it do? *New Yorker.* 2007:86-101.
3. Haynes AB, Weiser TG, Berry WR, et al; Safe Surgery Saves Lives Study Group. A surgical safety checklist to reduce morbidity and mortality in a global population. *N Engl J Med.* 2009;360:491-499.
4. Stevens PE, Levin A, Kidney Disease: Improving Global Outcomes Chronic Kidney Disease Guideline Development Work Group Members. Evaluation and management of chronic kidney disease: synopsis of the kidney disease: improving global outcomes 2012 clinical practice guideline. *Ann Intern Med.* 2013;158:825-830.
5. Peralta CA, Norris KC, Li S, et al; KEEP Investigators. Blood pressure components and end-stage renal disease in persons with chronic kidney disease: the kidney early evaluation program (KEEP). *Arch Intern Med.* 2012;172:41-47.
6. Fox CH, Swanson A, Kahn LS, Glaser K, Murray BM. Improving chronic kidney disease care in primary care practices: an upstate New York practice-based research network (UNYNET) study. *J Am Board Fam Med.* 2008;21:522-530.

Retinopathy and Progression of CKD: The CRIC Study

Grunwald JE, the Chronic Renal Insufficiency Cohort Study Investigators (Univ of Pennsylvania, Philadelphia; et al)

Clin J Am Soc Nephrol 9:1217-1224, 2014

Background and Objectives.—Retinal abnormalities may be associated with changes in the renal vasculature. This study assessed the association between retinopathy and progression of kidney disease in participants of the Chronic Renal Insufficiency Cohort (CRIC) study.

Design, Setting, Participants, & Measurements.—This was a prospective study in which patients with CKD enrolled in CRIC had nonmydriatic fundus photographs of both eyes. All CRIC participants in six clinical sites in which fundus cameras were deployed were offered participation. Photographs were reviewed at a reading center. The presence and severity of retinopathy and vessel calibers were assessed using standard protocols by graders masked to clinical information. The associations of retinal features with changes in eGFR and the need for RRT (ESRD) were assessed.

Results.—Retinal images and renal progression outcomes were obtained from 1852 of the 2605 participants (71.1%) approached. During follow-up (median 2.3 years), 152 participants (8.2%) developed ESRD. Presence and severity of retinopathy at baseline were strongly associated with the risk of subsequent progression to ESRD and reductions in eGFR in unadjusted analyses. For example, participants with retinopathy were 4.4 times (95% confidence interval [95% CI], 3.12 to 6.31) more likely to develop ESRD than those without retinopathy ($P < 0.001$). However, this association was not statistically significant after adjustment for initial eGFR and 24-hour proteinuria. Venular and arteriolar diameter calibers were not associated with ESRD or eGFR decline. The results showed a nonlinear relationship between mean ratio of arteriole/vein calibers and the risk of progression to ESRD; participants within the fourth arteriole/vein ratio quartile were 3.11 times (95% CI, 1.51 to 6.40) more likely to develop ESRD than those in the first quartile ($P < 0.001$).

Conclusions.—The presence and severity of retinopathy were not associated with ESRD and decline in eGFR after taking into account established risk factors.

▶ This is the first large, long-term, prospective, multicenter study to examine the association between retinopathy and kidney disease progression among individuals with established chronic kidney disease (CKD) who have been followed within a carefully defined and maintained database. This multicenter study followed a subset of the longitudinal cohort of the Chronic Renal Insufficiency Cohort over a median of 2.3 years.

The authors' previous cross-sectional study in 2012 showed a strong association between the degree of retinopathy and the level of kidney function.[1] Other population studies have suggested a correlation between renal disease progression and the degree of retinopathy.[2,3] The current study sought to further evaluate the relationship between retinal changes and renal disease progression. Patients underwent digital retinal photography, and the images were scored by trained, blinded specialists. An Early Treatment of Diabetic Retinopathy severity score was assigned for each eye.

The study was well conducted, the data were carefully analyzed, and the presence of underlying renal data made it possible to control for several confounding variables. With that, contrary to what may have intuitively seemed a certainty, the data show that after adjustment for estimated glomerular filtration rate (eGFR) at initiation and proteinuria, the presence and severity of retinopathy do not predict ESRD progression. In other words, both the presence and severity retinopathy are associated with the progression of CKD, but the prognostic information provided is the same as that provided by eGFR and the amount of 24-hour urine protein spillage.

These results are clinically quite important. They teach us that diabetic retinopathy is not additive but occurs along the same continuum as the renal injury. These findings support the idea that the retinovascular pathology may be a reflection of disease in other vascular beds, including the kidneys. Thus, we can advise patients to follow up with their ophthalmologist for the health of their eyes rather than as mirror to renal disease progression.

M. Brogan, MD

References

1. Grunwald JE, Alexander J, Ying GS; CRIC study group. Retinopathy and chronic kidney disease in the chronic renal insufficiency cohort (CRIC) study. *Arch Ophthalmol.* 2012;130:1136-1144.
2. Wong TY, Coresh J, Klein R, et al. Retinal microvascular abnormalities and renal dysfunction: the atherosclerosis risk in communities study. *J Am Soc Nephrol.* 2004;15:2469-2476.
3. Edwards MS, Wilson DB, Craven TE, et al. Associations between retinal microvascular abnormalities and declining renal function in the elderly population: the Cardiovascular Health Study. *Am J Kidney Dis.* 2005;46:214-224.

Chronic NSAID use and long-term decline of renal function in a prospective rheumatoid arthritis cohort study

Möller B, on behalf of the Swiss Clinical Quality Management in Rheumatic Diseases (SCQM) Foundation (Univ Hosp Bern, Switzerland; et al)
Ann Rheum Dis 74:718-723, 2015

Objectives.—Non-steroidal anti-inflammatory drugs (NSAIDs) may cause kidney damage. This study assessed the impact of prolonged NSAID exposure on renal function in a large rheumatoid arthritis (RA) patient cohort.

Methods.—Renal function was prospectively followed between 1996 and 2007 in 4101 RA patients with multilevel mixed models for longitudinal data over a mean period of 3.2 years. Among the 2739 'NSAID users' were 1290 patients treated with cyclooxygenase type 2 selective NSAIDs, while 1362 subjects were 'NSAID naive'. Primary outcome was the estimated glomerular filtration rate according to the

Cockroft–Gault formula ($eGFR_{CG}$), and secondary the Modification of Diet in Renal Disease and Chronic Kidney Disease Epidemiology Collaboration formula equations and serum creatinine concentrations. In sensitivity analyses, NSAID dosing effects were compared for patients with NSAID registration in ≤/>50%, ≤/>80% or ≤/>90% of assessments.

Findings.—In patients with baseline $eGFR_{CG}$ >30 mL/min, $eGFR_{CG}$ evolved without significant differences over time between 'NSAID users' (mean change in $eGFR_{CG}$ −0.87 mL/min/year, 95% CI −1.15 to −0.59) and 'NSAID naive' (−0.67 mL/min/year, 95% CI −1.26 to −0.09, $p = 0.63$). In a multivariate Cox regression analysis adjusted for significant confounders age, sex, body mass index, arterial hypertension, heart disease and for other insignificant factors, NSAIDs were an independent predictor for accelerated renal function decline only in patients with advanced baseline renal impairment ($eGFR_{CG}$ <30 mL/min). Analyses with secondary outcomes and sensitivity analyses confirmed these results.

Conclusions.—NSAIDs had no negative impact on renal function estimates but in patients with advanced renal impairment.

▶ Nonsteroidal antiinflammatory drugs (NSAIDS) are useful in the treatment of many inflammatory disorders. Acute adverse effects of NSAIDS on renal function have been well described.[1] It is presumed that their actions as prostaglandin inhibitors theoretically increase the risk of adverse renal effects in chronic users as well. It is assumed that this risk would be significantly higher in patients with chronic kidney disease (CKD). Therefore, it has been recommended that patients with CKD and estimated glomerular filtration rate (eGFR) < 60 avoid long-term use of these agents if at all possible.[2] Unfortunately, for many these drugs afford the only effective relief from their underlying painful conditions.

This study by Möller et al assessed the impact of prolonged NSAID use on renal function in a large cohort of patients with rheumatoid arthritis. This was a longitudinal cohort study nested within a Swedish quality database (SCQM). Renal function was monitored prospectively for 10 years in more than 4000 patients; 2739 were using NSAIDS, and 1362 were NSAID-naive.

After a mean follow-up of 3.2 years, outcome measures, creatinine clearance (Ccr), and serum creatinine levels, were evaluated. Overall Ccr decreased by 0.83 mL/min/year in the total population. However, the difference in slope of Ccr decline was statistically insignificant when comparing NSAID users to the NSAID-naive patients (−0.87 vs −0.67, $P = .63$). Overall the patients with CKD stage 4 with 5 mL/min demonstrated a steeper slope of decline in Ccr compared with those with CKD stage 3 and CKD stage 1 and 2 (9.98 vs 1.27 vs 1.04 mL/min/yr). When comparing NSAID users to NSAID-naive patients, it was only those with Ccr < 30 mL/min who demonstrated significantly faster declines in renal function, whereas those with Ccr > 30 mL/min demonstrated identical rates of decline irrespective of NSAID exposure.

This study is helpful because it suggests that NSAID use is safer than previously suspected. It opens up avenues of treatment previously presumed closed to patients with mild renal disease. An important caveat, however, is the need to consider the other drugs and over-the-counter agents that a patient consumes. For example, the simultaneous use of a diuretic, an angiotensin-converting enzyme inhibitor or angiotensin II receptor blocker, a proton pump inhibitor, and an NSAID would likely have a negative impact on the renal risk assessment for an individual patient, and this should be considered as part of patient-centered care. The authors propose a change to the recommendations that would limit the contraindication for chronic NSAID use to those with Ccr < 30 mL/min.

M. Klein, MD

References

1. Clive DM, Stoff JS. Renal syndromes associated with nonsteroidal antiinflammatory drugs. *N Engl J Med.* 1984;310:563-572.
2. Eknoyan G, Lameire N. KDIGO 2012 clinical practice guideline for the evaluation and management of chronic kidney disease. *Kidney Int.* 2013;3:5-14.

Predictors of Autosomal Dominant Polycystic Kidney Disease Progression

Schrier RW, Brosnahan G, Cadnapaphornchai MA, et al (Univ of Colorado School of Medicine, Aurora; et al)

J Am Soc Nephrol 25:2399-2418, 2014

Autosomal dominant polycystic kidney disease is a genetic disorder associated with substantial variability in its natural course within and between affected families. Understanding predictors for rapid progression of this disease has become increasingly important with the emergence of potential new treatments. This systematic review of the literature since 1988 evaluates factors that may predict and/or effect autosomal dominant polycystic kidney disease progression. Predicting factors associated with early adverse structural and/or functional outcomes are considered. These factors include *PKD1* mutation (particularly truncating mutation), men, early onset of hypertension, early and frequent gross hematuria, and among women, three or more pregnancies. Increases in total kidney volume and decreases in GFR and renal blood flow greater than expected for a given age also signify rapid disease progression. Concerning laboratory markers include overt proteinuria, macroalbuminuria, and perhaps, elevated serum copeptin levels in affected adults. These factors and others may help to identify patients with autosomal dominant polycystic kidney disease who are most likely to benefit from early intervention with novel treatments.

► Autosomal dominant polycystic kidney disease (ADPKD) is one of the most common genetic causes of end-stage renal disease (ESRD) with a prevalence of 1:400 to 1000 births.[1] Mutations in genes on chromosomes 16 and 4, leading to *PKD1* and *PKD2*, respectively, are responsible for the progressive growth of cysts and the ultimate loss of kidney function. Treatment is largely directed at minimizing the clinical effects of declining kidney function, with few treatments actually inhibiting cyst growth and halting progression to ESRD.[2] Because of genetic heterogeneity, there is wide variability and inherent unpredictability in renal functional decline due to ADPKD[3]; hence it is difficult to know who is at greatest risk. It would be most helpful, both for counseling patients as well as for the design of much-needed therapeutic trials, to know which patients exhibit higher risk profiles for progression and other unfavorable outcomes.

Schrier et al reviewed 666 articles on both *PKD1* and *PKD2* looking for predictors of rapid progression. They also evaluated genetic, demographic, familial, clinical, and radiographic predictors of disease progression. Their article includes an all-inclusive review of the relevant prospective and cross-sectional retrospective studies analyzing and validating predictors and outcomes of ADPKD progression.

Major predictors of rapid disease progression were found to include early onset of hypertension, gross hematuria, early decrease in GFR, increased total kidney volume, decreased renal blood flow, and presence of PKD1 mutations—especially with truncating mutations. Other predictors for disease progression were the presence of proteinuria and elevated copeptin levels. Various urinary biomarkers were reviewed as well (eg, NGAL, KIM-1, and others). In looking at predictors of cardiovascular disease in ADPKD, their review also suggests improvement in left ventricular hypertrophy and other cardiovascular outcomes with improvement in Blood pressure control, especially using renin-angiotensin system inhibitors. Finally, they reviewed the data on environmental factors affecting disease progression, such as low birth weight, caffeine intake, smoking, and water intake and protein restriction.

This wonderfully comprehensive study may be very helpful as a reference for clinicians to assess the risks of disease progression and to help target novel therapies to those most likely to derive benefit in treating ADPKD.

M. Klein, MD

References

1. Torres VE, Harris PC. Mechanisms of disease: autosomal dominant and recessive polycystic kidney diseases. *Nat Clin Pract Nephrol*. 2006;2:40-55.
2. Belibi FA, Edelstein CL. Novel targets for the treatment of autosomal dominant polycystic kidney disease. *Expert Opin Investig Drugs*. 2010;19:315-328.
3. Magistroni R, He N, Wang K, et al. Genotype-renal function correlation in type 2 autosomal dominant polycystic kidney disease. *J Am Soc Nephrol*. 2003;14:1164-1174.

CKD and the Risk of Incident Cancer

Lowrance WT, Ordoñez J, Udaltsova N, et al (Univ of Utah, Salt Lake City; Kaiser Permanente Oakland Med Ctr, CA; Kaiser Permanente Northern California, Oakland; et al)

J Am Soc Nephrol 25:2327-2334, 2014

Previous studies report a higher risk of cancer in patients with ESRD, but the impact of less severe CKD on risk of cancer is uncertain. Our objective was to evaluate the association between level of kidney function and subsequent cancer risk. We performed a retrospective cohort study of 1,190,538 adults who were receiving care within a health care delivery system, had a measurement of kidney function obtained between 2000 and 2008, and had no prior cancer. We examined the association between level of eGFR and the risk of incident cancer; the primary outcome was renal cancer, and secondary outcomes were any cancer and specific cancers (urothelial, prostate, breast, lung, and colorectal). During 6,000,420 person-years of follow-up, we identified 76,809 incident cancers in 72,875 subjects. After adjustment for time-updated confounders, lower eGFR (in milliliters per minute per 1.73 m^2) was associated with an increased risk of renal cancer (adjusted hazard ratio [HR], 1.39; 95% confidence interval [95% CI], 1.22 to 1.58 for eGFR = 45–59; HR, 1.81; 95% CI, 1.51 to 2.17 for eGFR = 30–44; HR, 2.28; 95% CI, 1.78 to 2.92 for eGFR <30). We also observed an increased risk of urothelial cancer at eGFR <30 but no significant associations between eGFR and prostate, breast, lung, colorectal, or any cancer overall. In conclusion, reduced eGFR is associated with an independently higher risk of renal and urothelial cancer but not other cancer types.

▶ To date, this is the largest single study evaluating the relationship between cancer risk and chronic kidney disease (CKD). The study excluded patients with end-stage renal disease (ESRD) and focused solely on the spectrum of all stages of CKD. Prior studies have yielded variable results with regard to the risk of cancer in patients with underlying CKD.[1-3] Studies[1,2,4] looking at whether the stage of CKD influences the risk of cancer or the specific site of cancer occurrence have shown that an estimated glomerular filtration rate (eGFR) of under 30 mL/min independently increased the risk of cancer. The main sites were nonprostate urinary cancers and lung cancers. The risk increased in a linear fashion among men with lower baseline eGFRs. Higher albumin-to-creatinine ratios[1] were also associated with a higher incidence of cancer (especially bladder and renal cancer).

The explanation for this association is less certain. Several lines of investigation suggest that kidney dysfunction results in a state of chronic inflammation, oxidative stress, and relative immunodeficiency,[5-8] which may each increase the risk of cancer.

Although the authors were not able to adjust for all confounding variables such as family history, drug use, and comorbid conditions, unlike prior studies, they were able to adjust for some variables including hematuria and prior abdominal imaging, which helps support specificity of the role of reduced renal function in the pathogenesis of cancer occurrence. More than 1.5 million cases of cancer are diagnosed each year. The ability to increase the specificity of cancer screening among patients with CKD may improve our efforts to screen these patients in a timely and cost-effective manner.

A. Kapoor, MD

References

1. Jørgensen L, Heuch I, Jenssen T, Jacobsen BK. Association of albuminuria and cancer incidence. *J Am Soc Nephrol.* 2008;19:992-998.
2. Wong G, Hayen A, Chapman JR, et al. Association of CKD and cancer risk in older people. *J Am Soc Nephrol.* 2009;20:1341-1350.
3. Wong G, Zoungas S, Lo S, et al. The risk of cancer in people with diabetes and chronic kidney disease. *Nephrol Dial Transplant.* 2012;27:3337-3344.

4. Christensson A, Savage C, Sjoberg DD, et al. Association of cancer with moderately impaired renal function at baseline in a large, representative, population-based cohort followed for up to 30 years. *Int J Cancer.* 2013;133:1452-1458.
5. Shlipak MG, Fried LF, Crump C, et al. Elevations of inflammatory and procoagulant biomarkers in elderly persons with renal insufficiency. *Circulation.* 2003;107:87-92.
6. Weng PH, Hung KY, Huang HL, Chen JH, Sung PK, Huang KC. Cancer specific mortality in chronic kidney disease: longitudinal follow-up of a large cohort. *Clin J Am Soc Nephrol.* 2011;6:1121-1128.
7. Giacchino F, Alloatti S, Quarello F, Bosticardo GM, Giraudo G, Piccoli G. The immunological state in chronic renal insufficiency. *Int J Artif Organs.* 1982;5:237-242.
8. Coussens LM, Werb Z. Inflammation and cancer. *Nature.* 2002;420:860-867.

Ultrasonography versus Computed Tomography for Suspected Nephrolithiasis

Smith-Bindman R, Aubin C, Bailitz J, et al (Univ of California, San Francisco; Washington Univ School of Medicine, St. Louis, MO; Rush Univ Med Ctr, Chicago, IL)
N Engl J Med 371:1100-1110, 2014

Background.—There is a lack of consensus about whether the initial imaging method for patients with suspected nephrolithiasis should be computed tomography (CT) or ultrasonography.

Methods.—In this multicenter, pragmatic, comparative effectiveness trial, we randomly assigned patients 18 to 76 years of age who presented to the emergency department with suspected nephrolithiasis to undergo initial diagnostic ultrasonography performed by an emergency physician (point-of-care ultrasonography), ultrasonography performed by a radiologist (radiology ultrasonography), or abdominal CT. Subsequent management, including additional imaging, was at the discretion of the physician. We compared the three groups with respect to the 30-day incidence of high-risk diagnoses with complications that could be related to missed or delayed diagnosis and the 6-month cumulative radiation exposure. Secondary outcomes were serious adverse events, related serious adverse events (deemed attributable to study participation), pain (assessed on an 11-point visual-analogue scale, with higher scores indicating more severe pain), return emergency department visits, hospitalizations, and diagnostic accuracy.

Results.—A total of 2759 patients underwent randomization: 908 to point-of-care ultrasonography, 893 to radiology ultrasonography, and 958 to CT. The incidence of high-risk diagnoses with complications in the first 30 days was low (0.4%) and did not vary according to imaging method. The mean 6-month cumulative radiation exposure was significantly lower in the ultrasonography groups than in the CT group ($P < 0.001$). Serious adverse events occurred in 12.4% of the patients assigned to point-of-care ultrasonography, 10.8% of those assigned to radiology ultrasonography, and 11.2% of those assigned to CT ($P = 0.50$). Related adverse events were infrequent (incidence, 0.4%) and similar across groups. By 7 days, the average pain score was 2.0 in each group ($P = 0.84$). Return emergency department visits, hospitalizations, and diagnostic accuracy did not differ significantly among the groups.

Conclusions.—Initial ultrasonography was associated with lower cumulative radiation exposure than initial CT, without significant differences in high-risk diagnoses with complications, serious adverse events, pain scores, return emergency department visits, or hospitalizations.

▶ Currently, kidney stones are typically diagnosed with high sensitivity and specificity via a CT scan of the abdomen and pelvis.[1] Will, or should, the results of this large, geographically diverse, randomized, multicenter, trial be viewed as establishing the "comparative therapeutic equivalence" of these tools and thereby alter our diagnostic approach to suspected nephrolithiasis? To answer this question, we must carefully understand the results of this study.

To evaluate the relative effectiveness of various imaging modalities, eligible patients were randomized to either receive ultrasonography by an ultrasound-certified emergency physician, a radiologist, or an abdominal CT. The diagnostic accuracy was assessed via either stone passage or a patient report of surgical stone removal.

The key primary outcome was not diagnostic accuracy per se but rather focused on missed predefined high-risk diagnoses, complications potentially related to a delay in diagnosis (occurring within 30 days of examination), and the cumulative radiation exposure.

The number of high-risk diagnoses with complications was small, and although it tended to be slightly higher in the emergency department (ED) ultrasound group, it did not reach statistical significance, nor did any of the other outcome parameters studied.

The statistics were handled using an intention-to-treat model. Ultimately, about 41% of the patients in the ED ultrasound group and about 27% of the patients in the radiology ultrasound group required CT imaging to establish a diagnosis of stone disease. When this is taken into account, the sensitivity of ultrasonography to detect renal stones is less than that of CT at 54% (95% confidence interval [CI]: 48-60); for point-of-care ultrasonography, it is 57% for radiology ultrasonography (95% CI: 51-64), and 88% for CT (95% CI: 84-92; $P < .001$).

Thus, there are several important caveats to this study. First, as the authors clearly point out, their results do not suggest that at-risk patients should undergo only ultrasound imaging. Instead, their findings suggested that ultrasonography is the most appropriate initial diagnostic imaging test for the detection of renal stones. Additional images may be required based on the clinical judgment of the physician.

The second caveat is that eligibility criteria were carefully defined. Several groups of patients were deemed ineligible for inclusion. These included anyone being evaluated for an alternative diagnosis such as appendicitis, cholecystitis, or aneurysm, and patients who were obese, pregnant, had a solitary kidney, were receiving dialysis, or had a prior transplantation. The third is that the ED physicians performing the study were certified in ultrasonography, and therefore the results may not be generalizable to other clinical settings.

Nonetheless, the results of the study are important. CT imaging and stone evaluations can involve significant exposure to ionizing radiation. In fact, Ferrandino and colleagues found that the typical acute stone evaluation at an academic medical center (which included an intravenous pyelogram, an abdominal radiograph, and an CT of the abdomen and pelvis) had a mean radiation exposure of 29.7 mSv.[2] The International Commission on Radiation Exposure recommends a total annual exposure of under 50 mSv.[3] In addition to using ultrasonography as a first-line approach to the diagnosis of stone disease, the applicability of low-dose CT[4,5] scans should continue to be explored.

R. Garrick, MD

References

1. Coursey CA, Casalino DD, Reimer EM, et al. ACR appropriateness criteria: acute onset flank pain—suspicion of stone disease. *Ultrasound Q*. 2012;28:227-233.
2. Ferrandino MN, Bagrodia A, Pierre SA, et al. Radiation exposure in the acute and short-term management of urolithiasis with biases at two academic centers. *J Urol*. 2009;181:668-672.
3. National Research Council. *Health Risks from Exposure to Low Levels of Ionizing Radiation: BEIR VII Phase 2*. Washington, DC: National Academies Press; 2006.
4. Ciaschini MW, Remer EM, Baker ME, Lieber M, Herts BR. Urinary calculi: radiation dose reduction of 50% and 75% at CT—effect on sensitivity. *Radiology*. 2009;251:105-111.
5. Poletti PA, Platon A, Rutschmann OT, Schmidlin FR, Iselin CE, Becker CD. Low dose versus standard-dose CT protocol in patients with clinically suspected renal colic. *AJR Am J Roentgenol*. 2007;188:927-933.

Effect of Sodium Zirconium Cyclosilicate on Potassium Lowering for 28 Days Among Outpatients With Hyperkalemia: The HARMONIZE Randomized Clinical Trial

Kosiborod M, Rasmussen HS, Lavin P, et al (Saint Luke's Mid America Heart Inst, Kansas City, MO; ZS Pharma, Coppell, TX; Boston Biostatistics Research Foundation, Framingham, MA; et al)

JAMA 312:2223-2233, 2014

Importance.—Hyperkalemia is a common electrolyte abnormality that may be difficult to manage because of a lack of effective therapies. Sodium zirconium cyclosilicate is a nonabsorbed cation exchanger that selectively binds potassium in the intestine.

Objective.—To evaluate the efficacy and safety of zirconium cyclosilicate for 28 days in patients with hyperkalemia.

Design, Setting, and Participants.—HARMONIZE was a phase 3, multicenter, randomized, double-blind, placebo-controlled trial evaluating zirconium cyclosilicate in outpatients with hyperkalemia (serum potassium

≥5.1 mEq/L) recruited from 44 sites in the United States, Australia, and South Africa (March-August 2014).

Interventions.—Patients (n = 258) received 10 g of zirconium cyclosilicate 3 times daily in the initial 48-hour open-label phase. Patients (n = 237) achieving normokalemia (3.5-5.0 mEq/L) were then randomized to receive zirconium cyclosilicate, 5 g (n = 45 patients), 10 g (n = 51), or 15 g (n = 56), or placebo (n = 85) daily for 28 days.

Main Outcomes and Measures.—The primary end point was mean serum potassium level in each zirconium cyclosilicate group vs placebo during days 8-29 of the randomized phase.

Results.—In the open-label phase, serum potassium levels declined from 5.6 mEq/L at baseline to 4.5 mEq/L at 48 hours. Median time to normalization was 2.2 hours, with 84% of patients (95% CI, 79%-88%) achieving normokalemia by 24 hours and 98% (95% CI, 96%-99%) by 48 hours. In the randomized phase, serum potassium was significantly lower during days 8-29 with all 3 zirconium cyclosilicate doses vs placebo (4.8 mEq/L [95% CI, 4.6-4.9], 4.5 mEq/L [95% CI, 4.4-4.6], and 4.4 mEq/L [95% CI, 4.3-4.5] for 5 g, 10 g, and 15 g; 5.1 mEq/L [95% CI, 5.0-5.2] for placebo; $P < .001$ for all comparisons). The proportion of patients with mean potassium <5.1 mEq/L during days 8-29 was significantly higher in all zirconium cyclosilicate groups vs placebo (36/45 [80%], 45/50 [90%], and 51/54 [94%] for the 5-g, 10-g, and 15-g groups, vs 38/82 [46%] with placebo; $P < .001$ for each dose vs placebo). Adverse events were comparable between zirconium cyclosilicate and placebo, although edema was more common in the 15-g group (edema incidence: 2/85 [2%], 1/45 [2%], 3/51 [6%], and 8/56 [14%] patients in the placebo, 5-g, 10-g, and 15-g groups). Hypokalemia developed in 5/51 (10%) and 6/56 patients (11%) in the 10-g and 15-g zirconium cyclosilicate groups, vs none in the 5-g or placebo groups.

Conclusions and Relevance.—Among outpatients with hyperkalemia, open-label sodium zirconium cyclosilicate reduced serum potassium to normal levels within 48 hours; compared with placebo, all 3 doses of zirconium cyclosilicate resulted in lower potassium levels and a higher proportion of patients with normal potassium levels for up to 28 days. Further studies are needed to evaluate the efficacy and safety of zirconium cyclosilicate beyond 4 weeks and to assess long-term clinical outcomes.

Trial Registration.—clinicaltrials.gov Identifier: NCT02088073.

▶ Hyperkalemia is potentially fatal and frequently encountered in patients with chronic kidney disease and is usually due to the decreased renal excretion of potassium.[1] This risk is increased by the use of angiotensin-converting enzyme inhibitors (ACE-I) and angiotensin II receptor blockers (ARBs), which are used in this population for the treatment of concomitant cardiac disease, hypertension with proteinuria, or diabetes.[2] Currently available therapies include temporizing agents, which rapidly drive extracellular potassium intracellularly, such as intravenous insulin and inhaled B-2 agonists. These therapies are not practical in the outpatient setting. The other class of medications include exchange resins such as patiromer and sodium polystyrene sulfate (SPS) which act by exchanging K for either Na (SPS) or Ca (patiromer).[3,4] However, the use of SPS (especially with sorbitol) has been associated with bowel necrosis, and other studies have questioned its overall efficacy. Hence, the results of the recent HARMONIZE trial are very interesting. It showed that using zirconium cyclosilicate (ZS-9) can effectively and acutely lower K and maintain a lower level for an extended time. The potassium-lowering effect of ZS-9 was observed immediately (1 hour after first dose) and was consistent across all patient subgroups; further, normal potassium levels were achieved in 84% of patients within 24 hours and in 98% within 48 hours of treatment. The majority of the study population had heart failure, diabetes, or both, and about 70% were on ACE-I or ARBs. ZS-9 works through the gut and selectively binds potassium with almost 9 times the affinity of SPS.[5] The major adverse event was increased peripheral edema.

Therapeutic caution is needed, however. The long-term effects of ZS-9 are not yet established in the general population at risk, and the results must be replicated in the end-stage renal disease population. Moreover, its onset of action is likely still too long to support its use as the sole immediate therapy for hyperkalemia-associated arrhythmias. However, even with these considerations in hand, the current findings may usher in a new era in which the risk-reduction benefit of ACEi/ARBs therapy can be extended to include even those patients at risk for hyperkalemia.

R. Morey, MD

References

1. Einhorn LM, Zhan M, Walker LD, et al. The frequency of hyperkalemia and its significance in chronic kidney disease. *Arch Intern Med.* 2009;169:1156-1162.
2. Raebel MA. Hyperkalemia associated with use of angiotensin-converting enzyme inhibitors and angiotensin receptor blockers. *Cardiovasc Ther.* 2012;30: e156-e166.
3. Jain N, Kotla S, Little BB, et al. Predictors of hyperkalemia and death in patients with cardiac and renal disease. *Am J Cardiol.* 2012;109:1510-1513.
4. Harel Z, Harel S, Shah PS, Wald R, Perl J, Bell CM. Gastrointestinal adverse events with sodium polystyrene sulfonate (Kayexalate) use: a systematic review. *Am J Med.* 2013;126:264.e9-264.e24.
5. Yang A, Leon A, Nuttall M, et al. In vitro ion exchange capacity and selectivity of ZS-9, a novel, selective cation trap for the treatment of hyperkalemia. *Am J Kidney Dis.* 2014;63:A115.

Association of Anti-PLA_2R Antibodies with Outcomes after Immunosuppressive Therapy in Idiopathic Membranous Nephropathy

Bech AP, Hofstra JM, Brenchley PE, et al (Radboud Univ Med Centre, Nijmegen, The Netherlands; Manchester Inst of Nephrology and Transplantation, UK)

Clin J Am Soc Nephrol 9:1386-1392, 2014

Background.—The optimal timing and duration of immunosuppressive therapy for idiopathic membranous nephropathy (iMN) have been debated. This study aimed to evaluate whether measuring the antibody against the phospholipase A_2 receptor (PLA_2R-ab) at start and end of therapy predicts long-term outcome and therefore may inform this debate.

Design, Setting, Participants, & Measurements.—This observational study included all consecutive high-risk patients with progressive iMN observed from 1997 to 2005 and treated with oral cyclophosphamide (CP) or mycophenolate mofetil (MMF) in combination with corticosteroids for 12 months. Patients were prospectively followed, and outcome was ascertained up to 5 years after completion of immunosuppressive therapy. Serum samples were collected before and after completion of therapy. PLA_2R antibodies were determined retrospectively in stored samples using ELISA.

Results.—In total, 48 patients (37 men) were included. The median age was 55 years (range, 34–75), and the median serum creatinine level was 1.60 mg/dl (range, 0.98–3.37 mg/dl). Twenty-two patients received MMF and 26 received CP. At baseline, PLA_2R-abs were present in 34 patients (71%). Baseline characteristics and outcome did not significantly differ between patients negative or positive for PLA_2R-ab. In PLA_2R-ab–positive patients, treatment resulted in a rapid decrease of antibodies: median anti–PLA_2R-ab, 428 U/ml (range, 41–16,260 U/ml) at baseline and 24 U/ml (range, 0–505 U/ml) after 2 months. The PLA_2R-ab levels at baseline did not predict initial response, but antibody status at end of therapy predicted long-term outcome: After 5 years, 14 of 24 (58%) antibody-negative patients were in persistent remission compared with 0 of 9 (0%) antibody-positive patients ($P = 0.003$).

Conclusions.—These data suggest that in PLA_2R-ab–positive patients, measuring PLA_2R-abs at the end of therapy predicts the subsequent course.

► The current study is important because it might help clinicians devise an optimal therapeutic approach for a common clinical condition. Membranous nephropathy is one of the most common causes of the nephrotic syndrome, and definitive diagnosis usually requires a renal biopsy. It can be idiopathic or occur secondarily, in association with various underlying conditions. In animal models, the pathogenesis is well documented and is related to a circulating antigen, Megalin.[1] In human studies, various similar antigens have been identified, and the most important appears to be the M-type phospholipase A_2 receptor (PLA_2R),[2] which has been found in up to 70% studies in patients with idiopathic membranous nephropathy.[3,4] These studies have shown the following: (1) anti-PLA_2R strongly correlated with clinical status, (2) lower anti-PLA_2R titers were associated with a higher rate of spontaneous remission, (3) a decline in anti-PLA_2R predicted the clinical response to immunosuppressive therapy, and (4) $aPLA_2R$ becomes negative during a remission and positive during a relapse.

Treatment of membranous nephropathy is tricky because it is difficult to predict which patients will have remissions and which will require long-term immunosuppressive therapy. The investigators looked at the predictive utility of $aPLA_2R$ levels pre- and posttreatment. They prospectively studied 48 patients with idiopathic membranous nephropathy treated with mycophenolate mofetil or cyclophosphamide and discovered that post–induction-therapy levels, but not baseline levels, predict long-term outcome. After 5 years, 14 of 24 (58%) antibody-negative patients were in persistent remission compared with 0 of 9 (0%) antibody-positive patients ($P = .003$). They also confirmed that the $aPLA_2R$ levels fall before the decline in proteinuria, suggesting that negative $aPLA_2R$ levels rather than the elimination of proteinuria might be useful for guiding therapy. The study does have limitations. The sample size is small, and $aPLA_2R$ can be found in membranous nephropathy with concurrent diseases such as lupus and hepatitis B, so it cannot be used to establish a diagnosis of idiopathic disease. The effect of calcineurin inhibitors on a PLA_2R levels has not been established, so the results should not be generalized. However, the study does open avenues for new research, and these antibodies may help establish diagnosis and treatment options for membranous glomerular disease.

S. Chugh, MD

References

1. Farquhar MG, Saito A, Kerjaschki D, et al. The Heymann nephritis antigenic complex: megalin (gp330) and RAP. *J Am Soc Nephrol.* 1995;6:35-47.
2. Beck LH Jr, Bonegio RG, Lambeau G, et al. M-type phospholipase A_2 receptor as target antigen in idiopathic membranous nephropathy. *N Engl J Med.* 2009;361: 11-21.
3. Hoxha E, Harendza S, Zahner G, et al. An immunofluorescence test for phospholipase-A_2-receptor antibodies and its clinical usefulness in patients with membranous glomerulonephritis. *Nephrol Dial Transplant.* 2011;26:2526-2532.
4. Beck LH, Fervenza FC, Beck DM, et al. Rituximab-induced depletion of anti-PLA_2R autoantibodies predicts response in membranous nephropathy. *J Am Soc Nephrol.* 2011;22:1543-1550.

34 Issues in Severe CKD and Dialysis

ESRD and Death after Heart Failure in CKD

Sud M, Tangri N, Pintilie M, et al (Univ of Toronto, Ontario, Canada; Univ of Manitoba, Winnipeg, Canada; Univ Health Network, Toronto, Ontario, Canada; et al)

J Am Soc Nephrol 26:715-722, 2015

CKD is a risk factor for heart failure, but there is no data on the risk of ESRD and death after recurrent hospitalizations for heart failure. We sought to determine how interim heart failure hospitalizations modify the subsequent risk of ESRD or death before ESRD in patients with CKD. We retrospectively identified 2887 patients with a GFR between 15 and 60 ml/min per 1.73 m^2 referred between January of 2001 and December of 2008 to a nephrology clinic in Toronto, Canada. We ascertained interim first, second, and third heart failure hospitalizations as well as ESRD and death before ESRD outcomes from administrative data. Over a median follow-up time of 3.01 (interquartile range = 1.56–4.99) years, interim heart failure hospitalizations occurred in 359 (12%) patients, whereas 234 (8%) patients developed ESRD, and 499 (17%) patients died before ESRD. Compared with no heart failure hospitalizations, one, two, or three or more heart failure hospitalizations increased the adjusted hazard ratio of ESRD from 4.89 (95% confidence interval [95% CI], 3.21 to 7.44) to 10.27 (95% CI, 5.54 to 19.04) to 14.16 (95% CI, 8.07 to 24.83), respectively, and the adjusted hazard ratio death before ESRD from 3.30 (95% CI, 2.55 to 4.27) to 4.20 (95% CI, 2.82 to 6.25) to 6.87 (95% CI, 4.96 to 9.51), respectively. We conclude that recurrent interim heart failure is associated with a stepwise increase in the risk of ESRD and death before ESRD in patients with CKD.

▶ Previously, the atherosclerosis risk in Community study demonstrated that chronic kidney disease is an independent risk for heart failure.[1] In turn, heart failure, especially when hospitalization is required, is associated with an increased risk of death.[2] The current study is drawn from coded (administrative) data on 6255 patients tracked in an electronic medical record database in outpatient nephrology clinic in Toronto, Ontario. Patients with an estimated glomerular filtration rate >15 and <60 mL/min/1.73 m^2 were followed to determine the risk of end-stage renal disease (ESRD) and death after recurrent hospitalizations for heart failure. The data demonstrate that in patients with underlying chronic kidney disease (CKD), the occurrence of sequential episodes of heart failure, results in a graded (4-, 10-, and 14-fold) increase in ESRD risk and an increase in mortality risk (3-, 4-, and 6-fold) before reaching ESRD compared with CKD patients without a history of, or hospitalizations related to, heart failure.

This study was well done. The major limitation was its reliance on coded (administrative) data rather than audited chart data, although typically administrative heart failure codes do achieve high validation scores. A second limitation was the inability to standardize the data for the precise use of cardioprotective medications. The authors did, however, do multiple sensitivity analyses, including corrections for possible confounding caused by interim myocardial infarction and stroke hospitalization.

These overlapping Venn diagrams are substantial. Approximately 24 million Americans have CKD,[2] and another 5.7 million suffer from heart failure.[3] The combined effect of these 2 chronic conditions is remarkably lethal.

These findings have important clinical implications. Other studies among patients with heart failure have demonstrated that hospital readmission rates and 30-day postdischarge mortality rates can be reduced by early postdischarge follow-up.[4] Whether the same type of vigilant follow-up will favorably affect these CKD/congestive heart failure mortality statistics will require further study.

R. Garrick, MD

References

1. Kottgen A, Russell SD, Loehr LR, et al. Reduced kidney function as a risk factor for incident heart failure: the atherosclerosis risk in communities (ARIC) study. *J Am Soc Nephrol.* 2007;18:1307-1315.
2. Solomon SD, Dobson J, Pocock S, et al; Candesartan in Heart failure: Assessment of Reduction in Mortality and morbidity (CHARM) Investigators. Influence of nonfatal hospitalization for heart failure on subsequent mortality in patients with chronic heart failure. *Circulation.* 2007;116:1482-1487.
3. Roger VL, Go AS, Lloyd-Jones DM, et al; American Heart Association Statistics Committee and Stroke Statistics Subcommittee. Heart disease and stroke statistics—2012 update: a report from the American Heart Association. *Circulation.* 2012;125:e2-e220.
4. McAlister FA, Youngson E, Bakal JA, Kaul P, Ezekowitz J, van Walraven C. Impact of physician continuity on death or urgent readmission after discharge among patients with heart failure. *CMAJ.* 2013;185:E681-E689.

Meta-Analysis of Methicillin-Resistant *Staphylococcus aureus* Colonization and Risk of Infection in Dialysis Patients

Zacharioudakis IM, Zervou FN, Ziakas PD, et al (Rhode Island Hosp, Providence; Warren Alpert Med School of Brown Univ, Providence, RI)
J Am Soc Nephrol 25:2131-2141, 2014

Patients undergoing dialysis are particularly vulnerable to methicillin-resistant *Staphylococcus aureus* (MRSA) infections. We performed a meta-analysis of published studies to estimate the prevalence of MRSA colonization in dialysis patients, time trends, and long-term risk of subsequent MRSA infections. Our search of the PubMed and Embase databases returned 5743 nonduplicate citations, from which we identified 38 relevant studies that included data on 5596 dialysis patients. The estimated prevalence of MRSA colonization was 6.2% (95% confidence interval [95% CI], 4.2% to 8.5%). The prevalence increased over time but remained stable after 2000. Stratification of patients according to dialysis modality and setting revealed that 7.2% (95% CI, 4.9% to 9.9%) of patients on hemodialysis were colonized with MRSA compared with 1.3% (95% CI, 0.5% to 2.4%) of patients on peritoneal dialysis ($P = 0.01$), and that a statistically significant difference existed in the percentage of colonized inpatients and outpatients (14.2% [95% CI, 8.0% to 21.8%] versus 5.4% [95% CI, 3.5% to 7.7%], respectively; $P = 0.04$). Notably, the risk of developing MRSA infections increased among colonized hemodialysis patients compared with noncolonized patients (relative risk, 11.5 [95% CI, 4.7 to 28.0]). The long-term (6–20 months) probability of developing a MRSA infection was 19% among colonized hemodialysis patients compared with only 2% among noncolonized patients. In summary, 6.2% of dialysis patients are MRSA colonized, and the average prevalence of colonization has remained stable since 2000. Colonization in hemodialysis patients is associated with increased risk of MRSA infection.

► Infection is second only to cardiovascular disease as a cause of death among patients on dialysis,[1] and methicillin-resistant *Staphylococcus aureus* (MRSA) is a key pathogen among this population. This large, well-constructed meta-analysis highlights that a significant percentage of patients with end-stage renal disease are colonized with MRSA. The presence of this colonization substantially increases the risk of systemic infection. The prevalence of colonization is greater among hemodialysis patients than peritoneal dialysis patients (7.2% vs 1.3%).

MRSA colonization has increased over a 30-year period from 1980 to 2010. Since 2010, the prevalence has appeared to be stabilized, but of note, the prevalence among hospitalized patients is 3 times greater than among outpatients. This may reflect the high rate of readmission of dialysis patients, which increases their opportunity for MRSA exposure and colonization. The risk of developing MRSA infection is approximately 11.5-fold higher in hemodialysis patients colonized with MRSA compared with noncolonized patients. Based on the available data, the authors estimate that approximately 1 in 5 dialysis patients colonized with MRSA will develop an active infection within 6 to 20 months.

These data are compelling. In addition, in most of the studies included here, MRSA colonization was detected via culture rather than polymerase chain reaction, so is possible these data underestimate the true level of colonization. Clearly steps should be taken to reduce MRSA colonization. Intranasal mupirocin ointment has been shown to be effective. However, to avoid the emergence of resistant strains, its use should be selectively confined to patients with documented colonization.[2] The use of chlorhexidine skin preparations, avoidance of catheter use, and the selective use of antibiotics have all been demonstrated to reduce MRSA colonization.[3,4]

M. Brogan, MD

References

1. US Renal Data System. *2013 Annual Data Report: Atlas of Chronic Kidney Disease and End-Stage Renal Disease in the United States.* Bethesda, MD: National Institutes of Health National Institute of Diabetes and Digestive and Kidney Diseases; 2013.
2. Kaur DC, Narayan A. Mupirocin serum resistance and nasal carriage of *Staphylococcus aureus* among healthcare workers of a tertiary care hospital. *Indian J Crit Care Med.* 2014;18:716-772.
3. Forster AJ, Oake N, Roth V, et al. Patient-level factors associated with methicillin-resistant *Staphylococcus aureus* carriage at hospital admission: a systematic review. *Am J Infect Control.* 2013;41:214-220.
4. Nguyen DB, Lessa FC, Belflower R, et al; Active Bacterial Core Surveillance (ABCs) MRSA Investigators of the Emerging Infections Program. Invasive methicillin-resistant *Staphylococcus aureus* infections among patients on chronic dialysis in the United States, 2005–2011. *Clin Infect Dis.* 2013;57:1393-1400.

Cognitive Function and All-Cause Mortality in Maintenance Hemodialysis Patients

Drew DA, Weiner DE, Tighiouart H, et al (Tufts Med Ctr, Boston, MA; et al)
Am J Kidney Dis 65:303-311, 2015

Background.—Cognitive impairment is common in hemodialysis patients and is associated with significant morbidity. Limited information exists about whether cognitive impairment is associated with survival and whether the type of cognitive impairment is important.

Study Design.—Longitudinal cohort.

Setting & Participants.—Cognitive function was assessed at baseline and yearly using a comprehensive battery of cognitive tests in 292 prevalent hemodialysis patients.

Predictor.—Using principal component analysis, individual test results were reduced into 2 domain scores, representing memory and executive function. By definition, each score carried a mean of 0 and SD of 1.

Outcomes.—Association of each score with all-cause mortality was assessed using Cox proportional hazards models adjusted for demographics and dialysis and cardiovascular (CV) risk factors.

Results.—Mean age of participants was 63 years, 53% were men, 23% were African American, and 90% had at least a high school education. During a median follow-up of 2.1 (IQR, 1.1-3.7) years, 145 deaths occurred. Each 1-SD better executive function score was associated with a 35% lower hazard of mortality (HR, 0.65; 95% CI, 0.55-0.76). In models adjusting for demographics and dialysis-related factors, this relationship was partially attenuated but remained significant (HR, 0.81; 95% CI, 0.67-0.98), whereas adjustment for CV disease and heart failure resulted in further attenuation (HR, 0.87; 95% CI, 0.72-1.06). Use of time-dependent models showed a similar unadjusted association (HR, 0.62; 95% CI, 0.54-0.72), with the relationship remaining significant after adjustment for demographics and dialysis and CV risk factors (HR, 0.79; 95% CI, 0.66-0.94). Better memory was associated with lower mortality in univariate analysis (HR per 1 SD, 0.82; 95% CI, 0.69-0.96), but not when adjusting for demographics (HR, 1.00; 95% CI, 0.83-1.19).

Limitations.—Patients with dementia were excluded from the full battery, perhaps underestimating the strength of the association.

Conclusions.—Worse executive function and memory are associated with increased risk of mortality. For memory, this association is explained by patient demographics, whereas for executive function, this relationship may be explained in part by CV disease burden.

▶ Prior studies based on billing data have suggested that dementia may be a risk factor for mortality among patients with end-stage renal disease (ESRD).[1,2] The current longitudinal study used well-described, standardized tests of cognitive function and evaluated whether memory and executive functions influence mortality in patients with ESRD.

Patients with worse cognitive function were older, less educated, and more likely to have cardiovascular disease (CVD), diabetes, and hypertension. Adjusted analyses showed complete attenuation for memory function after adjusting for demographic factors, whereas for executive function, partial attenuation occurred when adjusting for CVD and heart failure. That changes in executive function persisted after correction for patient demographics may reflect the high burden of subclinical cerebrovascular disease in these patients. In turn, the time-dependent analyses suggested that this reduced executive function may be an independent risk factor for mortality.

One limitation of the study was that a portion of the testing was done during the dialysis treatment, and it is possible that the dialysis treatment itself can alter a patients' ability to attend to cognitive function testing. Nonetheless, that would not be expected to alter the mortality data. These findings are clinically important because the data suggest that changes in executive function increase mortality, reduce quality of life, and may directly affect the ability of patients with renal disease to understand and participate in their care. Patient care, and potentially clinical outcomes, may be improved if providers are aware of these findings and take steps to evaluate patients' cognitive function. If limitations are present, steps should be taken to improve the care paradigm by using memory aides and by engaging the help of family members, if available.

A. Kapoor, MD

References

1. Rakowski DA, Caillard S, Agodoa LY, Abbott KC. Dementia as a predictor of mortality in dialysis patients. *Clin J Am Soc Nephrol.* 2006;1:1000-1005.
2. Kurella M, Mapes DL, Port FK, Chertow GM. Correlates and outcomes of dementia among dialysis patients: the dialysis outcomes and practice patterns study. *Nephrol Dial Transplant.* 2006;21:2543-2548.

Utilization of Acute Care among Patients with ESRD Discharged Home from Skilled Nursing Facilities

Hall RK, Toles M, Massing M, et al (Durham Veterans Affairs Geriatric Research, Education, and Clinical Ctr, NC; Univ of North Carolina at Chapel Hill; et al)

Clin J Am Soc Nephrol 10:428-434, 2015

Background and Objectives.—Older adults with ESRD often receive care in skilled nursing facilities (SNFs) after an acute hospitalization; however, little is known about acute care use after SNF discharge to home.

Design, Setting, Participants, & Measurements.—This study used Medicare claims for North and South Carolina to identify patients with ESRD who were discharged home from a SNF between January 1, 2010 and August 31, 2011. Nursing Home Compare data were used to ascertain SNF characteristics. The primary outcome was time from SNF discharge to first acute care use (hospitalization or emergency department visit) within 30 days. Cox proportional hazards models were used to identify patient and facility characteristics associated with the outcome.

Results.—Among 1223 patients with ESRD discharged home from a SNF after an acute hospitalization, 531 (43%) had at least one rehospitalization or emergency department visit within 30 days. The median time to first acute care use was 37 days. Characteristics associated with a shorter time to acute care use were black race (hazard ratio [HR], 1.25; 95% confidence interval [95% CI], 1.04 to 1.51), dual Medicare-Medicaid coverage (HR, 1.24; 95% CI, 1.03 to 1.50), higher Charlson comorbidity score (HR, 1.07; 95% CI, 1.01 to 1.12), number of hospitalizations during the 90 days before SNF admission (HR, 1.12; 95% CI, 1.03 to 1.22), and index hospital discharge diagnoses of cellulitis, abscess, and/or skin ulcer (HR, 2.59; 95% CI, 1.36 to 4.45). Home health use after SNF discharge was associated with a lower rate of acute care use (HR, 0.72; 95% CI, 0.59 to 0.87). There were no statistically significant associations between SNF characteristics and time to first acute care use.

Conclusions.—Almost one in every two older adults with ESRD discharged home after a post–acute SNF stay used acute care services within 30 days of discharge. Strategies to reduce acute care utilization in these patients are needed.

► Hall and colleagues have identified an important clinical care issue. The 30-day readmission rate of dialysis patients residing and skilled nursing facility approaches 50%. By identifying and addressing the risk factors that commonly characterize these readmissions, we might improve the transition of care between the hospital and nursing home and mitigate the risk of readmission. Based on Medicare claims data, and Nursing Home Facility Compare data, they identified that acute care was required for 7% of patients within 24 hours of discharge and for 66% of patients within 90 days of skilled nursing facility (SNF) discharge.[1] The key predictors for readmission were socioeconomic status (those with dual Medicare/Medicaid were more likely to be readmitted), a high Charleston comorbidity index; Black race; the number of hospitalizations in the 90 days prior to the index SNF stay, and an emergency department visit postdischarge. Among patients who were readmitted, discharge diagnoses of cellulitis and skin abscess or ulcer were almost twice common compared with the control cohort. Of added interest is that 65% of SNFs have between 2 and 9 patients with end-stage renal disease (ESRD), suggesting that many facilities may have little experience in caring for patients on dialysis, and templates and checklists may help standardize the approach to their care.

This is the first study describing acute care use among ESRD patients residing in SNFs. The study was based on claims data, and 1 limitation is that other areas, such as medication reconciliation, that have been identified as a potential risk factor for readmission were not captured as part of this evaluation. However, this is a beginning. For nephrologists, primary care providers, and both dialysis facilities and SNFs, these findings highlight an important issue and offer an early roadmap to help identify those at risk for readmissions.

R. Garrick, MD

Reference

1. Pennsylvania Patient Safety Advisory. Hemodialysis administration: strategies to ensure safe patient care. *Pa Patient Saf Advis.* 2010;7:87–96, http://patientsafetyauthority.org/ADVISORIES/AdvisoryLibrary/2010/Sep7(3)/Pages/87.aspx. Accessed December 28, 2014.

CKD in Elderly Patients Managed without Dialysis: Survival, Symptoms, and Quality of Life

Brown MA, Collett GK, Josland EA, et al (St. George Hosp, Sydney, Australia; et al)

Clin J Am Soc Nephrol 10:260-268, 2015

Background and Objectives.—Survival, symptom burden, and quality of life (QOL) are uncertain for elderly patients with advanced CKD managed without dialysis. We examined these outcomes in patients managed with renal supportive care without dialysis (RSC-NFD) and those planned for or commencing dialysis.

Design, Setting, Participants, & Measurements.—In this prospective observational study, symptoms were measured using the Memorial Symptom Assessment Scale and the Palliative care Outcomes Scale - Symptoms (renal) inventory and QOL was measured using the Short Form-36 survey. This study comprised 273 predialysis patients who had usual nephrology care and 122 nondialysis pathway patients who also attended a renal supportive care clinic adding the skills of a palliative medicine team. A further 72 patients commenced dialysis during this period without attending either clinic.

Results.—Nondialysis patients were older than the predialysis group (82 versus 67 years; $P < 0.001$) but had similar eGFR at the first clinic visit

(16 ml/min per 1.73 m^2; $P = 0.92$). Of the predialysis patients, 92 (34%) commenced dialysis. Compared with the RSC-NFD group, the death rate was lower in the predialysis group who did not require dialysis (hazard ratio, 0.23; 95% confidence interval, 0.12 to 0.41) and in those requiring dialysis (0.30; 0.13 to 0.67) but not in dialysis patients who had not attended the predialysis clinic (0.60; 0.35 to 1.03). Median survival in RSC-NFD patients was 16 (interquartile range, 9, 37) months and 32% survived >12 months after eGFR fell below 10 ml/min per 1.73 m^2. For the whole group, age, serum albumin, and eGFR <15 ml/min per 1.73 m^2 were associated with poorer survival. Of the nondialysis patients, 57% had stable or improved symptoms over 12 months and 58% had stable or improved QOL.

Conclusions.—Elderly patients who choose not to have dialysis as part of shared decision making survive a median of 16 months and about one-third survive 12 months past a time when dialysis might have otherwise been indicated. Utilizing the skills of palliative medicine helps provide reasonable symptom control and QOL without dialysis.

► In 1999 and 2010 the Renal Physicians Association published "shared decision making" guidelines to encourage patients and their caregivers to make rational choices regarding initiation or maintenance of dialysis services.[1,2] To be sure, these must be informed decisions based on empiric evidence, if available. Sadly, good predictive evidence regarding expected outcomes with versus without dialysis has been sparse. This study by Brown et al provides some valuable data from which to better inform these decisions.

In this prospective observational study, 467 stage 4/5 chronic kidney disease patients were prospectively and consecutively enrolled from a single center. This comprised 273 predialysis patients (HD+) and 122 patients who opted to forgo dialysis while receiving supportive palliative care (HD−). An additional 72 incident patients received no counseling and were started on dialysis without assignment to either group.

Assessments of various clinical parameters, comorbidities, and renal function were done at baseline. Symptom assessments were made using validated quality of life (QOL) surveys. The 72 unassigned incident patients were unable to have preassessment. Patients in the HD− group, on average, were 15 years older than the HD+ group and were significantly more likely to have dementia and more than 2 comorbidities (57% vs 40%). This group also suffered comparatively more malnutrition than the HD+ group (66% vs 36%).

Mean patient survival in the HD+ group was longer than in the HD− group (33 vs 20 months) with 34% actually starting dialysis. Survival was greater within the HD+ group than the HD− group regardless of whether they actually started dialysis. The primary cause of death in the HD− group was "renal failure" versus "cardiac failure" in the HD+ group. In patients older than 75 years, the mean survival was 19 months in the HD− group versus 31 months in the HD+ group and 34 months in all patients that started dialysis. One-year survival was much higher in the HD+ group than in the HD− group (93% vs 53%). Survival in the "no counseling" group was 81%. Notably, 100% of the voluntary withdrawals from dialysis, a full 30% of the total dialysis deaths, were drawn from this uncounseled group. No significant survival difference between the dialysis patients and the HD− group was seen in patients older than 75 and with 2 or more comorbidities, including cardiac disease. Change in QOL and physical function scores over the observation period was identical between the 2 groups, although the HD− group had more symptoms before the observation period.

This study is important because it demonstrates that survival may be longer in patients who opt for dialysis rather than palliative care, but this survival advantage may be due to higher comorbidity and age factors driving the election of palliation versus dialysis. What was clear is that those over age 75 with more than 2 comorbidities had no survival benefit on dialysis. In addition, selecting dialysis treatment did not result in any measurable differences in QOL over time. Also notable is that the dialysis patients who did not get counseling comprised 100% of the dialysis withdrawals in this study, stressing the importance of predialysis counseling as part of a comprehensive ESRD treatment plan.

M. Klein, MD

References

1. *Renal Physicians Association and American Society of Nephrology: Shared Decision-Making in the Appropriate Initiation of and Withdrawal from Dialysis. Rockville, MD: Renal Physicians Association; 2000.*
2. Moss AH. Revised dialysis clinical practice guideline promotes more informed decision-making. *Clin J Am Soc Nephrol.* 2010;5:2380-2383.

PART FIVE

PULMONARY DISEASE

JAMES A. BARKER, MD

35 Asthma, Allergy, and Cystic Fibrosis

Asthma: pathogenesis and novel drugs for treatment
Olin JT, Wechsler ME (Natl Jewish Health, Denver, CO)
BMJ 349:g5517, 2014

Asthma affects almost 20 million people in the United States and more than 300 million people worldwide. Of these, 10-15% have severe asthma, which is refractory to commonly available drugs. New drugs are needed because those that are currently available cannot control symptoms and exacerbations in all patients and can cause adverse reactions. In the past 10 years, there have been substantial advances in the understanding of asthma genetics, airway biology, and immune cell signaling. These advances have led to the development of small molecule therapeutics and biologic agents that may improve asthma care in the future. Several new classes of asthma drugs—including ultra long acting β agonists and modulators of the interleukin 4 (IL-4), IL-5, IL-13, and IL-17 pathways—have been evaluated in randomized controlled trials. Other new drug classes—including dissociated corticosteroids, CXC chemokine receptor 2 antagonists, toll-like receptor 9 agonists, and tyrosine kinase inhibitors—remain in earlier phases of development. Despite some preliminary efficacy data, there is insufficient evidence to make strong recommendations about the use of these newer agents. Future research on the clinical efficacy of these biologic agents, the effect of newer agents on severe asthma in pediatric patients, and the biology of non-eosinophilic and corticosteroid resistant asthma is needed to reduce the morbidity of asthma worldwide (Figs 1 and 2).

▶ This state-of-the-art review is a must read for all clinicians caring for patients with asthma. Figs 1 and 2 provide an update on currently understood mechanisms for pathophysiology of asthma and potential new target for antiasthma

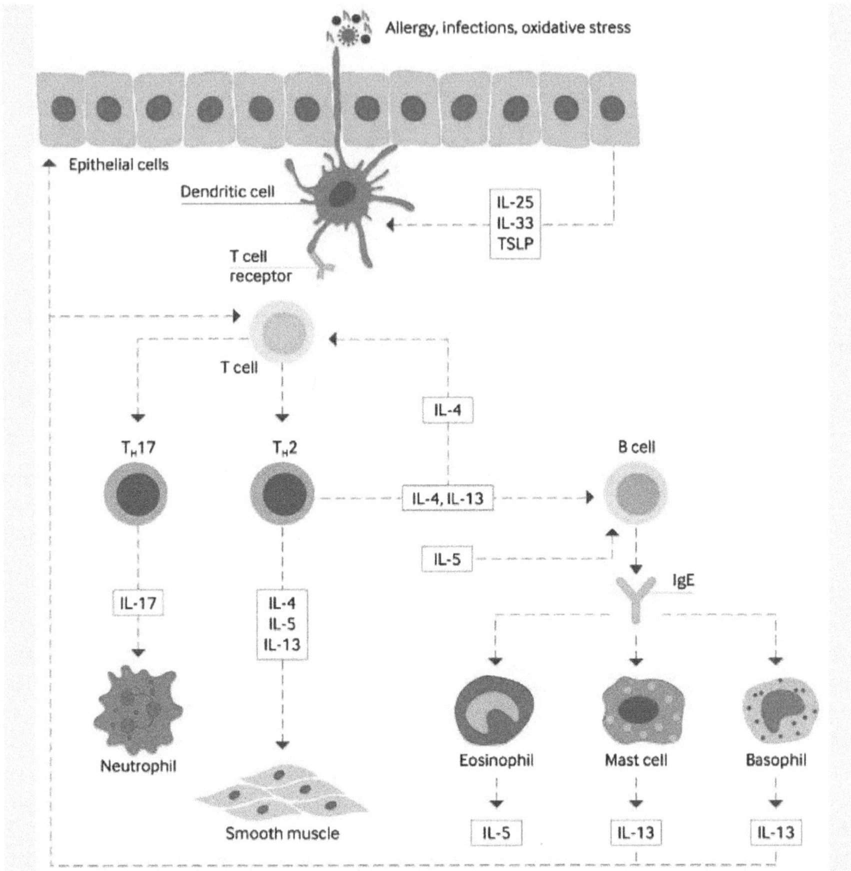

FIGURE 1.—Important host responses in the pathogenesis of asthma. Several asthma drugs in clinical trials target the cytokines (or their receptors) that are central to these pathways, including interleukin 4 (IL-4), IL-5, IL-13, and IL-17. TSLP = thymic stromal lymphopoietin. (Reprinted from Olin JT, Wechsler ME. Asthma: pathogenesis and novel drugs for treatment. *BMJ*. 2014;349:g5517, with permission from the BMJ Publishing Group Ltd.)

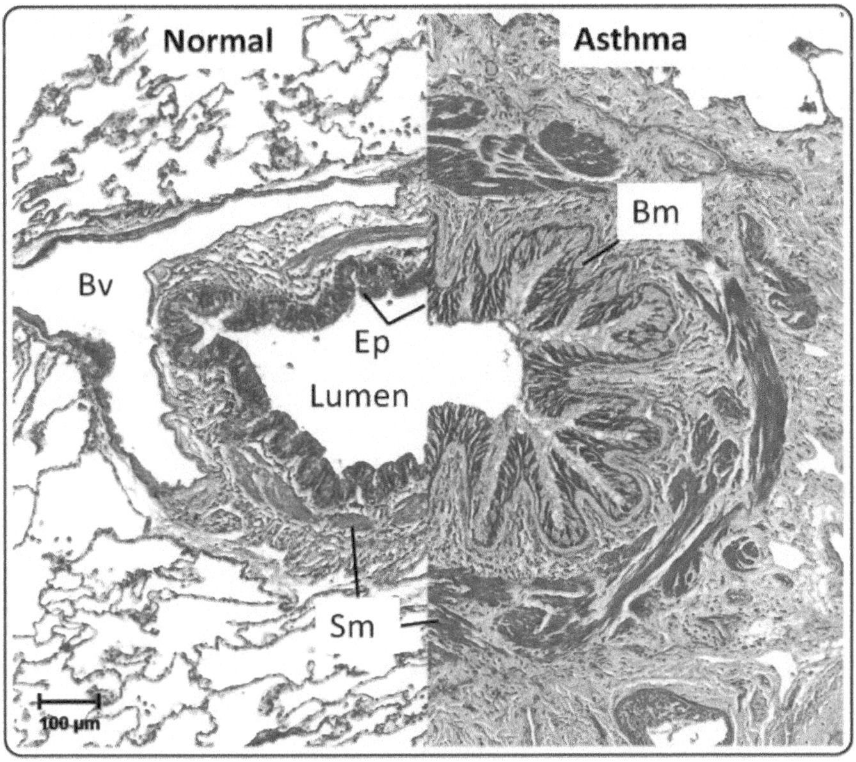

FIGURE 2.—The airways in asthma undergo substantial structural remodeling. Histological section of a medium sized airway from a person without asthma and a patient with severe asthma stained with Movat's pentachrome stain. In asthma the epithelium (Ep) shows mucus hyperplasia and hypersecretion (blue), and thickening of the basement membrane (Bm). Smooth muscle (Sm) volume is also increased in asthma. Bv = blood vessel. Reproduced, under an open access agreement, from Wadsworth and colleagues. IL-13, asthma, and glycosylation in airway epithelial repair. In: Chang C, ed. Carbohydrates—comprehensive studies on glycobiology and glycotechnology. InTech, 2012[67]. *Editor's Note*: Please refer to original journal article for full references. For interpretation of the references to color in this figure legend, the reader is referred to web version of this article. (Reprinted from Olin JT, Wechsler ME. Asthma: pathogenesis and novel drugs for treatment. *BMJ*. 2014;349:g5517, with permission from the BMJ Publishing Group Ltd.)

therapeutics. Succinct and well written, this review makes a good case as to why additional therapeutics are needed.

S. K. Willsie, DO, MA

Management of acute loss of asthma control in the yellow zone: A practice parameter

Dinakar C, Oppenheimer J, Portnoy J, et al ()
Ann Allergy Asthma Immunol 113:143-159, 2014

Asthma action plans have been recommended for all patients with asthma since the 1991 publication of the first National Heart, Lung, and Blood Institute (NHLBI) guidelines for the diagnosis and management of asthma. Establishment of a patient-provider partnership was a key component of the guidelines and the asthma action plan helped create this relationship by empowering patients to monitor their asthma status and take action when control deteriorated. The most recent iteration of the guidelines, the Expert Panel Report 3 (EPR3): Guidelines for the Diagnosis and Management of Asthma (EPR3), was developed by an expert panel commissioned by the National Asthma Education and Prevention Program Coordinating Committee, coordinated by the NHLBI of the National Institutes of Health. The EPR3 emphasized attainment of asthma control and recommended strategies to treat variations in symptoms that occur over a timeframe of months.

In addition to long-term variability of asthma control, most patients with asthma experience intermittent loss of control in response to exposure to acute triggers occurring over a shorter timeframe, such as hours to days. An asthma action plan is the logical tool to instruct patients on how to recognize and respond to such rapid changes in control that occur in a setting outside a supervised medical facility, such as the home. A typical asthma action plan includes written instructions regarding treatment recommendations in the green zone (asthma doing well), the yellow zone (asthma deterioration detected, intervention needed), and the red zone (asthma exacerbation requiring urgent treatment). Responding to the symptoms of acute loss of control in the yellow zone with effective interventions can help prevent deterioration to the red zone, necessitating use of systemic corticosteroids and/or urgent medical care.

The EPR3 recommends increasing administration of inhaled SABA (such as 2–6 puffs of albuterol) every 3 to 4 hours for 24 to 48 hours to treat home exacerbations of asthma. If there is insufficient improvement, it recommends adding a short course of oral systemic corticosteroids (Figure 5–4 of the EPR3). In other words, the intervention recommended in the yellow zone by the EPR3 is to increase the frequency of reliever SABA therapy. Guidelines providing evidence-based therapeutic options to manage patients who experience short-term loss of control are therefore lacking, and this practice parameter was written with the intent of addressing the gap. This document attempts to define criteria that indicate acute loss of control into the yellow zone and reviews therapeutic maneuvers to regain asthma control and prevent further progression into the red zone. These recommendations are based on a meticulous and critical review of the medical literature, and in situations where data are lacking, options are presented.

The first recommendation in this practice parameter is that patients with asthma should be given a written and/or electronic asthma action plan. Although the format may vary, action plans most commonly follow the traffic light model. The green zone indicates asthma that is controlled, the yellow zone forewarns acute loss of control and an impending exacerbation, and the red zone indicates onset of a severe exacerbation requiring a course of systemic corticosteroids and contact with a healthcare provider. The action plans may be based on symptoms or on symptoms and peak expiratory flow (PEF), depending on the preference of the provider and the patient.

The second summary statement describes criteria for recognition of a yellow zone episode. In particular, patients should be advised to take action when they experience an increase in asthma symptoms, increased use of reliever medications, a decrease in their PEF (if they monitor it), or the onset of nocturnal symptoms. In addition, patients with a history of loss of control in response to respiratory tract infections (RTIs) are advised to take action.

The specific action to be taken is dependent on the severity of the episode and the individual response to previous episodes with those interventions. The ideal intervention should provide quick relief of symptoms, prevent progression to the red zone, be safe enough to initiate at home, be convenient and practical for self-administration, be portable so that it is always available, and be cost effective. Obviously, the perfect intervention does not exist; however, some potential interventions have been studied and are discussed below.

Potential interventions for yellow zone treatment include repetitive use of inhaled SABA administered through a metered dose inhaler or nebulizer, scheduled step-up of an ICS, and symptom-driven use of controller with reliever therapy, otherwise known as dynamic dosing or adjustable maintenance dosing (AMD). The regular scheduled use of SABA as the sole treatment for symptoms in the yellow zone is discouraged because it does not consistently prevent progression to the red zone and might increase the risk of progression.

Patients who are treated with daily ICS therapy can be advised to increase their total 24-hour ICS dose, for example, by 4-fold. Increase in the frequency of ICS administration over 24 hours also may result in improved efficacy. The EPR2 guidelines had recommended doubling the dose of ICS; however, EPR3 discouraged the use of doubling ICS doses and instead mentioned that preliminary evidence indicates that quadrupling the dose of an ICS for 7 days, starting at the first appearance of worsening symptoms, may prevent exacerbations requiring oral systemic corticosteroids. The key concept acknowledged in this practice parameter is that each yellow zone episode may require a different amount of supplemental ICS dose to prevent progression. For that reason, symptom-driven ICS use and dynamic dosing are attractive alternative options. In this model, patients receive a larger amount of ICS as they experience increasing loss of asthma control and a smaller amount of ICS as control is achieved. The evidence for dynamic dosing appears to be more consistent to that supporting the scheduled use of increased ICS dose in 24 hours.

Methods for administration of dynamic dosing include (1) separate use of reliever (ie, SABA) and controller inhalers in combination and (2) use of single inhalers that contain a reliever (SABA or quick-onset long-acting β agonists [LABA] such as formoterol) and a controller that is used for symptom relief (with accompanying escalation in controller therapy). Although the 2 approaches are effective, the use of a single inhaler with a reliever (ie, formoterol) and controller (ie, AMD) is more convenient and has been widely studied and used in other countries. A recent evidence-based review demonstrated that the AMD strategy can decrease exacerbations requiring oral corticosteroids (OCSs) compared with current best-practice strategies, although the authors do not recommend use of this approach in children and adolescents younger than 18 years because large-scale studies have not been conducted in this age group. Notably, although inhalers with the desired properties (ie, ICS with formoterol) are available in the United States, the FDA has not approved those inhalers for dynamic dosing or AMD therapy. In fact, the FDA specifically cautions against initiating use, or increasing the dose, of these inhalers during periods of acutely worsening asthma symptoms. As a result, these treatment options for yellow zone management of patients with asthma would be considered off-label in the United States, to be prescribed at the discretion and medical judgment of the individual provider, with additional extra caution to be exercised when using them in patients younger than 18 years.

The practice parameter concludes by briefly discussing additional approaches with limited or no evidence. Although these approaches may be beneficial for individual patients in special circumstances, they are not recommended for general use.

It is the hope of the Yellow Zone Workgroup that routine use of an effective yellow zone intervention for patients as part of an action plan will lead to decreased morbidity and improved quality of life for individuals with asthma. This document also highlights evidence gaps in yellow zone asthma management and strongly recommends conducting clinical trials to further validate the approaches explored in this document and to examine other effective options.

▶ The publication of this new practice parameter addressing management of acute loss of asthma control represented by patients' asthma entering the yellow zone (referring to the Asthma Action Plan) was developed by the Joint Task Force on Practice Parameters, representing the American Academy of Allergy, Asthma and Immunology; the American College of Allergy, Asthma and Immunology; and the Joint Council of Allergy, Asthma and Immunology. Eight summary statements, with defined strength of recommendation and graded evidence, are provided for the healthcare practitioner, along with an exhaustive review of the literature. This document is a must read for all who care for patients with asthma, because entry into the yellow zone represents acute loss of asthma control, and prompt and adequate intervention at this stage offers the opportunity to mitigate the need for entry into the red zone, the need for emergency department visits or hospitalization, and potentially the end result of reduced morbidity and mortality. Kudos to the working group for the labor put into this excellent work product; it is timely indeed and should be the topic of journal clubs in all academic settings, reiterated at all regional/national meetings and a required portion of online continuing medical education courses.

S. K. Willsie, DO, MA

Comprehensive efficacy of omalizumab for severe refractory asthma: a time-series observational study

Tajiri T, Niimi A, Matsumoto H, et al (Kyoto Univ, Japan)

Ann Allergy Asthma Immunol 113:470-475, 2014

Background.—Omalizumab, a humanized anti-IgE monoclonal antibody, is reportedly an effective treatment for severe allergic asthma. However, there have been few comprehensive analyses of its efficacy, including assessments of small airways or airway remodeling.

Objective.—To comprehensively evaluate the efficacy of omalizumab, including its effects on small airways and airway remodeling, in adult patients with severe refractory asthma.

Methods.—In this prospective, time-series, single-arm observational study, 31 adult patients with severe refractory asthma despite the use of multiple controller medications, including high-dose inhaled corticosteroids (1,432 ± 581 μg/d of fluticasone propionate equivalent), were enrolled. Clinical variables, including Asthma Quality of Life Questionnaire, asthma exacerbations, exhaled nitric oxide, pulmonary function, methacholine airway responsiveness, induced sputum, and chest computed tomogram, were assessed at baseline and after 16 and 48 weeks of treatment with omalizumab.

Results.—Twenty-six of the 31 patients completed 48 weeks of treatment. For these patients, Asthma Quality of Life Questionnaire scores and peak expiratory flow values significantly and continuously improved throughout the 48 weeks ($P < .001$ for all comparisons). Unscheduled physician visits, asthma exacerbations requiring systemic corticosteroids, fractional exhaled nitric oxide at 50 mL/s and alveolar nitric oxide levels, sputum eosinophil proportions, and airway-wall thickness as assessed by computed tomography significantly decreased at 48 weeks ($P < .05$ for all comparisons).

Conclusion.—Omalizumab was effective for adult patients with severe refractory asthma. Omalizumab may have anti-inflammatory effects on small airways and reverse airway remodeling.

Trial Registration.—UMIN000002389 (Figs 2-4, Tables 2-4).

▶ Omalizumab, an anti-immunoglobulin E (IgE) monoclonal antibody approved for adjunctive treatment of severe allergic asthma, was prospectively administered every 2 to 4 weeks in addition to stable inhaled corticosteroid doses and other asthma therapy for 48 weeks to 31 subjects with severe refractory asthma. Twenty-six subjects complete the study, which included frequent detailed assessments throughout the study, including pulmonary function: Asthma Quality of Life Questionnaires (AQLQ), asthma exacerbations, exhaled nitric oxide (ENO), methacholine (MC) airway responsiveness, serum IgE levels, induced sputum, and chest computed tomography (CT). Table 2 depicts changes at baseline, 16 weeks, and 48 weeks in the AQLQ, which demonstrated statistically significant and maintained improvement over the 48-week period ($P < .05$). Figs 2-4 depict changes in the rate of unscheduled clinic visits and asthma exacerbations requiring systemic steroids for at least 3 days; changes in fractional ENO vs alveolar NO over time, all statistically significant; and changes across time in peak expiratory flow showing significant improvement ($P < .001$), respectively. Table 3 depicts the results of pulmonary function that did not significantly improve over time, and Table 4 demonstrates the

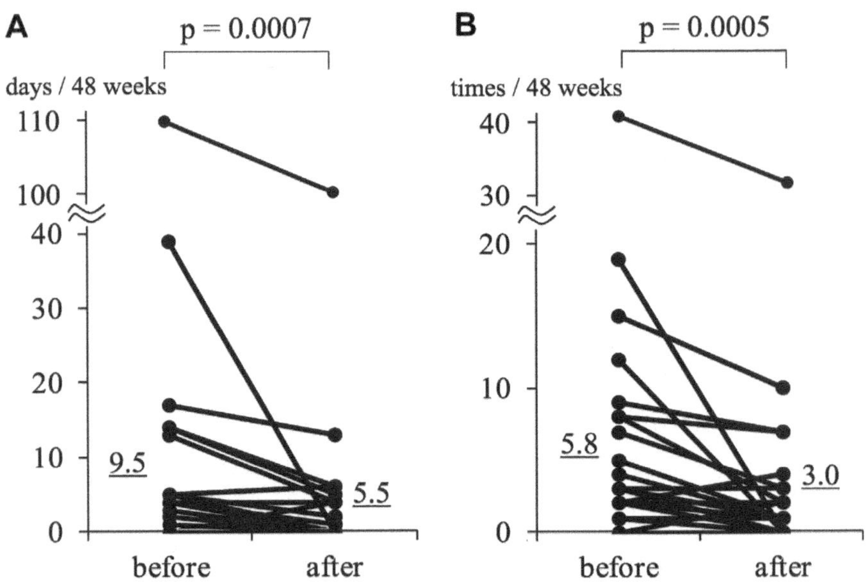

FIGURE 2.—Changes from 48 weeks before treatment to 48 weeks after treatment in *(A)* the rate of unscheduled physician visits and *(B)* the rate of asthma exacerbations that required systemic corticosteroids for at least 3 days. Each point represents a single patient and values indicate means. (Reprinted from Annals of Allergy, Asthma and Immunology. Tajiri T, Niimi A, Matsumoto H, et al. Comprehensive efficacy of omalizumab for severe refractory asthma: a time-series observational study. *Ann Allergy Asthma Immunol.* 2014;113:470-475, Copyright 2014, with permission from American College of Annals of Allergy, Asthma & Immunology.)

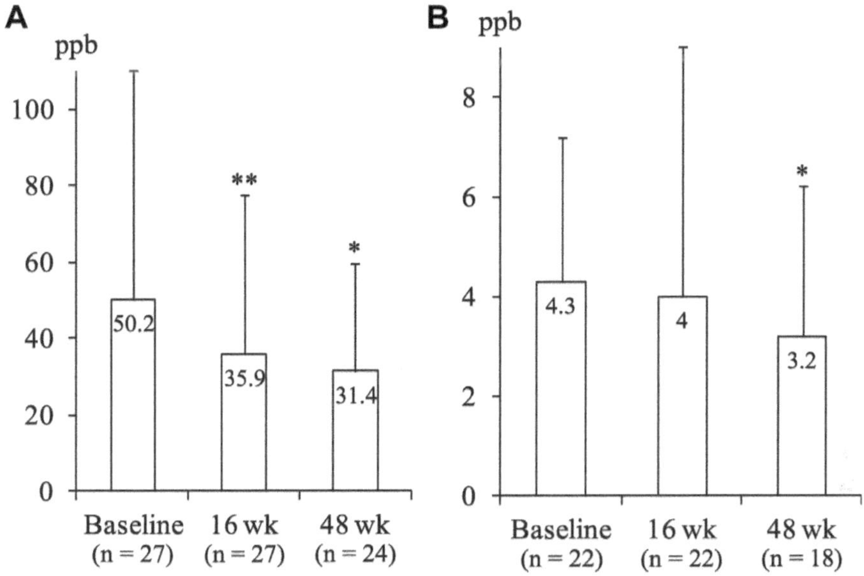

FIGURE 3.—Changes from baseline to 48 weeks of treatment in *(A)* fractional exhaled nitric oxide at 50-mL/s levels and *(B)* alveolar nitric oxide levels. **P* < .05, ***P* < .01 compared with baseline values. Values and bars indicate means and SDs. (Reprinted from Annals of Allergy, Asthma and Immunology. Tajiri T, Niimi A, Matsumoto H, et al. Comprehensive efficacy of omalizumab for severe refractory asthma: a time-series observational study. *Ann Allergy Asthma Immunol.* 2014;113:470-475, Copyright 2014, with permission from American College of Annals of Allergy, Asthma & Immunology.)

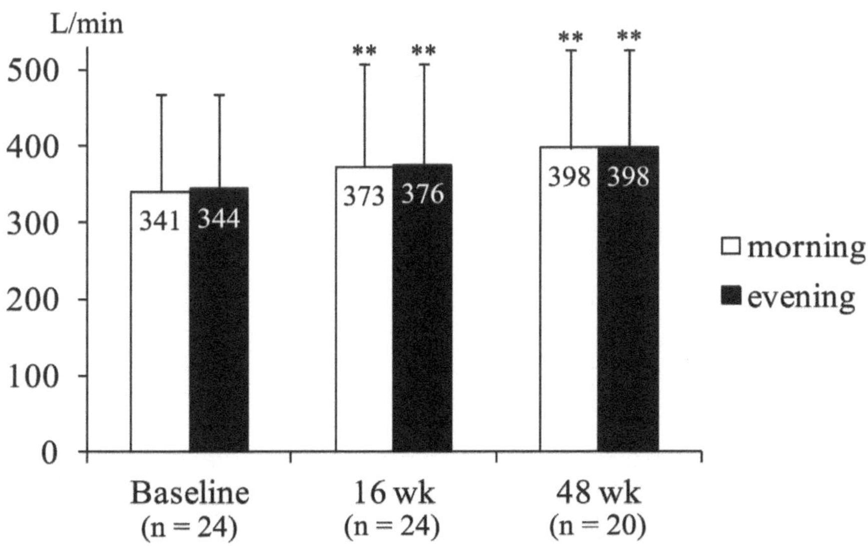

FIGURE 4.—Changes from baseline to 48 weeks of treatment in peak expiratory flow values in the morning and evening. ***P* < .001 compared with baseline values. Values and bars indicate means and SDs. (Reprinted from Annals of Allergy, Asthma and Immunology. Tajiri T, Niimi A, Matsumoto H, et al. Comprehensive efficacy of omalizumab for severe refractory asthma: a time-series observational study. *Ann Allergy Asthma Immunol.* 2014;113:470-475, Copyright 2014, with permission from American College of Annals of Allergy, Asthma & Immunology.)

TABLE 2.—Changes From Baseline and 16 Weeks in SGRQ, AQLQ, and ACQ Scores[a]

Questionnaire and Domain	Baseline (n = 31)	Baseline vs 16 wk (n = 31)	16 vs 48 wk (n = 26)	Baseline vs 48 wk (n = 26)
SGRQ				
Symptoms	65.7 ± 24.1	−10.08[b]	−12.45[c]	−22.49[d]
Activities	51.6 ± 27.8	−4.31	−12.04[b]	−14.41[d]
Impact	40.6 ± 23.4	−9.81[c]	−9.70[c]	−19.08[d]
Total	48.1 ± 23.1	−4.88[b]	−14.81[c]	−18.24[d]
AQLQ				
Symptoms	4.3 ± 1.6	0.97[d]	0.66[c]	1.74[d]
Activities	4.1 ± 1.4	0.59[b]	0.48[c]	1.07[d]
Emotions	4.4 ± 1.6	0.86[c]	0.42[b]	1.29[d]
Environment	4.5 ± 1.7	0.62[b]	0.47[b]	1.09[d]
Overall	4.2 ± 1.4	0.81[c]	0.50[b]	1.36[d]
ACQ				
Total	2.0 ± 1.0	−0.62[c]	−0.37[b]	−1.11[d]

Abbreviations: ACQ, Asthma Control Questionnaire; AQLQ, Asthma Quality of Life Questionnaire; SGRQ, St George's Respiratory Questionnaire.

[a]Values at baseline are presented as mean ± SD. Values at 16 and 48 weeks are average changes in score from baseline values.

[b]$P < .05$ compared with baseline by paired *t* test.

[c]$P < .01$ compared with baseline by paired *t* test.

[d]$P < .001$ compared with baseline by paired *t* test.

Reprinted from Annals of Allergy, Asthma and Immunology. Tajiri T, Niimi A, Matsumoto H, et al. Comprehensive efficacy of omalizumab for severe refractory asthma: a time-series observational study. Ann Allergy Asthma Immunol. 2014;113:470-475, Copyright 2014, with permission from American College of Annals of Allergy, Asthma & Immunology.

TABLE 3.—Effects of Omalizumab on Pulmonary Function[a]

Variables	Baseline (n = 29)	Time Points 16 wk (n = 29)	48 wk (n = 25)	*P* Value[b]
Pulmonary function				
VC (L)	3.02 ± 0.73	3.13 ± 0.75[c]	3.05 ± 0.61	.07
FVC (L)	2.93 ± 0.68	3.02 ± 0.71	2.96 ± 0.61	.41
FEV_1 (L/s)	2.17 ± 0.53	2.25 ± 0.56	2.24 ± 0.55	.09
$FEF_{25\text{-}75}$ (L/s)	1.86 ± 1.01	1.85 ± 1.03	1.89 ± 1.13	.09
RV/TLC (%)	32.1 ± 8.1	31.2 ± 5.6	30.7 ± 6.3	.61
ΔN2	2.52 ± 2.85	2.17 ± 1.95	1.78 ± 1.37	.06
Impulse oscillometry				
R5 (kPa/L/s)	0.41 ± 0.23	0.40 ± 0.22	0.36 ± 0.20	.06
R20 (kPa/L/s)	0.30 ± 0.10	0.29 ± 0.09	0.28 ± 0.10	.07
R5−R20 (kPa/L/s)	0.11 ± 0.15	0.11 ± 0.15	0.08 ± 0.12	.16
AX (kPa/L)	1.13 ± 1.96	1.19 ± 2.09	0.91 ± 1.68	.47

Abbreviations: AX, integrated area of low-frequency reactance; ΔN_2, slope of phase 3 of nitrogen single-breath washout curve; $FEF_{25\text{-}75}$, forced expiratory flow at 25% to 75%; FEV_1, forced expiratory volume in 1 second; FVC, forced vital capacity; R20, respiratory resistance at 20 Hz; R5, respiratory resistance at 5 Hz; R5−R20, difference in respiratory resistance between 5 and 20 Hz; RV, residual volume; TLC, total lung capacity; VC, vital capacity.

[a]Values are presented as mean ± SD.

[b]*P* values for baseline vs 48 weeks by paired *t* test.

[c]$P < .05$ compared with baseline by paired *t* test.

Reprinted from Annals of Allergy, Asthma and Immunology. Tajiri T, Niimi A, Matsumoto H, et al. Comprehensive efficacy of omalizumab for severe refractory asthma: a time-series observational study. Ann Allergy Asthma Immunol. 2014;113:470-475, Copyright 2014, Copyright 2014, with permission from American College of Annals of Allergy, Asthma & Immunology.

TABLE 4.—Effects of Omalizumab on Computed Tomographic Indices[a]

	Time Points			
	Baseline	16 wk[b]	48 wk	*P* Value[c]
Airway dimensions	21	21	14	
WA (mm^2)	30.3 ± 12.6	29.5 ± 12.5	26.0 ± 7.6	.09
WA/BSA (mm^2/m^2)	18.6 ± 8.2	18.1 ± 7.9	11.0 ± 3.3	.09
WA%	62.0 ± 7.2	60.6 ± 7.3	57.1 ± 6.2	.002
Ao (mm^2)	49.7 ± 21.7	48.9 ± 21.5	45.6 ± 13.1	.51
Ao/BSA (mm^2/m^2)	30.6 ± 13.8	30.1 ± 13.5	27.9 ± 7.2	.54
Ai (mm^2)	19.5 ± 9.8	19.4 ± 9.9	19.6 ± 6.6	.024
Ai/BSA (mm^2/m^2)	12.0 ± 6.1	12.0 ± 6.2	12.1 ± 4.0	.025
Lung density	24	24	17	
LAA% of inspiratory scans	22.2 ± 7.6	22.4 ± 6.5	24.8 ± 5.1	.07
LAA% of expiratory scans	9.8 ± 4.9	10.4 ± 6.6	9.9 ± 4.6	.43
E/I ratio of LAA%	0.51 ± 0.51	0.46 ± 0.27	0.39 ± 0.15	.89
MLD of inspiratory scans (HU)	−859.7 ± 35.6	−863.4 ± 28.4	−874.0 ± 16.9	.10
MLD of expiratory scans (HU)	−761.6 ± 58.9	−762.6 ± 62.6	−764.8 ± 50.3	.71
E/I ratio of MLD	0.89 ± 0.06	0.88 ± 0.06	0.87 ± 0.05	.78

Abbreviations: Ai, luminal area; Ao, outer area of bronchus; BSA, body surface area; E/I ratio, percentage of low-attenuation area to lung area and mean lung density on inspiratory and expiratory computed tomographic scans and the ratios of these values at expiration to the respective values at inspiration; LAA%, percentage of low-attenuation area to lung area; MLD, mean lung density; WA%, percentage of wall area equal to wall area divided by outer area of bronchus multiplied by 100; WA, wall area.

[a]Values are presented as number of patients or mean ± SD.

[b]$P > .05$ for all indices compared with baseline by paired t test.

[c]P value for baseline vs 48 weeks by paired t test.

results of chest CT, which showed evidence of statistically significant increase in luminal area and wall area/outer area of bronchus (%WA) at 48 weeks but not at 16 weeks. The reduced %WA seen at 48 weeks was associated with a reduced ENO and sputum eosinophil numbers. These same type of CT changes have been suggested to be associated with possible reversal in airway remodeling.[1] These results add to the body of knowledge related to using this drug in severe refractory asthma. The data regarding the potential for reversal of airway remodeling, albeit in limited numbers of subjects, holds potential promise for the future, pending confirmation by larger prospective, randomized studies.

S. K. Willsie, DO, MA

Reference

1. Niimi A, Matsumoto H, Amitani R, et al. Effect of short-term treatment with inhaled corticosteroid on airway wall thickening in asthma. *Am J Med.* 2004; 116:725-731.

Impact of exhaled nitric oxide measurements on treatment decisions in an asthma specialty clinic

LaForce C, Brooks E, Herje N, et al (North Carolina Clinical Res, Raleigh; Reimbursement Principles, Littleton, CO; Aerocrine, Inc, Morrisville, NC; et al)

Ann Allergy Asthma Immunol 113:619-623, 2014

Background.—Asthma management in an outpatient setting is best accomplished by clinical evaluation coupled with spirometry and symptom evaluation, but these assessments do not provide information about airway inflammation. Exhaled nitric oxide (fraction of exhaled nitric oxide [FeNO]) measures T-helper cell type 2–mediated airway inflammation and may be a useful adjunct in asthma management.

Objective.—To determine whether the use of FeNO in the specialist management of asthma results in more effective and cost-effective treatment decisions.

Methods.—Fifty subjects 7 to 60 years old with established asthma participated in this observational study. Subjects were evaluated by clinical examination, spirometry, and symptom assessment using the Asthma Control Test, and clinicians estimated airway inflammation and made treatment decisions based on these assessments. Then, FeNO was measured, and changes in therapy based on FeNO levels were documented. The estimated cost impact of using FeNO was calculated presuming ongoing FeNO use in patient management.

Results.—Without FeNO, the clinician's assessment of airway inflammation was incorrectly classified in 50% of subjects. FeNO results substantially altered treatment decisions in more than one third of subjects, notably medication augmentation in 10 (20%) and medication decreases in 8 (16%). Use of FeNO in addition to standard of care was estimated to save $629 per subject per year.

Conclusion.—Measurement of FeNO augments routine clinical assessment of asthma by measuring airway inflammation. Knowledge of FeNO affects medication treatment decisions to augment or decrease pharmacotherapy, which has important long-term asthma management implications, most notably the potential to lower the costs and morbidity associated with asthma exacerbation.

Trial Registration.—ClinicalTrials.gov identifier NCT01729247 (Tables 2, 4 and 6).

► Previous investigations have indicated that high levels of exhaled nitric oxide (ENO) portend uncontrolled asthma and increased risk of deterioration and potential for future deterioration.[1-3] This interesting single-center, single-observation study of children and adults with asthma measured ENO after completion of clinician assessment of asthma stability. The clinician was not provided with the results of the ENO levels until all medical decision making had been completed. Table 2 compares and depicts measured ENO vs clinician appraisal of inflammatory status and expected ENO level in each subject. In more than 50% of the cases, the level of severity/inflammation was underestimated

TABLE 2.—Airway Inflammation: Subjects Categorized by Clinical Appraisal vs Observed FeNO Levels

Observed FeNO Level of Airway Inflammation	Clinical Appraisal of Airway Inflammation Low	Intermediate	High	Total
Low	21 (42%)	7 (14%)	1 (2%)	29 (58%)
Intermediate	7 (14%)	3 (6%)	0	10 (20%)
High	6 (12%)	4 (8%)	1 (2%)	11 (22%)
Total	34 (68%)	14 (28%)	2 (4%)	

Abbreviation: FeNO, fraction of exhaled nitric oxide.

based on spirometry, Asthmas Control Test questionnaire, and clinician assessment. Table 4 details medication changes made by the clinician after being provided with the measured ENO levels for each asthmatic. Thirty-six percent of subjects had a medication change made by the clinician following review of the ENO level review: 20% of subjects had their inhaled corticosteroid (ICS) dose increased; 2 subjects who were on moderate to high doses of ICS had leukotriene modifiers added to their medication regimen. Table 6 provides estimated annual asthma management costs per subjects in the case of using ENO levels at each visit; note that the overall asthma cost saves shows that

TABLE 4.—Asthma Medication Changes Based on FeNO Results

	Overall (N = 50)
Overall	
No change	32 (64%)
Added medication or increased medication dose	10 (20%)
Subtracted medication or decreased medication dose	8 (16%)
OCS	
No change	50 (100%)
Added or increased dose	0
Subtracted or decreased dose	0
ICS-LABA	
No change	46 (92%)
Added or increased dose	3 (6%)
Subtracted or decreased dose	1 (2%)
ICS	
No change	35 (70%)
Added or increased dose	8 (16%)
Subtracted or decreased dose	7 (14%)
LTRA	
No change	47 (94%)
Added or increased dose	2 (4%)
Subtracted or decreased dose	1 (2%)

Abbreviations: ICS, inhaled corticosteroid; ICS-LABA, inhaled corticosteroid plus long-acting β agonist; LTRA, leukotriene receptor antagonist; OCS, oral corticosteroid.

TABLE 6.—Estimated Annual Asthma Management Costs (per Subject)

	Maintenance Medications (US$)	Exacerbations (US$)[a]	Scheduled Physician Office Visits (US$)[b]	All Asthma-Related Care (US$)
Standard guidelines	1,601.16	864.37	281.68	2,747.21
FeNO in addition to standard guidelines	1,376.30	410.90	331.48	2,118.38

Abbreviation: FeNO, fraction of exhaled nitric oxide.
[a]Includes direct payer costs of unscheduled physician office visits, outpatient visits, hospital emergency department visits, inpatient hospitalizations, FeNO testing, spirometry, and rescue medications.
[b]Includes level III physician office visits, FeNO testing, and spirometry.

utilization of ENO would actually lead to significant cost savings related to reduced exacerbation costs, increase in scheduled office visits, and overall reduction in all asthma-related care. Unstated in the table's depiction is the overall reduction of asthma morbidity due to fewer cases of emergency department visits and hospitalizations related to underestimation of asthma severity. It's time that point-of-care testing for ENO becomes routine in the care of asthma.

S. K. Willsie, DO, MA

References

1. Agache I, Ciobanu C. Predictive value of lung function trend and FENO for difficult asthma in children. *J Investig Allergol Clin Immunol.* 2012;22:419-426.
2. Dweik RA, Sorkness RL, Wenzel S, et al. Use of exhaled nitric oxide measurement to identify a reactive, at risk phenotype among patients with asthma. *Am J Respir Crit Care Med.* 2010;181:1033-1041.
3. van Veen IH, Ten Brinke A, Sterk PJ, et al. Exhaled nitric oxide predicts lung function decline in difficult to treat asthma. *Eur Resp J.* 2008;32:344-349.

36 Chronic Obstructive Pulmonary Disease

The association between childhood asthma and adult chronic obstructive pulmonary disease

Tai A, Tran H, Roberts M, et al (Women's and Children's Hosp, Adelaide, South Australia, Australia; Murdoch Children's Res Inst, Melbourne, Victoria, Australia; Royal Children's Hosp Melbourne, Victoria, Australia; et al)

Thorax 69:805-810, 2014

Introduction.—There is epidemiological evidence to suggest that events in childhood influence lung growth and constitute a significant risk for adult COPD. The aim of the study is to evaluate for an association between childhood asthma and adult COPD.

Methods.—This longitudinal, prospective study of 6–7-year-old children with asthma has been regularly reviewed every 7 years to the current analysis at 50 years of age. Participants completed respiratory questionnaires and lung function spirometry with postbronchodilator response. At the age of 50, subjects were classified to the following subgroups: non-asthmatics, asthma remission, current asthma and COPD which was defined by FEV_1 to FVC ratio postbronchodilator of less than 0.7.

Results.—Of the remaining survivors, 346 participated in the current study (participation rate of 76%) of whom 197 completed both questionnaire and lung function testing. As compared with children without symptoms of wheeze to the age of 7, (non-asthmatics) children with severe asthma had an adjusted 32 times higher risk for developing COPD (95% CI 3.4 to 269). In this cohort, 43% of the COPD group had never smoked. There was no evidence of a difference in the rate of decline in FEV_1 (mL/year, 95th CI) between the COPD group (17, 10 to 23) and the other groups: non-asthmatics (16, 12 to 21), asthma remission (20, 16 to 24) and current asthma (19, 13 to 25).

Conclusions.—Children with severe asthma are at increased risk of developing COPD.

► Adult chronic obstructive pulmonary disorder (COPD) is an amalgam of many diseases, the most common of which are tobacco-related, inhalation of toxic materials, and genetic mutations. It has long been suggested that another determinant of adult lung obstruction is airway disease as a child. In a large cohort of adults older than 20 years and followed for 20 years from the

American Southwest, the presence of childhood asthma had a large impact on the development of subsequent obstructive disease in adulthood.[1] This report is of a study of children started more than 40 years ago. The cohort of asthmatic children has been reviewed every 7 years until age 50. At age 50, of the 34 patients with severe asthma as children, nearly half had a diagnosis of COPD. This represented a far greater percentage of patients progressing to COPD than any other group with lesser degrees of asthma or wheezing. In fact, children with these lesser degrees of airway disease did not appear to be at increased risk of adult obstructive disease. Forty plus years ago, of course, the medications available for managing asthma and the general approach to management were much less effective than today's antiinflammatory/bronchodilator approach. Hopefully, current management with good control will reduce the impact of childhood on adult lung health.

J. R. Maurer, MD

Reference

1. Silva GE, Sherrill DL, Guerra S, Barbee RA. Asthma as a risk factor for COPD in a longitudinal study. *Chest.* 2004;126:59-65.

Pneumothorax Risk Factors in Smokers with and without Chronic Obstructive Pulmonary Disease

Hobbs BD, the COPDGene Investigators (Brigham and Women's Hosp and Harvard Med School, Boston, MA; et al)
Ann Am Thorac Soc 11:1387-1394, 2014

Rationale.—The demographic, physiological, and computed tomography (CT) features associated with pneumothorax in smokers with and without chronic obstructive pulmonary disease (COPD) are not clearly defined.

Objectives.—We evaluated the hypothesis that pneumothorax in smokers is associated with male sex, tall and thin stature, airflow obstruction, and increased total and subpleural emphysema.

Methods.—The study included smokers with and without COPD from the COPDGene Study, with quantitative chest CT analysis. Pleural-based emphysema was assessed on the basis of local histogram measures of emphysema. Pneumothorax history was defined by subject self-report.

Measurements and Main Results.—Pneumothorax was reported in 286 (3.2%) of 9,062 participants. In all participants, risk of prior pneumothorax was significantly higher in men (odds ratio [OR], 1.55; 95% confidence interval [CI], 1.08–2.22) and non-Hispanic white subjects (OR, 1.90; 95% CI, 1.34–2.69). Risk of prior pneumothorax was associated with increased percent CT emphysema in all participants and participants with COPD (OR, 1.04 for each 1% increase in emphysema; 95% CI,

1.03–1.06). Increased pleural-based emphysema was independently associated with risk of past pneumothorax in all participants (OR, 1.05 for each 1% increase; 95% CI, 1.01–1.10). In smokers with normal spirometry, risk of past pneumothorax was associated with non-Hispanic white race and lifetime smoking intensity (OR, 1.20 for every 10 pack-years; 95% CI, 1.09–1.33).

Conclusions.—Among smokers, pneumothorax is associated with male sex, non-Hispanic white race, and increased percentage of total and subpleural CT emphysema. Pneumothorax was not independently associated with height or lung function, even in participants with COPD.

Clinical trial registered with www.clinicaltrials.gov (NCT00608764).

▶ Pulmonary lore surrounding the occurrence of primary spontaneous pneumothoraces (not those occurring in the context of diseases that predispose to pneumothorax, such as lymphangioleiomyomatosis or chronic obstructive pulmonary disease [COPD]) is that they occur in tall, thin males; smokers; and in the presence of atmospheric pressure changes. Studies have identified subpleural blebs as well as decreased lung density on computed tomography (CT) in many of the patients who develop spontaneous pneumothoraces.[1,2] Secondary spontaneous pneumothoraces occur in the context of known disease, most commonly COPD. In COPD, severe disease has been reported to be associated with more pneumothoraces, which can be a devastating complication.[3] However, these anecdotal risk factors have not previously been verified by a large, population-based study. In this report, the investigators looked at a population of more than 9000 patients in the COPD Genetic Epidemiology (COPDGene) Study to get a more complete and accurate view of the demographics of pneumothorax and the associated risk factors. This included a large population of smokers with a broad range of lung function values. The authors were particularly interested in the difference in risk factors for pneumothorax in patients with COPD compared with those with normal spirometry. Their hypothesis was to test the traditionally held beliefs about the demographics of patients who develop pneumothorax in this large population. In addition, they hypothesized that quantitative CT measures of pleural-based emphysema would be associated with histories of pneumothorax. The results were mixed. To start, the entire population smoked, so these are risk factors within smokers. Risk factors included male sex and increased percentage of total and subpleural emphysematous changes. However, neither height nor lung function were supported as risk factors, the latter contradicting previous cohort studies. In smokers with normal spirometry, risk of pneumothorax increased with increased pack-years of smoking. Of particular interest was the finding that non-Hispanic white patients had a greater risk than African-Americans in that two-thirds of the population was non-Hispanic white, but 80% of the pneumothoraces occurred in that group. This latter finding was noted both in patients with normal and abnormal spirometry and deserves more investigation.

J. R. Maurer, MD

References

1. Casali C, Stefani A, Ligabue G, et al. Role of blebs and bullae detected by high-resolution computed tomography and recurrent spontaneous pneumothorax. *Ann Thorac Surg*. 2013;95:249-255.
2. Lesur O, Delorme N, Fromaget JM, Bernadac P, Polu JM. Computed tomography in the etiologic assessment of idiopathic spontaneous pneumothorax. *Chest*. 1990; 98:341-347.
3. Sahn SA, Heffner JE. Spontaneous pneumothorax. *N Engl J Med*. 2000;342: 868-874.

Prognostic evaluation of COPD patients: GOLD 2011 versus BODE and the COPD comorbidity index COTE

de Torres JP, Casanova C, Marín JM, et al (Clínica Universidad de Navarra, Pamplona, Spain; Hospital Ntra Sra de Candelaria, Tenerife, Spain; Hospital Universitario Miguel Servet, Zaragoza, Spain; et al)

Thorax 69:799-804, 2014

Background.—The Global Obstructive Lung Disease (GOLD) 2011 revision recommends the multidimensional assessment of COPD including comorbidities and has developed a disease categories system (ABCD) attempting to implement this strategy. The added value provided by quantifying comorbidities and integrating them to multidimensional indices has not been explored.

Objective.—Compare the prognostic value of the GOLD ABCD categories versus the BMI, Obstruction, Dyspnea, Exercise (BODE) index, and explore the added prognostic value of comorbidities evaluation to this multidimensional assessment.

Methods.—From the patients who have been enrolled in the BODE study, we selected the most recent ones who had the available information needed to classify them by the ABCD GOLD categories. Cox proportional hazards ratios for all-cause mortality were performed for GOLD categories and BODE index. The added value of the comorbidity Copd cOmorbidity TEst (COTE) index was also explored using receiver operating curves (ROC) values.

Results.—707 patients were followed for 50 ± 30 months including all degrees of airway limitation and BODE index severity. ABCD GOLD predicted global mortality (HR: 1.47; 95% CI 1.28 to 1.70) as did the BODE index (HR: 2.02; 95% CI 1.76 to 2.31). Area under the curve (AUC) of ROC for ABCD GOLD was 0.68; (95% CI 0.64 to 0.73) while for the BODE index was 0.71 (95% CI 0.67 to 0.76). The C statistics value was significantly higher for the observed difference. Adding the COTE index to the BODE index improved its AUC to 0.81 (95% CI 0.77 to 0.85), ($\chi^2 = 40.28$, $p < 0.001$).

Conclusions.—In this population of COPD patients, the BODE index had a better survival prediction than the ABCD GOLD categories. Adding the COTE to the BODE index was complimentary and significantly improved outcome prediction.

▶ De Torres and colleagues present an interesting study in which they used chronic obstructive pulmonary disease (COPD) patients from the BODE (body mass index, obstruction, dyspnea, and exercise capacity) cohort to compare prognostic value of the GOLD 2011 guidelines to the BODE index.[1,2] In 2011, the Global Obstructive Lung Disease guidelines were changed to include not only degree of airway obstruction but also the phenotype or clinical components of the disease in the individual patient. Four groupings reflected a combination of either more or less airway obstruction in conjunction with more or fewer symptoms/hospitalizations. Although this change in the GOLD guidelines was designed to assist in appropriate management of COPD and not to serve as a prognostic tool, a number of studies have tried to compare the prognostic value (in terms of survival) of this enhanced model with the traditional approach that classified patients only by degree of airway obstruction. The traditional approach was notoriously poor at predicting survivals. However, the multifactorial BODE mode has been much better at this. De Torres et al assess the prognostic value of the GOLD model against the prognostic value of BODE and find the BODE index to be slightly better across the severity classifications of COPD in predicting survival. The most interesting part of this study is not the comparison of BODE versus GOLD, but rather the addition of patient medical comorbidities into the predictive model. The investigators used a comorbidity index called COTE (COPD Comorbidity Test Index) developed by many of this same group of investigators and published by Divo et al.[3] The COTE index includes 12 comorbidities that were shown previously in the BODE cohort of COPD patients to be associated with increased mortality. A scoring system was developed to incorporate these comorbidities into the overall prediction algorithm. Adding the COTE score to the BODE index greatly improved the ability to estimate prognosis (Fig 3 in the original article). The authors apparently did not try adding COTE to the GOLD categories, so the predictive value of GOLD + COTE is not known. The addition of comorbidities is a critical piece in understanding the progression of COPD through patients' disease, as is illustrated here. The approach to COPD patients has tended to be disease-specific and not whole-person oriented. That has often led to inadequate management of comorbidities such as coronary artery disease, heart failure, and depression, possibly contributing to earlier deaths. We need more prospective evaluation of the most beneficial whole-person management approaches to the COPD patient.

J. R. Maurer, MD

References

1. Celli BR, Cote C, Marin JM, et al. The body mass index, airflow obstruction, dyspnea, exercise performance (BODE) index in chronic obstructive pulmonary disease. *N Engl J Med.* 2004;350:1005-1012.

2. GOLD. Documents and resources. http://www.goldcopd.org/Guidelines/guidelines-resources.html. Accessed December 29, 2014.
3. Divo M, Cote C, de Torres JP, et al; BODE Collaborative Group. Comorbidities and risk of mortality in patients with chronic obstructive pulmonary disease. *Am J Respir Crit Care Med.* 2012;186:155-161.

Performance of the BODE index in patients with α_1-antitrypsin deficiency-related COPD

Thabut G, Mornex J-F, Pison C, et al (APHP, Paris, France; Hospices Civils de Lyon, France; Clinique Universitaire de Pneumologie CHU Grenoble, France; et al)
Eur Respir J 44:78-86, 2014

The BODE (body mass index, airflow obstruction, dyspnoea and exercise capacity) index is used to decide on referral and transplantation of patients with chronic obstructive pulmonary disease (COPD). The BODE index has not been validated in patients with α_1-antitrypsin deficiency, who account for 15% of COPD patients undergoing lung transplantation. We sought to validate the BODE index in α_1-antitrypsin deficiency-related COPD.

We assessed the prognostic value of the BODE index in 191 patients followed from 2006 to 2012 in a French prospective cohort of patients with α_1-antitrypsin deficiency.

20 patients died during follow-up and 22 underwent lung transplantation. Survival (95% CI) was 93.0% (91.7–94.3%) at 3 years and 76.0% (72.9–79.1%) at 5 years. The 3-year survival was 97.4% (96.6–98.2%), 98.0% (96.7–99.3%), 87.7% (84.5–90.9%) and 75.3% (66.0–84.6%) for patients with BODE index 0–2, 3–4, 5–6 and 7–10, respectively. Survival discrimination of the BODE index was better than with both forced expiratory volume in 1 s and Global Initiative for Chronic Obstructive Lung Disease classification. Regarding calibration, expected survival by BODE index was noticeably lower than observed survival.

The BODE index showed very good survival discrimination in patients with α_1-antitrypsin deficiency-related COPD. Larger studies are needed to support its use to drive patient referral for lung transplantation.

▶ The BODE index (using measures of body mass index, obstruction, dyspnea, and exercise capacity) was the first multidimensional and now well-validated model designed to predict the progression and approximate survival of patients with chronic obstructive pulmonary disorder (COPD).[1] The value of the index is that it takes into account not only the patient's lung function but also elements of the multisystem nature of the disease, such as exercise capacity and nutritional status. BODE was, however, developed and validated primarily in patients who had smoking-related disease. That cohort of COPD patients is generally at least a decade older than patients with alpha-1 antitrypsin deficiency disease, and they have many of the comorbidities related to smoking such as coronary artery disease. However, because the BODE index has been the most useful and best validated prognosticator for COPD patients, it is often used for alpha-1 antitrypsin-deficient patients to determine when to refer them to transplant centers. Despite the use of BODE in this population, some have suspected that it is not as accurate a prognostic tool as in tobacco-related disease. This study, which is ongoing, uses a national cohort of alpha-1 antitrypsin-deficient emphysema patients and is longitudinally following the cohort with BODE measurements. Although BODE was much better at predicting survival that lung function alone, it was not as sensitive in this population as in the original test populations; the BODE index underestimated survival and will probably require changes to be of optimal use in alpha-1 antitrypsin-deficient patients.

Another study, published this year, authored by Ringbaek et al followed a national cohort of all patients with COPD started on long-term oxygen therapy between January 1994 and December 2010.[2] Alpha-1 antitrypsin-deficient patients in this cohort were on average 17 years younger than other COPD patients and had significantly fewer medical comorbidities. Even adjusting for the comorbidities, however, as well as age and gender, alpha-1 antitrypsin-deficient patients had a significantly lower risk of death. Both types of COPD are systemic diseases in different ways; however, the ubiquitous effects of tobacco clearly result in the greatest whole-body morbidity.

J. R. Maurer, MD

References

1. Celli BR, Cote CG, Marin JM, et al. The body-mass index, airflow obstruction, dyspnea, and exercise capacity index in chronic obstructive pulmonary disease. *N Engl J Med.* 2004;350:1005-1012.
2. Ringbaek TJ, Seersholm N, Perch M, Iversen M, Lange P. Prognosis of patients with alpha1-antitrypsine deficiency on long-term oxygen therapy. *Respir Med.* 2014;108:1189-1194.

Physical Activity as a Predictor of Thirty-Day Hospital Readmission after a Discharge for a Clinical Exacerbation of Chronic Obstructive Pulmonary Disease

Chawla H, Bulathsinghala C, Tejada JP, et al (Univ of Connecticut, Farmington)
Ann Am Thorac Soc 11:1203-1209, 2014

Rationale.—Because physical inactivity in chronic obstructive pulmonary disease (COPD) predicts health care use and mortality, we prospectively evaluated the relationship of this variable to the frequency of 30-day readmissions after a hospitalization for an exacerbation.

Methods.—Consented patients discharged after an exacerbation of COPD were asked to wear a GT3X+ accelerometer (ActiGraph, Pensacola, FL) continuously on the wrist for 30 days after hospital discharge. Vector magnitude units (VMU), the sum of movements in three planes over each minute of use, were recorded. Higher physical activity for each minute was defined by a VMU threshold of at least 3,000 counts.

Those patients with fewer than 60 minutes/day over the first week were considered inactive.

Measurements and Main Results.—Fifty-four study patients were discharged from the hospital and 38 underwent activity testing. In the latter subgroup, all-cause hospital readmissions within 30 days occurred in 12 patients (32%). Minutes of higher physical activity per day over the first week after discharge were considerably lower in those eventually readmitted than in those who remained as outpatients: 42 ± 14 (SE) versus 114 ± 19 minutes, respectively ($P = 0.02$). In addition, physical activity decreased over time in those who were eventually readmitted, but increased in those who were not readmitted. Those with lower physical activity over Week 1 after discharge were more likely to have 30-day all-cause readmissions than those with higher activity: odds ratio, 6.7, $P = 0.02$. In multivariate testing, both physical inactivity and a history of two or more hospitalizations for exacerbations in the preceding year predicted 30-day readmission.

Conclusions.—These findings underscore the importance of physical activity as a predictor of this type of health care use outcome.

▶ The finding that higher levels of physical activity is an independent predictor of better survivals has recently been reported for a number of chronic illnesses ranging from cancer to cardiac disease to diabetes.[1-3] Exercise capacity measured by a 6-minute walk in 1 of the 4 components of the BODE (body mass index, airway obstruction, dyspnea, and exercise capacity) is one of the best prognostic tools for expected survival in chronic obstructive pulmonary disease (COPD).[4] Furthermore, several studies have consistently identified low levels of physical activity with exacerbations and mortality.[5] This study by Chawla et al identified lower levels of physical activity, probably not surprisingly, as predictive of that group of recently discharged COPD patients who would require readmission. In addition to low levels of activity, decreasing levels of activity postdischarge also predicted both pulmonary and all-cause admissions. This is an important finding because it can identify those patients likely to fall within Medicare's Hospital Readmission Reduction Program, which penalizes hospitals for excessive readmissions within 30 days of discharge. Early identification of at-risk patients should allow increased interventions aimed at increasing levels of activity and keeping them out of hospital—a win-win both for the patient and for the hospitals! However, to achieve this goal, it is important to understand the determinants of physical activity in COPD patients. Although that may seem like a simple task, there is an incomplete understanding of the determinants of physical activity in these patients. A recent systematic review aimed to identify and summarize studies assessing associations between physical activity and its determinants and/or outcomes in COPD patients. Almost all of the 86 studies included in the review were based on low- or very low-quality evidence and often were cross-sectional.[5] Although moderate-level evidence was found relating the impact of low physical activity on mortality and exacerbations, only poor-quality evidence was identified regarding determinants of low physical activity, including the impact of attempted treatments.

To design successful interventions to improve physical activity in these patients, much more research is required into the underlying determinants, likely multifactorial, of this problem.

J. R. Maurer, MD

References

1. Nocon M, Hiemann T, Müller-Riemenschneider F, Thalau F, Roll S, Willich SN. Association of physical activity with all-cause and cardiovascular mortality: a systematic review and meta-analysis. *Eur J Cardiovasc Prev Rehabil.* 2008;15:239-246.
2. Cassileth BR, Yarett I, Lemanne D. Fitness: can exercise lengthen survival in patients with cancer? *The ASCO Post.* 2013;6, http://www.ascopost.com. Accessed December 29, 2014.
3. Sigal RJ, Kenny GP, Wasserman DH, Castaneda-Sceppa C. Physical activity/exercise and type 2 diabetes. *Diabetes Care.* 2004;27:2518-2534.
4. Celli BR, Cote CG, Marin JM, et al. The body-mass index, airflow obstruction, dyspnea, exercise capacity index in chronic obstructive pulmonary disease. *N Engl J Med.* 2004;350:1005-1012.
5. Gimeno-Santos E, Frei A, Steurer-Stey C, on behalf of PROactive consortium. Determinants and outcomes of physical activity in patients with COPD: a systematic review. *Thorax.* 2014;69:731-739.

Coronary artery calcification is increased in patients with COPD and associated with increased morbidity and mortality

Williams MC, for the Evaluation of COPD Longitudinally to Identify Predictive Surrogate Endpoints (ECLIPSE) investigators (Univ of Edinburgh/British Heart Foundation Centre for Cardiovascular Science, UK; et al)
Thorax 69:718-723, 2014

Background.—Coronary artery calcification is pathognomonic of coronary artery disease (CAD). Whether CAD in patients with COPD is linked to lung function, functional capacity and/or clinically relevant outcomes is unknown. The objective was to assess the association between CAD and disease severity, functional capacity and outcomes in patients with COPD.

Methods.—Coronary artery calcium score (CACS; Agatston score) was measured using chest CT in patients with COPD, smokers with normal spirometry and nonsmokers from the Evaluation of COPD Longitudinally to Identify Predictive Surrogate Endpoints (ECLIPSE) study.

Results.—CACS was measured in 942 subjects: 672 with COPD (mean age ± SD, 63 ± 7 years; FEV1 49 ± 16% predicted), 199 smokers with normal spirometry (54 ± 9 years; FEV_1 110 ± 12% predicted) and 71 nonsmokers (55 ± 9 years; FEV_1 114 ± 14% predicted). CACS was higher in patients with COPD than smokers or non-smokers (median (IQR), 128 (492) vs 0 (75) vs 0 (3) Agatston units (AU), $p < 0.001$). In patients with COPD, CACS correlated with age, pack-years, 6 min walking distance, modified Medical Research Council Dyspnoea score and circulating levels of interleukin (IL)-6, IL-8, Clara Cell protein 16, surfactant protein D and peripheral blood neutrophil count, but not with emphysema, exacerbation frequency, % predicted FEV1 or decline in FEV1. CACS was higher in patients with COPD who died than in those who survived until 3-year follow-up (CACS 406 vs 103 AU, $p < 0.001$), and was associated with mortality in a Cox proportional hazards model ($p = 0.036$).

Conclusions.—Patients with COPD have more CAD than controls and this is associated with increased dyspnoea, reduced exercise capacity and increased mortality. These data indicate that the presence of CAD in patients with COPD is associated with poor clinical outcomes (Fig 1).

▶ Cardiac disease is widely recognized as one of the most common medical comorbidities in patients with chronic obstructive pulmonary disease (COPD). Indeed, the primary differential diagnosis in patients presenting with a respiratory decompensation in their health status is often COPD exacerbation versus heart failure. The coexistence of cardiac disease and COPD is not surprising because both have tobacco as a common causative agent.

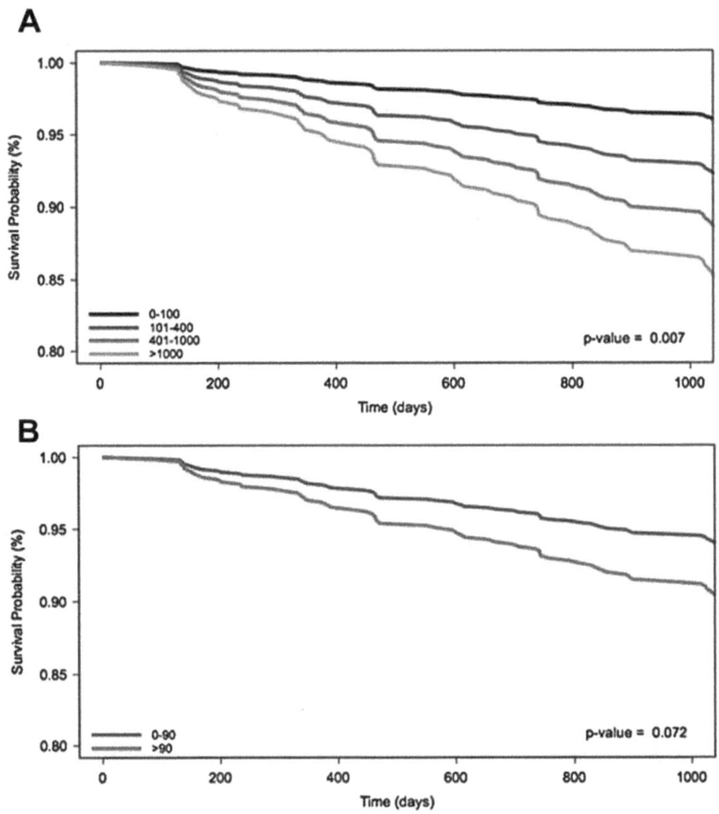

FIGURE 1.—Cox proportional hazards model for patients with COPD and (A) coronary artery calcium score (CACS) (Agatston score)adjusted for age, gender, pack-years, severity of COPD and self-reported cardiovascular disease and (B) CACSP adjusted for pack-years. (Reproduced from Thorax. Williams MC, for the Evaluation of COPD Longitudinally to Identify Predictive Surrogate Endpoints (ECLIPSE) investigators. Coronary artery calcification is increased in patients with COPD and associated with increased morbidity and mortality. *Thorax.* 2014;69:718-723, with permission from the BMJ Publishing Group Ltd.)

Nevertheless, the relationship between cardiac disease and COPD is complex and poorly studied or understood. For example, COPD remains an independent predictor of coronary artery disease once adjustments are made for smoking and other cardiovascular risk factors.[1] Smoking and coronary disease are associated with low-grade inflammation, oxidative stress, and the downstream effects of circulating inflammatory markers. One way to assess and better define coronary artery disease in COPD patients is to look at coronary artery calcium scores (CACS) on computed tomography (CT) scans. CACS are pathognomonic of coronary artery disease and can help determine the prevalence of coronary artery disease among patients. CACS, although associated with increased mortality in smokers,[2] have not been clearly associated with inflammatory markers.[3] However, CACS are useful in stratifying risk for coronary disease, and this has not been done systematically in COPD patients. The authors sought to determine whether there was a relationship between CACS in these patients and long-term outcomes such as mortality, exacerbations, and FEV_1 (forced expiratory volume in 1 second) decline. They used CT data gathered during the Evaluation of COPD Longitudinally to Identify Predictive Surrogate Endpoints (ECLIPSE) study to do this.[4] Not surprisingly, the incidence of coronary artery calcium was higher in COPD patients than in controls, and higher CACS (Fig 1), an indicator of comorbid coronary artery disease, had worse outcomes. Whether these poorer outcomes are related to COPD, cardiac events, or both is unknown; however, COPD patients are reported to have high cardiovascular disease morbidity and mortality.[5] Further, coronary artery disease is likely undertreated in many COPD patients. CACS may be a good screening test to alert physicians treating COPD to the presence of comorbid coronary artery disease.

J. R. Maurer, MD

References

1. Boschetto P, Beghé B, Fabbri LM, et al. The link between COPD and coronary artery disease—implication for clinical practice. *Respirology.* 2012;17:422-431.
2. Jacobs PC, Prokop M, van der Graaf Y, et al. Comparing coronary artery calcium and thoracic aorta calcium for prediction of all-cause mortality and cardiovascular events on low-dose non-gated computed tomography in a high-risk population of heavy smokers. *Atherosclerosis.* 2010;209:455-462.
3. Jenny NS, Brown ER, Detrano R, et al. Associations of inflammatory markers with coronary artery calcification: results from the Multi-Ethnic Study of Atherosclerosis. *Atherosclerosis.* 2010;209:226-229.
4. Vestbo J, Anderson W, Coxson HO, et al; ECLIPSE investigators. Evaluation of COPD Longitudinally to Identify Predictive Surrogate End-points (ECLIPSE). *Eur Respir J.* 2008;31:869-873.
5. Curkendall SM, Lanes S, de Luise C, et al. Chronic obstructive pulmonary disease severity and cardiovascular outcomes. *Eur J Epidemiol.* 2006;21:803-813.

37 Lung Cancer

Cancer Statistics, 2014

Siegel R, Ma J, Zou Z, et al (American Cancer Society, Atlanta, GA; Information Management Services, Inc, Silver Spring, MD; et al)

CA Cancer J Clin 64:9-29, 2014

Each year, the American Cancer Society estimates the numbers of new cancer cases and deaths that will occur in the United States in the current year and compiles the most recent data on cancer incidence, mortality, and survival. Incidence data were collected by the National Cancer Institute, the Centers for Disease Control and Prevention, and the North American Association of Central Cancer Registries and mortality data were collected by the National Center for Health Statistics. A total of 1,665,540 new cancer cases and 585,720 cancer deaths are projected to occur in the United States in 2014. During the most recent 5 years for which there are data (2006-2010), delay-adjusted cancer incidence rates declined slightly in men (by 0.6% per year) and were stable in women, while cancer death rates decreased by 1.8% per year in men and by 1.4% per year in women. The combined cancer death rate (deaths per 100,000 population) has been continuously declining for 2 decades, from a peak of 215.1 in 1991 to 171.8 in 2010. This 20% decline translates to the avoidance of approximately 1,340,400 cancer deaths (952,700 among men and 387,700 among women) during this time period. The magnitude of the decline in cancer death rates from 1991 to 2010 varies substantially by age, race, and sex, ranging from no decline among white women aged 80 years and older to a 55% decline among black men aged 40 years to 49 years. Notably, black men experienced the largest drop within every 10-year age group. Further progress can be accelerated by applying existing cancer control knowledge across all segments of the population (Fig 6).

► As has unfortunately been the case for several decades, lung cancer was the leading cause of cancer death in both men and women in the United States in 2014. Although more new cases of breast cancers in women and more new cases of prostate cancer in men were diagnosed, more people of both sexes died from lung cancer this year than from breast, prostate, and colorectal cancers combined. In 2014, lung cancer claimed an estimated 159 260 American lives—86 930 men and 72 330 women. Fig 6 demonstrates trends in death rates overall and for selected sites for men and women in the United States from 1930 to 2010. The total number of overall deaths has been decreasing steadily over the past 20 years (Fig 6, top panel), a substantial portion of

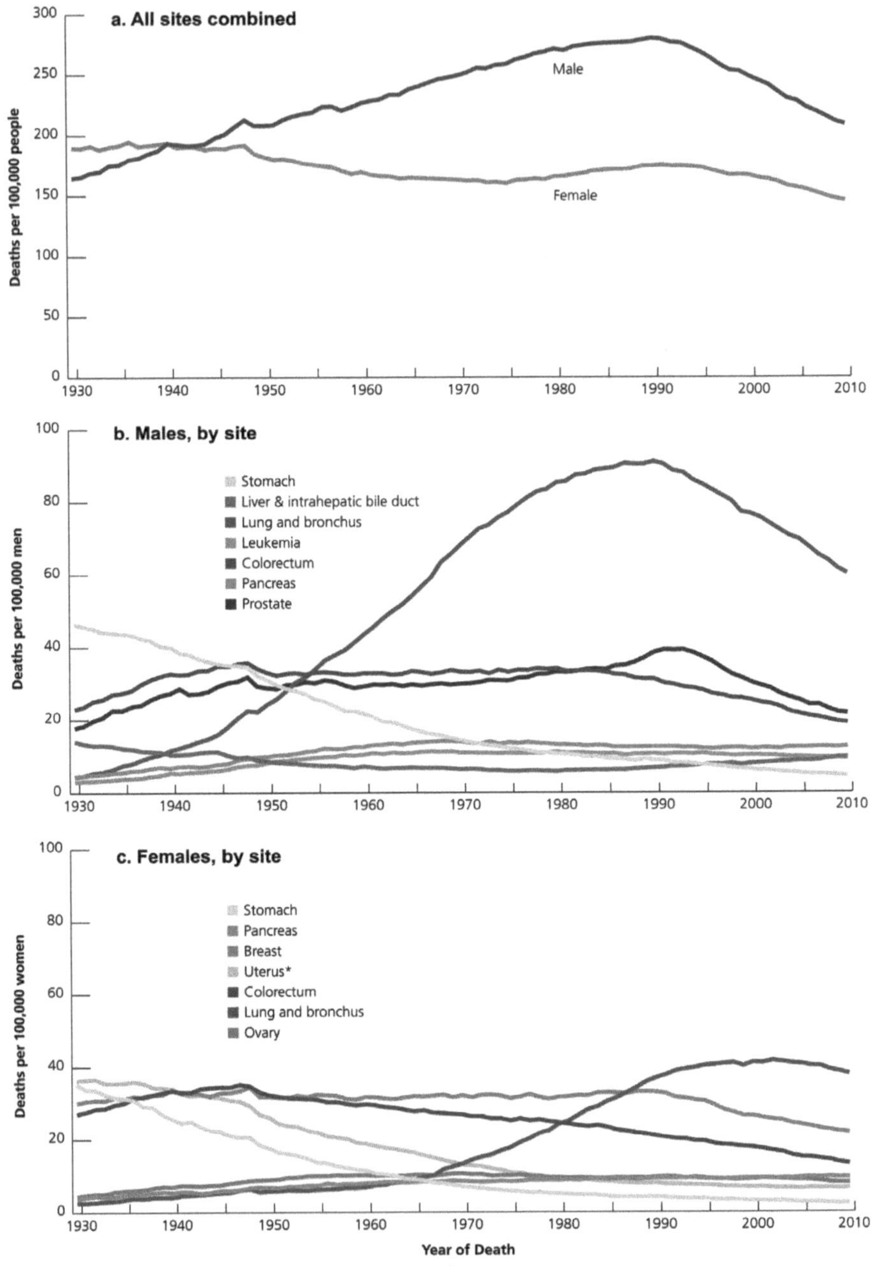

FIGURE 6.—Trends in Death Rates Overall and for Selected Sites by Sex, United States, 1930 to 2010. Rates are age adjusted to the 2000 US standard population. Due to changes in International Classification of Diseases (ICD) coding, numerator information has changed over time. Rates for cancers of the lung and bronchus, colorectum, liver, uterus, and ovary are affected by these changes. *Uterus includes uterine cervix and uterine corpus. (Reprinted from Siegel R, Ma J, Zou Z, et al. Cancer statistics, 2014. *CA Cancer J Clin*. 2014;64:9-29, with permission from CA: A Cancer Journal for Clinicians and John Wiley and Sons, www.interscience.wiley.com.)

which is the result of the steady decrease in lung cancer deaths in men (Fig 6, middle panel). In women, the lung cancer death rate does seem finally to be decreasing slightly (Fig 6, bottom panel). Notably, death rates for the 4 leading causes of cancer death—lung, breast, prostate, and colorectal—are now all declining. Although the reductions in lung cancer death rates among both men and women are largely due to reduction in tobacco use, reductions in death rates for breast, prostate, and colorectal cancers are generally attributed to early detection and treatment advances.[1-4] It will be interesting over the coming years to observe the impact of lung cancer screening on lung cancer incidence and death rates as screening is introduced into medical practice.[5]

L. T. Tanoue, MD

References

1. Jemal A, Thun MJ, Ries LA, et al. Annual report to the nation on the status of cancer, 1975–2005, featuring trends in lung cancer, tobacco use, and tobacco control. *J Natl Cancer Inst.* 2008;100:1672-1694.
2. Berry DA, Cronin KA, Plevritis SK, et al. Effect of screening and adjuvant therapy on mortality from breast cancer. *N Engl J Med.* 2005;353:1784-1792.
3. Etzioni R, Tsodikov A, Mariotto A, et al. Quantifying the role of PSA screening in the US prostate cancer mortality decline. *Cancer Causes Control.* 2008;19:175-181.
4. Edwards BK, Ward E, Kohler BA, et al. Annual report to the nation on the status of cancer, 1975–2006, featuring colorectal cancer trends and impact of interventions (risk factors, screening, and treatment) to reduce future rates. *Cancer.* 2010; 116:544-573.
5. Moyer VA. Screening for Lung Cancer: U.S. Preventive Services Task Force Recommendation Statement. *Ann Intern Med.* 2014;160:330-338.

Is Previous Respiratory Disease a Risk Factor for Lung Cancer?

Denholm R, Schüz J, Straif K, et al (International Agency for Res on Cancer, Lyon, France; et al)
Am J Respir Crit Care Med 190:549-559, 2014

Rationale.—Previous respiratory diseases have been associated with increased risk of lung cancer. Respiratory conditions often co-occur and few studies have investigated multiple conditions simultaneously.

Objectives.—Investigate lung cancer risk associated with chronic bronchitis, emphysema, tuberculosis, pneumonia, and asthma.

Methods.—The SYNERGY project pooled information on previous respiratory diseases from 12,739 case subjects and 14,945 control subjects from 7 case–control studies conducted in Europe and Canada. Multivariate logistic regression models were used to investigate the relationship between individual diseases adjusting for co-occurring conditions, and patterns of respiratory disease diagnoses and lung cancer. Analyses were stratified by sex, and adjusted for age, center, ever-employed in a high-risk occupation, education, smoking status, cigarette pack-years, and time since quitting smoking.

Measurements and Main Results.—Chronic bronchitis and emphysema were positively associated with lung cancer, after accounting for other respiratory diseases and smoking (e.g., in men: odds ratio [OR], 1.33; 95% confidence interval [CI], 1.20–1.48 and OR, 1.50; 95% CI, 1.21–1.87, respectively). A positive relationship was observed between lung cancer and pneumonia diagnosed 2 years or less before lung cancer (OR, 3.31; 95% CI, 2.33–4.70 for men), but not longer. Co-occurrence of chronic bronchitis and emphysema and/or pneumonia had a stronger positive association with lung cancer than chronic bronchitis "only." Asthma had an inverse association with lung cancer, the association being stronger with an asthma diagnosis 5 years or more before lung cancer compared with shorter.

Conclusions.—Findings from this large international case–control consortium indicate that after accounting for co-occurring respiratory diseases, chronic bronchitis and emphysema continue to have a positive association with lung cancer.

▶ This is a report from the SYNERGY project, which is a consortium of international lung cancer case-control studies that collected information on occupational and smoking histories. Thirteen of the participating SYNERGY centers also collected information on self-reported previous respiratory disease, including chronic bronchitis, emphysema, tuberculosis, pneumonia, and asthma. The study population included 12 739 case subjects and 14 945 controls. Of the respiratory diseases studied, emphysema had the strongest association with lung cancer. Pneumonia had a positive association, with the relationship being stronger if pneumonia were diagnosed less than 2 years before the lung cancer diagnosis. No association was observed between tuberculosis and lung cancer. For men, chronic bronchitis, emphysema, and pneumonia were associated with an increased risk of lung cancer, compared with persons with no previous respiratory diagnoses. For women, emphysema and pneumonia were associated with increased lung cancer risk.

One of the main points of this report is the observation that co-occurrence of chronic bronchitis, emphysema, and/or pneumonia was common. The presence of more than 1 of these diseases resulted in a stronger association with lung cancer than each individually. Co-occurrence of more than one respiratory disease was observed in 50% to 83% of cases and 40% to 83% of controls. Although previous respiratory disease is not at present a criterion for lung cancer screening, the identification of groups at higher risk may influence surveillance in the future.

L. T. Tanoue, MD

Global Effects of Smoking, of Quitting, and of Taxing Tobacco

Jha P, Peto R (Univ of Toronto, Ontario, Canada; Univ of Oxford, UK)

N Engl J Med 370:60-68, 2014

Background.—If current global smoking patterns continue, about 50% of all the young men and 10% of all the young women now living will become smokers and few will stop. As a result the annual number of deaths attributable to tobacco will increase from about 5 million in 2010 to over 10 million in a few decades. Tobacco will be associated with about 1 billion deaths in this century, mostly in low- and middle-income countries and half before these individuals reach age 70 years. The 2013 World Health Assembly issued a call to governments to reduce the prevalence of smoking by a third by 2015 and thereby avoid over 200 million deaths from tobacco. Such a reduction could be achieved if the inflation-adjusted price of cigarettes doubled, since price is a key factor in the initiation and cessation of smoking behavior. Without large price increases, it is unlikely that the desired reduction in smoking will be achieved.

Smoking Effects and Cessation.—Mortality among middle-aged cigarette smokers is two to three times that of similar persons who never smoked. Life span is reduced by an average of 10 years. Many of those who die are still in middle age and lose many years of life. The good news is that stopping smoking is an effective intervention. Persons who begin smoking in early adulthood but stop by age 30, 40, or even 50 years gain about 10, 9, and 6 years of life, respectively, compared to those who continue to smoke. Persons who stop smoking before age 40 years avoid more than 90% of the excess risk for death during the next few decades compared to those who continue to smoke.

Pricing Effects.—Tobacco-control programs that use price and non-price interventions can increase smoking cessation rates and discourage the initiation of smoking. The two pricing approaches are specific excise taxes on tobacco and ad valorem (added value) taxes. Of these, the specific excise taxes exert a substantial, rapid effect on cigarette consumption. Higher taxes are especially effective for poorer or less educated individuals and may prevent young persons from taking up the habit.

Smuggling can be a concern with higher tobacco taxes. Using specific excise taxes on tobacco, employing stronger tax administration strategies, and instituting efforts to control smuggling can limit the problem. Even with some smuggling, large tax increases tend to substantially reduce consumption while raising revenue, which can then be used in health-promotion activities.

Other effective interventions include bans on advertising, the use of plain packaging for tobacco products, and the removal of all brand images. Pictorial warnings can be placed on the packages to convey the danger of smoking even to illiterate persons, who account for half of the deaths from tobacco in India. Bans on advertising should be comprehensive and include all direct and indirect promotions. This has the added advantage of severing the media from any dependence on the tobacco industry. Among populations with many long-term smokers, low-cost epidemiologic studies showing linkages between tobacco use and premature death may inform political movements against tobacco use as well as provide information for individuals who smoke.

Conclusions.—Many countries use non-price interventions, but few use large increases in specific excise taxes on tobacco to reduce smoking. However, studies show that a key component of effective and realistic

strategies to significantly reduce smoking is a large increase in the price of cigarettes.

▶ Global mortality and morbidity related to cigarette smoking are staggering. In 2010, there were an estimated 5 million tobacco-attributable deaths in the world. On average, 50% of men and 10% of women begin smoking at young ages, and relatively few quit. The health burden of these individuals will increase as they age, with resultant morbidity and premature death. The World Health Organization (WHO) estimates that if current smoking prevalence continues, 1 billion persons during this century will die of tobacco-related diseases.[1,2]

In this review, Jha and Peto identify 3 key messages for smokers in the 21st century:

1. The risk is big, and there is a lot to lose. In middle age, mortality among smokers is 2 to 3 times what would be expected, leading to an average reduction in life span of about 10 years, as demonstrated in Fig 1 in the original article.
2. The loss is worse for those who die of tobacco-related disease in middle age. Those smokers who die in middle age have a loss of life expectancy of about 20 years of life compared with never smokers.
3. Quitting works. People who stop smoking at ages 30, 40, or 50 gain, on average, 10, 9, and 6 years of life expectancy, respectively, compared with people who continue smoking.[3]

The World Health Assembly of WHO estimates that a reduction in smoking prevalence by one-third by 2025 will save 200 million tobacco-related deaths over the rest of the century. The challenge is, how do we achieve that goal? Jha and Peto offer the following observations and recommendations on interventions that have reliably resulted in decreasing tobacco consumption:

1. Large increases in specific tobacco taxes are rapid and effective curbs.[4-6]
2. Taxes must consistently result in high cost to the consumer to achieve the desired effect.
3. Comprehensive curtailing advertising and plain packaging of cigarettes.
4. Bans on smoking in public places.
5. Raising political awareness.
6. Providing information, including data about premature death, to individual smokers.
7. Physician support, telephone- or Internet-based counseling.
8. Pharmacologic treatments.

As individual physicians and healthcare providers, we may not feel empowered to enact most of these interventions. Nonetheless, the combined voice is powerful, and we should lend ours to achieve these goals.

L. T. Tanoue, MD

References

1. Jha P. Avoidable global cancer deaths and total deaths from smoking. *Nat Rev Cancer.* 2009;9:655-664.
2. WHO Report on the Global Tobacco Epidemic, 2013. *Enforcing Bans on Tobacco Advertising, Promotion and Sponsorship.* Geneva, Switzerland: World Health Organization; 2013.
3. Pirie K, Peto R, Reeves GK, Green J, Beral VMillion Women Study Collaborators. The 21st century hazards of smoking and benefits of stopping: a prospective study of one million women in the UK. *Lancet.* 2013;381:133-141.
4. Effectiveness of Tax and Price Policies for Tobacco Control. *IARC Handbook of Cancer Prevention, Volume 14.* Lyon, France: International Agency for Research on Cancer; 2011.
5. Levy DT, Hyland A, Higbee C, Remer L, Compton C. The role of public policies in reducing smoking prevalence in California: results from the California tobacco policy simulation model. *Health Policy.* 2007;82:167-185.
6. Pizacani B, Mosbaek C, Hedberg K, et al. Decline in cigarette consumption following implementation of a comprehensive tobacco prevention and education program - Oregon, 1996—1998 (Reprinted from MMWR, vol 48, pg 140—143, 1999). *JAMA.* 1999;281:1483-1484.

Electronic Cigarettes: A Position Statement of the Forum of International Respiratory Societies

Schraufnagel DE, on behalf of the Forum of International Respiratory Societies (Univ of Illinois at Chicago; et al)

Am J Respir Crit Care Med 190:611-618, 2014

Background.—Awareness and usage of electronic cigarettes has exponentially increased during the last few years, especially among young people and women in some countries. The rapid acceptance of electronic cigarettes may be attributed in part to the perception created by marketing and the popular press that they are safer than combustible cigarettes.

Goals.—To alert and advise policy makers about electronic cigarettes and their potential hazards.

Methods.—Using The Union's position paper on electronic cigarettes as the starting template, the document was written using an iterative process. Portions of the manuscript have been taken directly from the position papers of participating societies.

Results.—Because electronic cigarettes generate less tar and carcinogens than combustible cigarettes, use of electronic cigarettes may reduce disease caused by those components. However, the health risks of electronic cigarettes have not been adequately studied. Studies looking at whether electronic cigarettes can aid smoking cessation have had inconsistent results. Moreover, the availability of electronic cigarettes may have an overall adverse health impact by increasing initiation and reducing cessation of combustible nicotine delivery products.

Conclusions.—The health and safety claims regarding electronic nicotine delivery devices should be subject to evidentiary review. The potential

benefits of electronic cigarettes to an individual smoker should be weighed against potential harm to the population of increased social acceptability of smoking and use of nicotine, the latter of which has addictive power and untoward effects. As a precaution, electronic nicotine delivery devices should be restricted or banned until more information about their safety is available. If they are allowed, they should be closely regulated as medicines or tobacco products.

▶ Electronic cigarettes have been rapidly introduced into the culture of our communities. Patients frequently ask me if it is "OK" to smoke electronic cigarettes to help them quit smoking. Recently, a patient wanted to know why he could not "vape" his electronic cigarette in our hospital healing garden. This statement by Schraufnagel and colleagues represents the stance on electronic cigarettes of the Forum of International Respiratory Societies (FIRS), whose member societies include the Asociación Latinoamericana del Tórax (ALAT), the American College of Chest Physicians (ACCP), the American Thoracic Society (ATS), the Asian Pacific Society of Respirology (APSR), the European Respiratory Society (ERS), the International Union Against Tuberculosis and Lung Disease (The Union), and the Pan African Thoracic Society (PATS). The FIRS statement summarizes all the relevant concerns about electronic cigarettes as follows:

- "The health risks of electronic cigarettes have not been adequately studied.
- The addictive power of nicotine and its untoward effects should not be underestimated.
- The potential benefits of electronic nicotine delivery devices, including harm reduction and as an aid to smoking cessation, have not been well studied.
- Potential benefits to an individual smoker should be weighed against harm to the population of increased social acceptability of smoking and use of nicotine.
- Health and safety claims regarding electronic nicotine delivery devices should be subject to evidentiary review.
- Adverse health effects for nonsmokers exposed to the emissions of electronic cigarettes cannot be excluded.
- Electronic nicotine delivery devices should be restricted or banned, at least until more information about their safety is available.
- If electronic nicotine delivery devices are permitted, they should be regulated as medicines and subject to the same evidentiary review as other medicines.
- If electronic nicotine delivery devices are not regulated as medicines, they should be regulated as tobacco products.
- Research, supported by sources other than the tobacco or electronic cigarette industry, should be performed to determine the impact of electronic nicotine delivery devices on health in a wide variety of settings.
- The patterns of use and the consequences at the population level of electronic nicotine delivery devices should be monitored.

- All information derived from this research should be conveyed to the public in a clear manner."

L. T. Tanoue, MD

Components Necessary for High Quality Lung Cancer Screening: American College of Chest Physicians and American Thoracic Society Policy Statement

Mazzone P, Powell CA, Arenberg D, et al (Cleveland Clinic, OH; Icahn School of Medicine at Mount Sinai, NY; Univ of Michigan, Ann Arbor; et al)
Chest 147:295-303, 2015

Lung cancer screening with a low dose chest CT scan can result in more benefit than harm when performed in settings committed to developing and maintaining high quality programs. This project aimed to identify the components of screening that should be a part of all lung cancer screening programs. To do so, committees with expertise in lung cancer screening were assembled by the Thoracic Oncology Network of the ACCP and the Thoracic Oncology Assembly of the ATS. Lung cancer program components were derived from evidence-based reviews of lung cancer screening, and supplemented by expert opinion. This statement was developed and modified based on iterative feedback of the committees. Nine essential components of a lung cancer screening program were identified. Within these components twenty one Policy Statements were developed and translated into criteria that could be used to assess the qualification of a program as a screening facility. Two additional Policy Statements related to the need for multi-society governance of lung cancer screening were developed. High quality lung cancer screening programs can be developed within the presented framework of nine essential program components outlined by our committees. This document has been formally endorsed by several professional organizations (ACCP, ATS, American Association of Thoracic Surgery, American Cancer Society, American Society of Preventive Oncology).

▶ Much of the controversy and concern relating to lung cancer screening with low-dose computed tomography (CT) scanning revolves around the balance between the benefit and potential harms of screening. The benefit is straightforward: Lung cancer screening performed properly in the appropriate population results in a reduction in mortality from lung cancer.[1,2] The potential harms are less straightforward, although well appreciated, the most prominent of which are a high rate of abnormal results of which the large majority are false-positive findings, the potential for complications of invasive and noninvasive testing related to those findings, the appreciation of the enormous potential cost of screening, and concern about cost-effectiveness.

This policy statement was generated by a committee of experts in lung cancer screening representing the American College of Chest Physicians (ACCP) and

American Thoracic Society (ATS). The committee identified nine essential components of a high-quality lung cancer screening program:

1. Who is offered lung cancer screening?
2. How often, and for how long, to screen?
3. How the CT is performed?
4. Lung nodule identification
5. Structured reporting
6. Lung nodule management algorithms
7. Smoking cessation
8. Patient and provider education
9. Data collection

Using the evidence base for each component, the committee developed policy statements outlining assessment criteria for measuring program quality. (See the table in article by Tanoue et al, reproduced here.) These policy statements may potentially inform the performance metrics by which the quality of a lung cancer screening program is measured. The committee already suggested 2 such metrics: 1) for component 1 (Who is offered lung cancer screening?), at least 90% of all screened subjects must match the program's stated policy, the evidence base for which indicates that screening should be limited to persons identified at high enough risk of developing lung cancer that potential benefit outweighs potential harm. These individuals would at a minimum meet the criteria of the National Lung Screening Trial cohort or the screening population recommended by the US Preventive Task Force.[1,3] For component 5 (Structured reporting), the selected structured CT scan reporting system identified by the screening program should be used for at least 90% of CT screen reports.

The components and policy statements are likely to serve as the platform informing the development of other metrics that will be used to measure quality and performance of screening programs. The policy statement has been endorsed by ACCP, ATS, the American Association of Thoracic Surgery, the American Cancer Society, and the American Society of Preventive Oncology.

L. T. Tanoue, MD

References

1. Aberle DR, Adams AM, Berg CD, et al. Reduced lung-cancer mortality with low-dose computed tomographic screening. *N Engl J Med.* 2011;365:395-409.
2. de Koning HJ, Meza R, Plevritis SK, et al. Benefits and harms of computed tomography lung cancer screening strategies: a comparative modeling study for the U.S. Preventive SERVICES Task Force. *Ann Intern Med.* 2014;160:311-320.
3. Moyer VA. Screening for lung cancer: U.S. Preventive Services Task Force recommendation statement. *Ann Intern Med.* 2014;160:330-338.

38 Pleural, Interstitial Lung, and Pulmonary Vascular Disease

Relationship of DNA Methylation and Gene Expression in Idiopathic Pulmonary Fibrosis

Yang IV, Pedersen BS, Rabinovich E, et al (Univ of Colorado School of Medicine, Aurora; Univ of Pittsburgh Med Ctr, PA; et al)

Am J Respir Crit Care Med 190:1263-1272, 2014

Rationale.—Idiopathic pulmonary fibrosis (IPF) is an untreatable and often fatal lung disease that is increasing in prevalence and is caused by complex interactions between genetic and environmental factors. Epigenetic mechanisms control gene expression and are likely to regulate the IPF transcriptome.

Objectives.—To identify methylation marks that modify gene expression in IPF lung.

Methods.—We assessed DNA methylation (comprehensive high-throughput arrays for relative methylation arrays [CHARM]) and gene expression (Agilent gene expression arrays) in 94 patients with IPF and 67 control subjects, and performed integrative genomic analyses to define methylation–gene expression relationships in IPF lung. We validated methylation changes by a targeted analysis (Epityper), and performed functional validation of one of the genes identified by our analysis.

Measurements and Main Results.—We identified 2,130 differentially methylated regions (DMRs; <5% false discovery rate), of which 738 are associated with significant changes in gene expression and enriched for expected inverse relationship between methylation and expression ($P < 2.2 \times 10^{-16}$). We validated 13/15 DMRs by targeted analysis of methylation. Methylation–expression quantitative trait loci (methyl-eQTL) identified methylation marks that control *cis* and *trans* gene expression, with an enrichment for *cis* relationships ($P < 2.2 \times 10^{-16}$). We found five *trans* methyl-eQTLs where a methylation change at a single DMR is associated with transcriptional changes in a substantial number of genes; four of these DMRs are near transcription factors (castor zinc finger 1 [CASZ1], FOXC1, MXD4, and ZDHHC4). We studied the *in vitro* effects of change in CASZ1 expression and validated its role in regulation of target genes in the methyl-eQTL.

Conclusions.—These results suggest that DNA methylation may be involved in the pathogenesis of IPF.

► In their study published in the Blue Journal, Yang and colleagues explored the role of DNA methylation in idiopathic pulmonary fibrosis (IPF) lungs. The authors assessed lung tissue from 94 patients with IPF and 67 controls. They identified 2130 differentially methylated regions, of which 738 were associated with regulation of gene expression, specifically reduction in expression.

DNA methylation results in down regulation of gene expression, particularly when it occur in or around promoter regions. Cigarette smoking and environmental factors are known to influence levels of methylation. Previous studies have identified suspect targets but were limited by sample size. This study, as pointed out by the authors, suffers from the limitation that samples were obtained from heterogeneous tissue and not specific cell types.

The authors reported that there were extensive alterations in DNA methylation, some of which were known to have strong associations with IPF. Additional areas of interest were also identified. The authors point out that these may prove promising future targets for therapy in IPF.

C. D. Spradley, MD

Randomized Trial of Acetylcysteine in Idiopathic Pulmonary Fibrosis

The Idiopathic Pulmonary Fibrosis Clinical Research Network (Univ of Michigan, Ann Arbor; Univ of Alabama at Birmingham; Duke Clinical Res Inst, Durham, NC; et al)

N Engl J Med 370:2093-2101, 2014

Background.—Acetylcysteine has been suggested as a beneficial treatment for idiopathic pulmonary fibrosis, although data from placebo-controlled studies are lacking.

Methods.—In our initial double-blind, placebo-controlled trial, we randomly assigned patients who had idiopathic pulmonary fibrosis with mild-to-moderate impairment in pulmonary function to receive a three-drug regimen of prednisone, azathioprine, and acetylcysteine; acetylcysteine alone; or placebo. The study was interrupted owing to safety concerns associated with the three-drug regimen. The trial continued as a two-group study (acetylcysteine vs. placebo) without other changes; 133 and 131 patients were enrolled in the acetylcysteine and placebo groups, respectively. The primary outcome was the change in forced vital capacity (FVC) over a 60-week period.

Results.—At 60 weeks, there was no significant difference in the change in FVC between the acetylcysteine group and the placebo group (−0.18 liters and −0.19 liters, respectively; $P = 0.77$). In addition, there were no significant differences between the acetylcysteine group and the placebo group in the rates of death (4.9% vs. 2.5%, $P = 0.30$ by the log-rank test) or acute exacerbation (2.3% in each group, $P > 0.99$).

Conclusions.—As compared with placebo, acetylcysteine offered no significant benefit with respect to the preservation of FVC in patients with idiopathic pulmonary fibrosis with mild-to-moderate impairment in lung function. (Funded by the National Heart, Lung, and Blood Institute and others; ClinicalTrials.gov number, NCT00650091.)

► In 1 of 3 studies published in the May 29 *New England Journal of Medicine*, The Idiopathic Pulmonary Fibrosis Clinical Research Network presented the results of the PANTHER-IPF trial. The original study design compared acetylcysteine alone to acetylcysteine plus prednisone plus azathioprine to placebo in a 1:1:1 randomization. The combination arm was discontinued early at the request of the data safety monitoring board. The resulting 2-arm study was the subject of this publication.

The primary endpoint was reduction in forced vital capacity, and multiple secondary endpoints were prespecified. There was no significant difference between the intervention and placebo arms at 60 weeks, making this a negative study (Fig 2 in the original article). There were trends toward improvement in the treatment arm for a number of secondary endpoints, but the final conclusion drawn was that acetylcysteine was not effective in preventing decline in forced vital capacity at 60 weeks compared with placebo in patients with mild to moderate idiopathic pulmonary fibrosis diagnosed by high-resolution computed tomography or biopsy.

C. D. Spradley, MD

A Phase 3 Trial of Pirfenidone in Patients with Idiopathic Pulmonary Fibrosis

King TE Jr, for the ASCEND Study Group (Univ of California; et al)
N Engl J Med 370:2083-2092, 2014

Background.—In two of three phase 3 trials, pirfenidone, an oral antifibrotic therapy, reduced disease progression, as measured by the decline in forced vital capacity (FVC) or vital capacity, in patients with idiopathic pulmonary fibrosis; in the third trial, this end point was not achieved. We sought to confirm the beneficial effect of pirfenidone on disease progression in such patients.

Methods.—In this phase 3 study, we randomly assigned 555 patients with idiopathic pulmonary fibrosis to receive either oral pirfenidone (2403 mg per day) or placebo for 52 weeks. The primary end point was the change in FVC or death at week 52. Secondary end points were the 6-minute walk distance, progression-free survival, dyspnea, and death from any cause or from idiopathic pulmonary fibrosis.

Results.—In the pirfenidone group, as compared with the placebo group, there was a relative reduction of 47.9% in the proportion of patients who had an absolute decline of 10 percentage points or more in the percentage of the predicted FVC or who died; there was also a relative increase of

132.5% in the proportion of patients with no decline in FVC ($P < 0.001$). Pirfenidone reduced the decline in the 6-minute walk distance ($P = 0.04$) and improved progression-free survival ($P < 0.001$). There was no significant between-group difference in dyspnea scores ($P = 0.16$) or in rates of death from any cause ($P = 0.10$) or from idiopathic pulmonary fibrosis ($P = 0.23$). However, in a prespecified pooled analysis incorporating results from two previous phase 3 trials, the between-group difference favoring pirfenidone was significant for death from any cause ($P = 0.01$) and from idiopathic pulmonary fibrosis ($P = 0.006$). Gastrointestinal and skin-related adverse events were more common in the pirfenidone group than in the placebo group but rarely led to treatment discontinuation.

Conclusions.—Pirfenidone, as compared with placebo, reduced disease progression, as reflected by lung function, exercise tolerance, and progression-free survival, in patients with idiopathic pulmonary fibrosis. Treatment was associated with an acceptable side-effect profile and fewer deaths. (Funded by InterMune; ASCEND ClinicalTrials.gov number, NCT01366209.)

▶ The ASCEND trial is the result of conflicting data from 2 previous randomized double-blind placebo-controlled trials comparing pirfenidone, a novel antifibrotic agent, to placebo for the treatment of mild to moderate idiopathic pulmonary fibrosis. Inclusion criteria were similar to the PANTHER-IPF study (see above), and the study included patients with mild to moderate disease. Unlike PANTHER-IPF, the ASCEND trial was a positive trial with the treatment arm outperforming the placebo arm when comparing the primary and a number of prespecified secondary endpoints (Fig 2 in the original article). Mortality benefit did not reach clinical significance, but pooled data including the 2 previous phase III trials (Table 2 in the original article) did show statistically significant benefit. There was a slight increase in mild to moderate gastrointestinal and skin side effects in the treatment arm, and the study drug was well tolerated.

The year 2014 will go down in history as a big year for lung disease with the Food and Drug Administration approval of 2 new drugs for the treatment of idiopathic pulmonary fibrosis. Patients will benefit from these new options for life-prolonging treatment for what just last year was thought of as an untreatable disease. Intermune, the manufacturer of pirfenidone and the sponsor of the ASCEND trial, will also undoubtedly benefit in light of the hefty reported 6-figure sticker price for a year of therapy.

C. D. Spradley, MD

Comparison of Pleural Pressure Measuring Instruments

Lee HJ, Yarmus L, Kidd D, et al (Johns Hopkins Univ, Baltimore, MD; et al)
Chest 146:1007-1012, 2014

Objective.—The objective of this study was to compare the accuracy of a handheld digital manometer (DM) and U-tube (UT) manometer with an electronic transducer (ET) manometer during thoracentesis.

Methods.—Thirty-three consecutive patients undergoing thoracentesis were enrolled in the study. Pleural pressure (Ppl) measurements were made using a handheld DM (Compass; Mirador Biomedical), a UT water manometer, and an ET (reference instrument). End-expiratory Ppl was recorded after catheter insertion, after each aspiration of 240 mL, and prior to catheter removal. Volume of fluid removed, symptoms during thoracentesis, pleural elastance, and pleural fluid chemistry were also evaluated.

Results.—A total of 594 Ppl measurements were made in 30 patients during their thoracenteses. There was a strong linear correlation coefficient between elastance for the DM and ET ($r = 0.9582$, $P < .001$). Correlation was poor between the UT and ET ($r = 0.0448$, $P = .84$). Among the 15 patients who developed cough, recorded ET pressures ranged from −9 to +9 cm H_2O at the time of symptom development, with a mean (SD) of −2.93 (4.89) cm H_2O. ET and DM measurements among those patients with cough had a low correlation between these measurements ($R^2 = 0.104$, $P = .24$). Nine patients developed chest discomfort and had ET pressures that ranged from −26 to +6 cm H_2O, with a mean (SD) of −7.89 (9.97) cm H_2O.

Conclusions.—The handheld DM provided a valid and easy-to-use method to measure Ppl during thoracentesis. Future studies are needed to investigate its usefulness in predicting clinically meaningful outcomes.

► In this small, unfunded study out of Johns Hopkins published in *Chest*, the authors compare 3 methods of pleural manometry: electronic transducer (ET), U-tube (UT), and a proprietary handheld digital manometer (DM) (Fig 1 in the original article). The authors performed 594 individual measurements on 30 consecutive patients. A measurement from each device was made at each point in drainage.

The authors found excellent correlation between the standard ET manometer and the DM manometer but not between the ET manometer and the UT manometer (Fig 2 in the original article). The digital manometer correctly predicted nonexpandable lung in 5 of 5 patients with end expiratory pleural pressures less than −20 cm H_2O. UT manometry was not predictive. Cough was associated with a pressure of −2.93 cm H_2O, and pain was associated with a pressure of −7.89.

The study demonstrated good correlation between the DM manometer and the more cumbersome gold standard ET manometer. This lays the groundwork for future studies addressing the clinical implications of manometry during thoracentesis. The authors point out, however, that the device costs about $40 and has no associated common procedural terminology code, thus disincentivizing its widespread use.

C. D. Spradley, MD

Pharmacologic Therapy for Pulmonary Arterial Hypertension in Adults: CHEST Guideline and Expert Panel Report

Taichman DB, Ornelas J, Chung L, et al (Univ of Pennsylvania, Philadelphia; CHEST, Glenview, IL; Stanford Univ and Palo Alto VA Health Care System; et al)

Chest 146:449-475, 2014

Objective.—Choices of pharmacologic therapies for pulmonary arterial hypertension (PAH) are ideally guided by high-level evidence. The objective of this guideline is to provide clinicians advice regarding pharmacologic therapy for adult patients with PAH as informed by available evidence.

Methods.—This guideline was based on systematic reviews of English language evidence published between 1990 and November 2013, identified using the MEDLINE and Cochrane Library databases. The strength of available evidence was graded using the Grades of Recommendations, Assessment, Development, and Evaluation methodology. Guideline recommendations, or consensus statements when available evidence was insufficient to support recommendations, were developed using a modified Delphi technique to achieve consensus.

Results.—Available evidence is limited in its ability to support high-level recommendations. Therefore, we drafted consensus statements to address many clinical questions regarding pharmacotherapy for patients with PAH. A total of 79 recommendations or consensus statements were adopted and graded.

Conclusions.—Clinical decisions regarding pharmacotherapy for PAH should be guided by high-level recommendations when sufficient evidence is available. Absent higher level evidence, consensus statements based upon available information must be used. Further studies are needed to address the gaps in available knowledge regarding optimal pharmacotherapy for PAH.

▶ In August, Taichman and colleagues published the CHEST Guideline and Expert Panel on pharmacologic treatment of pulmonary arterial hypertension (PAH). The guideline provides 79 separate graded recommendations, which are essentially the summary of clinical trial results available to date. It makes for a laborious read but does provide a "one-stop shop" for guidance concerning PAH therapy based on the evidence.

The authors emphasize the importance of early involvement of PAH experts in collaboration with local physicians. They also strongly endorse vasoreactivity testing and calcium-channel blockade in appropriate patients. They warn against advanced therapy in asymptomatic individuals and endorse the treatment of contributing factors such as sleep-disordered breathing. They advise the use of intravenous prostanoid therapy in patients presenting with class 4 symptoms.

Additional recommendations include the initiation of combination therapy in patients with inadequate clinical response (class III and IV) despite monotherapy, as well as consideration for triple therapy should the same scenario play out in combination. The guideline provides recommendations for most therapies currently available on the US market with the notable singular exception of oral treprostinil.

They endorse pregnancy prevention and referral to high-risk centers for those who get pregnant. The guideline also endorses oxygen supplementation when necessary at altitude, vaccination, and avoidance of elective surgical procedures. When necessary, surgeries should be performed at a PAH center using a multidisciplinary team including cardiac anesthesia.

The guideline provides a thorough and useful (if dry) reference for guiding clinical therapy in PAH.

C. D. Spradley, MD

39 Community-Acquired Pneumonia

Rates and Risk Factors for Recurrent Pneumonia in Patients Hospitalized With Community-Acquired Pneumonia: Population-Based Prospective Cohort Study With 5 Years of Follow-up

Dang TT, Eurich DT, Weir DL, et al (Univ of Alberta, Edmonton, Canada; et al)

Clin Infect Dis 59:74-80, 2014

Background.—The rates and risk factors for developing *recurrent* pneumonia following hospitalization with community-acquired pneumonia (CAP) are poorly understood.

Methods.—We examined a population-based cohort of patients with CAP who survived hospital admission and who were free of pneumonia for at least 3 months. We collected clinical, functional, and medication-related information and pneumonia severity index (PSI). Using linked databases we followed patients for 5 years and captured any clinical episode of pneumonia 90 days or more post-discharge. We used Cox proportional hazards models (adjusted for age, sex, PSI, functional status, medications) to determine rates and independent correlates of recurrent pneumonia.

Results.—The final cohort included 2709 inpatients; 43% were 75 years or older, 34% were not fully independent, and 56% had severe pneumonia. Over 5 years of follow-up, 245 (9%; 95% confidence interval [CI], 8%–10%) patients developed recurrent pneumonia, and 156 (64%) of these episodes required hospitalization. Rate of recurrence was 3.0/100 person-years and median time to recurrence was 317 days (interquartile range, 177–569); 32 (13%) patients had 2 or more recurrences. In multivariable analyses only age > 75 years (adjusted $P = .047$) and less than fully independent functional status (12% recurrence rate with impaired functional status vs 7% for fully independent; adjusted hazard ratio, 1.7; 95% CI, 1.3–2.2; $P < .001$) were significantly associated with recurrent pneumonia.

Conclusions.—One of 11 patients who survived CAP hospitalization had recurrent pneumonia over 5 years and those with impaired functional status were at particularly high risk. Recurrent pneumonia is common and more attention to preventive strategies at discharge and closer follow-up over the long-term seem warranted (Fig 1).

▶ The problem of recurrent community-acquired pneumonia (CAP) has been sparsely studied. The authors postulated that it would be valuable to have a more complete picture of the rates of and risks for recurrent pneumonia over a 5-year period. Existing studies of recurrent pneumonia were found to have limitations in terms of population size, nonrepresentative populations, lack of clinical detail, and short follow-up periods, among other things. The potential benefit of having a clearer picture of those at risk of recurrent disease would be 2-fold: to apprise patients of the risk and to put into place measures that might help prevent the recurrence. Only age > 75 years and impaired functional status were associated significantly with recurrent disease (Fig 1). Typical risk factors for an initial event of CAP include medical comorbidities or use of certain types of medications, but these were not identified as risks for recurrence. The authors point out that previous research has shown that it is relatively common to identify different risk factors for the recurrence of an event than for the initial episode.[1] An explanation for this is that a high percentage of the cohort would be defined as high risk for the initial event; those developing recurrence would likely fall within a subset of the initial risk factors. The median time to recurrence was almost a year. Within 90 days of discharge, 2% of patients had recurrences or relapses (and were excluded from this study); these tended to be in people with heart failure or chronic obstructive pulmonary disorder. The limitations of this study are that the data documenting recurrences were via an administrative database linked to the original episode's clinical radiographic documentation. Thus, detailed clinical information in reference to the recurrent episode was not used; recurrences could therefore have been miscoded or misclassified as pneumonia when, in fact, they were actually a different clinical condition. Finally, the risk factors were not updated during the 5-year follow-up, so patients may have developed new risks that are not recorded in the

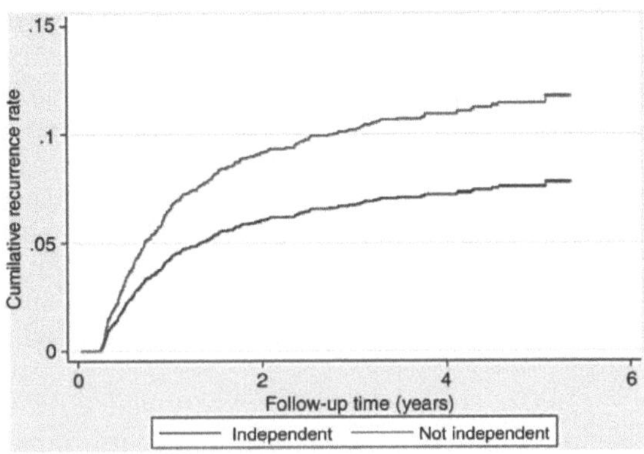

FIGURE 1.—Rates of recurrent pneumonia according to functional status: cumulative incidence curves. (Reprinted from Dang TT, Eurich DT, Weir DL, et al. Rates and risk factors for recurrent pneumonia in patients hospitalized with community-acquired pneumonia: population-based prospective cohort study with 5 years of follow-up. *Clin Infect Dis.* 2014;59:74-80, by permission of the Infectious Diseases Society of America.)

study. Nevertheless, this is the most complete study of recurrent CAP to date and will hopefully help physicians better manage their pneumonia patients.

J. R. Maurer, MD

Reference

1. Dahabreh IJ, Kent DM. Index event bias as an explanation for the paradoxes of recurrence risk research. *JAMA*. 2011;305:822-823.

Diagnoses of Early and Late Readmissions after Hospitalization for Pneumonia: A Systematic Review

Prescott HC, Sjoding MW, Iwashyna TJ (Univ of Michigan, Ann Arbor)
Ann Am Thorac Soc 11:1091-1100, 2014

Rationale.—Pneumonia is a frequent cause of hospitalization, yet drivers of post-pneumonia morbidity remain poorly characterized. Causes of hospital readmissions may elucidate important sources of morbidity and are of particular interest given the U.S. Hospital Readmission Reductions Program.

Objectives.—To review the primary diagnoses of early (≤30 d) and late (≥31 d) readmissions after pneumonia hospitalization.

Methods.—Systematic review of MEDLINE, Embase, and CINAHL databases. We identified original research studies of adults aged 18 years or older, hospitalized for pneumonia, and for whom cause-specific readmission rates were reported. Two authors abstracted study results and assessed study quality.

Measurements and Main Results.—Of the 1,243 citations identified, 12 met eligibility criteria. Included studies were conducted in the United States, Spain, Canada, Croatia, and Sweden. All-cause 30-day readmission rates ranged from 16.8 to 20.1% across administrative studies; the weighted average for the studies using chart review was 11.6% (15.6% in United States-based studies). Pneumonia, heart failure/cardiovascular causes, and chronic obstructive pulmonary disease/pulmonary causes are the most common reasons for early readmission after pneumonia hospitalization. Although it was the single most common cause for readmission, pneumonia accounted for only 17.9 to 29.4% of all 30-day readmissions in administrative studies and a weighted average of 23.0% in chart review studies. After accounting for study population, there was no clear difference in findings between claims-based versus chart-review studies. Few studies assessed readmissions beyond 30 days, although the limited available data suggest similar primary diagnoses for early and late readmissions. No studies assessed whether reasons for readmission were similar to patients' reasons for healthcare use before hospitalization.

Conclusions.—Pneumonia, heart failure/cardiovascular disease, and chronic obstructive pulmonary disease/pulmonary disease are the most common readmission diagnoses after pneumonia hospitalization. Although pneumonia was the most common readmission diagnosis, it accounted for only a minority of all readmissions. Late readmission diagnoses are less thoroughly described, and further research is needed to understand how hospitalization for pneumonia fits within the broader context of patients' health trajectory.

▶ The article in this section by Dang et al addresses timing and rates of recurrence of community-acquired pneumonia. This systematic review by Prescott et al asks a similar, but quite different, question: What are the diagnoses for which patients are readmitted after an admission for pneumonia? As has been noted in other studies[1-3] only a minority—less than one-third—of the readmissions either within 30 days of discharge or later after discharge are for recurrent or relapsed pneumonia. Many of the readmissions especially within the first 30 days of discharge are attributed to heart failure or other cardiac issues and preexisting pulmonary disease. In many cases, it is likely the physiological stress and inflammatory milieu of the pneumonia was a major contributor to the considerable worsening of these comorbid conditions that required admissions for management. Interestingly, the major reasons for readmission beyond 30 days was not different from readmissions within 30 days. With the Centers for Medicare and Medicaid Services' keen focus on readmission for any cause within 30 days and current penalties ranging up to $1 million for early readmissions, studies such as this help us better understand the importance of being aware of and addressing as optimally as possible all the patient comorbidities. However, sometimes deterioration is hard to predict, and so instituting early follow-up in patients with underlying heart and lung disease postdischarge is essential.

J. R. Maurer, MD

References

1. Dharmarajan K, Hsieh AF, Lin Z, et al. Diagnoses and timing of 30-day readmissions after hospitalization for heart failure, acute myocardial infarction, or pneumonia. *JAMA.* 2013;309:355-363.
2. Jasti H, Mortensen EM, Obrosky DS, Kapoor WN, Fine MJ. Causes and risk factors for rehospitalization of patients hospitalized with community-acquired pneumonia. *Clin Infect Dis.* 2008;46:550-556.
3. Dang TT, Eurich DT, Weir DL, Marrie TJ, Majumdar SR. Rates and risk factors for recurrent pneumonia in patients hospitalized with community-acquired pneumonia: population-based prospective cohort study with 5 years of follow-up. *Clin Infect Dis.* 2014;59:74-80.

Lower Respiratory Tract Virus Findings in Mechanically Ventilated Patients With Severe Community-Acquired Pneumonia

Karhu J, Ala-Kokko TI, Vuorinen T, et al (Oulu Univ Hosp, Finland; Univ of Turku, Finland)
Clin Infect Dis 59:62-70, 2014

Background.—The role of viral infections in the etiology of severe community-acquired pneumonia (SCAP) was prospectively evaluated from 2008 to 2012 at a university-level intensive care unit.

Methods.—Clinical data and microbiological tests were assessed: blood cultures, urine pneumococcal and legionella antigens, *Mycoplasma pneumoniae and Chlamydia pneumoniae* antibodies from paired serums, and respiratory virus detection by multiplex, real-time polymerase chain reaction (PCR) from nasopharyngeal swabs and lower tracheal specimens via intubation tube.

Results.—Of 49 mechanically ventilated SCAP patients (21 men and 28 women; median age, 54 years), the etiology was identified in 45 cases (92%). There were 21 pure bacterial infections (43%), 5 probably pure viral infections (10%), and 19 mixed bacterial-viral infections (39%), resulting in viral etiology in 24 patients (49%). Of 26 viruses, 21 (81%) were detected from bronchial specimens and 5 (19%) from nasopharyngeal swabs. Rhinovirus (15 cases, 58%) and adenovirus (4 cases, 15%) were the most common viral findings. The bacterial-viral etiology group had the highest peak C-reactive protein levels (median, 356 [25th-75th percentiles, 294-416], $P = .05$), whereas patients with probably viral etiology had the lowest peak procalcitonin levels (1.7 [25th-75th percentiles, 1.6–1.7]). The clinical characteristics of pure bacterial and mixed bacterial-viral etiologies were comparable. Hospital stay was longest among the bacterial group (17 vs 14 days; $P = .02$).

Conclusions.—Viral findings were demonstrated in almost half of the SCAP patients. Clinical characteristics were similar between the pure bacterial and mixed bacterial-viral infections groups. The frequency of viral detection depends on the availability of PCR techniques and lower respiratory specimens.

▶ Common bacterial pathogens in patients with community-acquired pneumonia (CAP) have been described and incorporated into the accepted guidelines for management of this disease.[1] The most common of these organisms is *Streptococcus* pneumonia. Most initial therapy is directed toward this organism and the organisms are common in younger patients, *Mycoplasma pneumonia* and *Chlamydia pneumonia*. Although viruses are thought to be responsible for a significant percentage of CAP cases, the epidemiology and distribution of these cases is less studied. Unless influenza is suspected, antiviral therapy is rarely used in initial treatment. More than 50% of CAP cases are treated in the outpatient setting, and many of those never receive a specific etiologic diagnosis. The more severe cases that are admitted to hospital—also many without a specific diagnosis—are generally aggressively treated with antibiotics. The assumption is that the vast majority of these are bacterial. In this study, an aggressive approach was taken to determine specific etiologies in the most severe CAP cases, those requiring mechanical ventilation. The surprising finding that up to half of these cases had pure viral or mixed bacterial-viral causes should encourage early use of sophisticated testing, such as molecular diagnostic approaches including polymerase chain reaction tests. Early identification of viral etiologies should help direct more appropriate therapy.

J. R. Maurer, MD

Reference

1. Mandell LA, Wunderink RG, Anzueto A, et al. Infectious Diseases Society of America/American Thoracic Society consensus guidelines on the management of community-acquired pneumonia in adults. *Clin Infect Dis.* 2007;44:S27-S72.

Association of Azithromycin With Mortality and Cardiovascular Events Among Older Patients Hospitalized With Pneumonia

Mortensen EM, Halm EA, Pugh MJ, et al (VA North Texas Health Care System, Dallas, TX; Univ of Texas Southwestern Med Ctr, Dallas; South Texas Veterans Health Care System, San Antonio, TX; et al)
JAMA 311:2199-2208, 2014

Importance.—Although clinical practice guidelines recommend combination therapy with macrolides, including azithromycin, as first-line therapy for patients hospitalized with pneumonia, recent research suggests that azithromycin may be associated with increased cardiovascular events.

Objective.—To examine the association of azithromycin use with all-cause mortality and cardiovascular events for patients hospitalized with pneumonia.

Design.—Retrospective cohort study comparing older patients hospitalized with pneumonia from fiscal years 2002 through 2012 prescribed azithromycin therapy and patients receiving other guideline-concordant antibiotic therapy.

Setting.—This study was conducted using national Department of Veterans Affairs administrative data of patients hospitalized at any Veterans Administration acute care hospital.

Participants.—Patients were included if they were aged 65 years or older, were hospitalized with pneumonia, and received antibiotic therapy concordant with national clinical practice guidelines.

Main Outcomes and Measures.—Outcomes included 30- and 90-day all-cause mortality and 90-day cardiac arrhythmias, heart failure, myocardial infarction, and any cardiac event. Propensity score matching was used to control for the possible effects of known confounders with conditional logistic regression.

Results.—Of 73, 690 patients from 118 hospitals identified, propensity-matched groups were composed of 31, 863 patients exposed to azithromycin and 31, 863 matched patients who were not exposed. There were no significant differences in potential confounders between groups after matching. Ninety-day mortality was significantly lower in those who received azithromycin (exposed, 17.4%, vs unexposed, 22.3%; odds ratio [OR], 0.73; 95% CI, 0.70-0.76). However, we found significantly increased odds of myocardial infarction (5.1% vs 4.4%; OR, 1.17; 95% CI, 1.08-1.25) but not any cardiac event (43.0% vs 42.7%; OR, 1.01; 95% CI, 0.98-1.05), cardiac arrhythmias (25.8% vs 26.0%; OR, 0.99; 95% CI, 0.95-1.02), or heart failure (26.3% vs 26.2%; OR, 1.01; 95% CI, 0.97-1.04).

Conclusions and Relevance.—Among older patients hospitalized with pneumonia, treatment that included azithromycin compared with other antibiotics was associated with a lower risk of 90-day mortality and a smaller increased risk of myocardial infarction. These findings are consistent with a net benefit associated with azithromycin use.

▶ Current guidelines for both outpatient-treated and more severe in-hospital treated community-acquired pneumonia (CAP) recommend macrolides either as single-drug therapy or in combination with other drugs.[1] However, the *New England Journal of Medicine* in 2012 published an article suggesting that azithromycin treatment compared with amoxicillin or ciprofloxacin in a Medicaid population resulted in a higher risk of cardiovascular and all-cause mortality.[2] However, other studies have shown no such association between azithromycin and cardiac mortality.[3,4] The purpose of the study reported here was to "assess the association of azithromycin use and outcomes within 90 days of hospital admission, including cardiovascular events... and mortality, for patients 65 and older who were hospitalized with pneumonia." The authors were particularly interested in trying to determine whether the potential benefits of azithromycin outweighed the potential harms. To do this, they used the Veterans Administration health care administrative and clinical databases of patients hospitalized with pneumonia between October 1, 2001, and September 30, 2012. This provided almost 64 000 almost entirely male patients (98%) over age 65 years, half of whom received azithromycin for their pneumonia and half of whom did not. The authors concluded that the significant survival benefit of azithromycin was a greater benefit than the potential harm of a small increased risk of myocardial infarction that was observed in azithromycin-treated patients. This study does not support the initial 2012 *New England Journal of Medicine* Medicaid study conclusions. However, although this study population was large, it was completely retrospective and therefore should be considered only a starting point for a more definitive randomized prospective study that will put this issue to rest. That study should include a more gender-balanced population that uses clinical data and does not rely solely on *International Classification of Diseases, Ninth Revision,* diagnoses, which are notoriously unreliable.

J. R. Maurer, MD

References

1. Mandell LA, Wunderink RG, Anzueto A, et al. Infectious Diseases Society of America/American Thoracic Society consensus guidelines on the management of community-acquired pneumonia in adults. *Clin Infect Dis.* 2007;44:S27-S72.
2. Ray WA, Murray KT, Hall K, Arbogast PG, Stein CM. Azithromycin and the risk of cardiovascular death. *N Engl J Med.* 2012;366:1881-1890.
3. Svanström H, Pasternak B, Hviid A. Use of azithromycin and death from cardiovascular causes. *N Engl J Med.* 2013;368:1704-1712.
4. O'Connor CM, Dunne MW, Pfeffer MA, et al; Investigators in the WIZARD Study. Azithromycin for the secondary prevention of coronary heart disease events: the WIZARD study: a randomized controlled trial. *JAMA.* 2003;290:1459-1466.

40 Sleep Disorders

Obstructive Sleep Apnea and Severe Maternal-Infant Morbidity/Mortality in the United States, 1998-2009

Louis JM, Mogos MF, Salemi JL, et al (Univ of South Florida, Tampa, FL; et al)

Sleep 37:843-849, 2014

Study Objectives.—A recent trend in increasing rates of severe maternal morbidity and mortality despite quality improvements has been noted. The goal of this study is to estimate the national prevalence of obstructive sleep apnea (OSA) in pregnant women and examine associations between OSA and pregnancy-related morbidities, including in-hospital maternal mortality.

Design.—A retrospective, cross-sectional analysis.

Setting.—A nationally representative sample of maternal hospital discharges from 1998-2009.

Patients or Participants.—The analytic sample included 55,781,965 pregnancy-related inpatient hospital discharges.

Interventions.—N/A.

Measurements and Results.—The Nationwide Inpatient Sample (NIS) database was used to identify hospital stays for women who were pregnant or gave birth. Among these women, we determined length of hospital stay, in-hospital mortality, and used International Classification of Diseases, Ninth Revision, Clinical Modification (ICD-9-CM) codes to identify OSA and other outcome measures. Multivariable logistic regression modeling was used to calculate adjusted odds ratios (OR) and 95% confidence intervals (CI) for the associations between OSA and each outcome. The overall rate of OSA was 3.0 per 10,000; however, the rate climbed substantially from 0.7 in 1998 to 7.3 in 2009, with an average annual increase of 24%. After controlling for obesity and other potential confounders, OSA was associated with increased odds of pregnancy-related morbidities including preeclampsia (OR, 2.5; 95% CI, 2.2–2.9), eclampsia (OR, 5.4; 95% CI, 3.3–8.9), cardiomyopathy (OR, 9.0; 95% CI, 7.5–10.9), and pulmonary embolism (OR, 4.5; 95% CI, 2.3–8.9). Women with OSA experienced a more than fivefold increased odds of in-hospital mortality (95% CI, 2.4–11.5). The adverse effects of OSA on selected outcomes were exacerbated by obesity.

Conclusions.—Obstructive sleep apnea is associated with severe maternal morbidity, cardiovascular morbidity, and in-hospital death. Targeted interventions may improve pregnancy outcomes in this group.

▶ Previous studies have shown an association between obstructive sleep apnea (OSA) and gestational diabetes, hypertension, and preeclampsia.[1] This study adds to the literature by examining the largest dataset of more than 55 million pregnancy-related hospital discharges. OSA is associated with increased odds of cardiomyopathy, pulmonary embolism, eclampsia, and in-hospital mortality. The odds risk range from 5.4 to 9 and was independent of comorbid obesity. The investigators noted an increased diagnosis of OSA and obesity over the course of the timeline, which is not surprising given that the rates of obesity are climbing. Women with OSA were more likely to be older, smoke, drink, and use illicit drugs along with being of lower socioeconomic status.

There are obvious limitations to doing research using datasets based on billing codes. However, the high odds ratio in this study should trigger providers and hospitals to focus on increased awareness of OSA in the pregnant women and goals to reduce the adverse outcomes to both mother and baby.

S. F. Jones, MD, FCCP, DABSM

Reference

1. Chen YH, Kang JH, Lin CC, Wang IT, Keller JJ, Lin HC. Obstructive sleep apnea and the risk of adverse pregnancy outcomes. *Am J Obstet Gynecol*. 2012;206: 136.e1-136.e5.

Role of Sleep Apnea and Continuous Positive Airway Pressure Therapy in the Incidence of Stroke or Coronary Heart Disease in Women

Campos-Rodriguez F, Martinez-Garcia MA, Reyes-Nuñez N, et al (Hospital Universitario de Valme, Seville, Spain; Hospital Universitario y Politecnico La Fe, Valencia, Spain; et al)

Am J Respir Crit Care Med 189:1544-1550, 2014

Rationale.—It is unknown whether obstructive sleep apnea (OSA) may be a risk factor for incident cardiovascular events in women.

Objectives.—We sought to investigate whether OSA increases the incidence of a composite of stroke or coronary heart disease (CHD) in women, and the role of continuous positive airway pressure (CPAP) treatment on this association.

Methods.—This was a prospective, observational study conducted in two Spanish teaching hospitals between 1998 and 2007. Consecutive women referred for suspected OSA and free of previous stroke and CHD were analyzed. Women with an apnea–hypopnea index (AHI) less than 10 comprised the control group, and those with an AHI greater than or equal to 10 were diagnosed with OSA and classified as CPAP-treated (adherence $\geq$ 4 h/d) or untreated (adherence $<$ 4 h/d or not prescribed). The follow-up ended in December 2010.

Measurements and Main Results.—A total of 967 women were studied (median follow-up, 6.8 yr; interquartile range, 5.2–8.2). The untreated OSA group showed a greater incidence rate of the composite outcome than the control group (2.19 vs. 0.54 per 100 person-years; $P < 0.0005$). Compared with the control group, the fully adjusted hazard ratios for the composite outcome incidence were 2.76 (95% confidence interval [CI], 1.35–5.62) for the untreated OSA group, and 0.91 (95% CI, 0.43–1.95) for the CPAP-treated group. When the type of cardiovascular event was separately assessed, untreated OSA showed a stronger association with incident stroke (adjusted hazard ratio, 6.44; 95% CI, 1.46–28.3) than with CHD (adjusted hazard ratio, 1.77; 95% CI, 0.76–4.09).

Conclusions.—In women, untreated OSA is associated with increased incidence of serious cardiovascular outcomes, particularly incident stroke. Adequate CPAP treatment seems to reduce this risk (Fig 2).

▶ Much of the known literature about the association between increased risk of cardiovascular events and stroke are from studies with little representation from

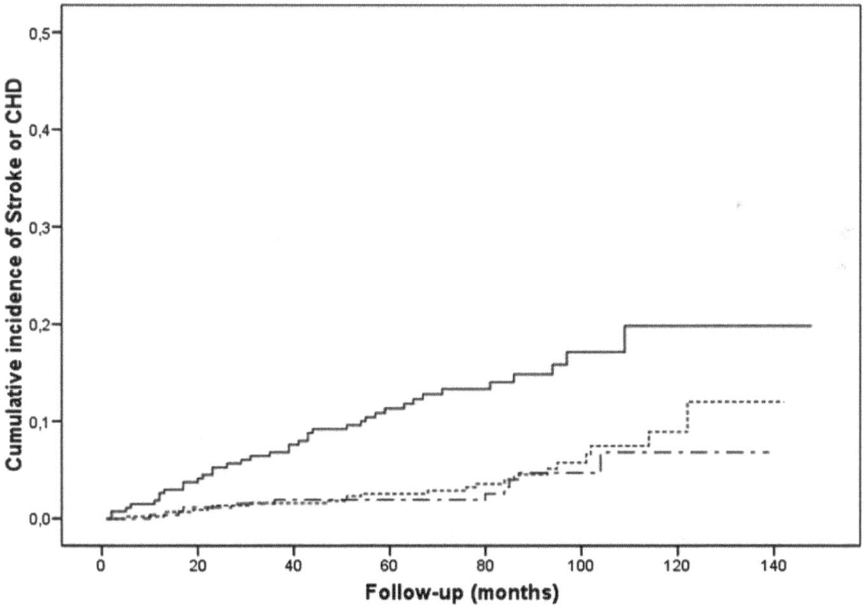

FIGURE 2.—Kaplan-Meier cardiovascular cumulative incidence curves for study groups. AHI = apnea–hypopnea index; CHD = coronary heart disease. *Dashed line*, AHI less than 10 (control group). *Dotted line*, AHI greater than or equal to 10 treated with continuous positive airway pressure. *Straight line*, AHI greater than or equal to 10 untreated. The cumulative incidence of stroke or CHD was significantly higher in the group of women with AHI greater than or equal to 10 and untreated compared with the control group (AHI < 10): $P < 0.0005$. (Reprinted from Campos-Rodriguez F, Martinez-Garcia MA, Reyes-Nuñez N, et al. Role of sleep apnea and continuous positive airway pressure therapy in the incidence of stroke or coronary heart disease in women. *Am J Respir Crit Care Med.* 2014;189:1544-1550, Official Journal of the American Thoracic Society. © 2014, American Thoracic Society, http://www.ajrccm.org.)

women. For this reason, we do not know if untreated obstructive sleep apnea (OSA) is associated with similar risk in women.

In this prospective observational clinical cohort study of nearly 1000 women conducted over a median follow-up of 82 months, investigators examined the role of OSA and positive airway pressure treatment on the incidence of stroke or coronary heart disease in women. Untreated sleep apnea is associated with increased risk of either first-time stroke or coronary heart disease, but a stronger association was found with stroke. Use of continuous positive airway pressure (CPAP) seems to mitigate the risk (Fig 2).

A major strength in this study is the duration of follow-up and that CPAP compliance was measured objectively using the download data. The limitation of this study is its observational nonrandomized design and its potential for selection bias. The authors address the limitations thoroughly.

The major impact of this study is that there is clearly an association between OSA and stroke or coronary heart disease in women (which is the number 1 leading cause of death in women). The results of this study shed light on the fact that OSA does not have gender bias. Education about the benefits of CPAP treatment is important and should be emphasized.

S. F. Jones, MD, FCCP, DABSM

Nocturnal intermittent hypoxia predicts prevalent hypertension in the European Sleep Apnoea Database cohort study

Tkacova R, on behalf of the European Sleep Apnoea Database study collaborators (P.J. Safarik Univ, Kosice, Slovakia; et al)

Eur Respir J 44:931-941, 2014

Systemic hypertension is associated with obstructive sleep apnoea syndrome (OSAS) but the pathophysiological mechanisms are incompletely understood. A collaborative European network of 24 sleep centres established a European Sleep Apnoea Database to evaluate cardiovascular morbidity associated with OSAS.

11 911 adults referred with suspected OSAS between March 2007 and September 2013 underwent overnight sleep studies, either cardiorespiratory polygraphy or polysomnography. We compared the predictive value of the apnoea–hypopnoea index (AHI) and 4% oxygen desaturation index (ODI) for prevalent hypertension, adjusting for relevant covariates including age, smoking, obesity, dyslipidaemia and diabetes.

Among patients (70% male, mean ± SD age 52 ± 12 years), 78% had AHI > 5 events$\cdot$h^{-1} and 41% systemic hypertension. Both AHI and ODI independently related to prevalent hypertension after adjustment for relevant covariates ($p < 0.0001$ for linear trend across quartiles (Q) of severity for both variables). However, in multiple regression analysis with both ODI and AHI in the model, ODI was, whereas AHI was not, independently associated with prevalent hypertension: odds ratios (95% CI) for Q4 *versus* Q1 regarding ODI were 2.01 (1.61–2.51) and regarding AHI were 0.92 (0.74–1.15) ($p < 0.0001$ and $p = 0.3054$, respectively).

This cross sectional study suggests that chronic intermittent hypoxia plays an important role in OSAS-related hypertension.

▶ The Wisconsin Sleep Cohort Study showed a dose-response relationship between apnea hypopnea index (AHI) and hypertension after adjusting for confounders.[1] The European Sleep Apnoea Database cohort study similarly evaluated cross-sectional data from nearly 12 000 adults. Although it too noted an independent relationship between the AHI and the oxygen desaturation index (ODI) to prevalent hypertension, after a multiple regression analysis, only the ODI was independently associated with hypertension.

The authors suggested that it is chronic intermittent hypoxia that plays a significant mechanism in the development of hypertension. This is in contrast to other studies that suggest a role of sympathetic activation and arousal in the mechanism.[2]

One of the limitations (and strengths) of the study is the varying methods of diagnosis OSA in this study, which uses both in laboratory and ambulatory methods. Although this obviously led to the study's large sample size, which is nearly 12 times the size of the Wisconsin Sleep Cohort Study, it also led to varying ways of scoring respiratory events. This could have generated the less than robust relationship between AHI and hypertension.

One of the implications of this study is the impact that only ODI carries a significant association with hypertension. If this is true, then scoring sleep studies becomes much more objective and simpler.

S. F. Jones, MD, FCCP, DABSM

References

1. Young T, Peppard P, Palta M, et al. Population-based study of sleep-disordered breathing as a risk factor for hypertension. *Arch Intern Med.* 1997;157: 1746-1752.
2. Prabhakar NR, Kumar GK. Mechanisms of sympathetic activation and blood pressure elevation by intermittent hypoxia. *Respir Physiol Neurobiol.* 2010;174: 156-161.

Diabetes Mellitus Prevalence and Control in Sleep-Disordered Breathing: The European Sleep Apnea Cohort (ESADA) Study

Kent BD, on behalf of the ESADA collaborators (St. Vincent's Univ Hosp, Dublin, Ireland; et al)

Chest 146:982-990, 2014

Background.—OSA is associated with an increased risk of cardiovascular morbidity. A driver of this is metabolic dysfunction and in particular type 2 diabetes mellitus (T2DM). Prior studies identifying a link between OSA and T2DM have excluded subjects with undiagnosed T2DM, and there is a lack of population-level data on the interaction between OSA and glycemic control among patients with diabetes. We assessed the relationship between OSA severity and T2DM prevalence and control in a large multinational population.

Methods.—We performed a cross-sectional analysis of 6,616 participants in the European Sleep Apnea Cohort (ESADA) study, using multivariate regression analysis to assess T2DM prevalence according to OSA severity, as measured by the oxyhemoglobin desaturation index. Patients with diabetes were identified by previous history and medication prescription, and by screening for undiagnosed diabetes with glycosylated hemoglobin (HbA1c) measurement. The relationship of OSA severity with glycemic control was assessed in diabetic subjects.

Results.—T2DM prevalence increased with OSA severity, from 6.6% in subjects without OSA to 28.9% in those with severe OSA. Despite adjustment for obesity and other confounding factors, in comparison with subjects free of OSA, patients with mild, moderate, or severe disease had an OR (95% CI) of 1.33 (1.04-1.72), 1.73 (1.33-2.25), and 1.87 (1.45-2.42) ($P < .001$), respectively, for prevalent T2DM. Diabetic subjects with more severe OSA had worse glycemic control, with adjusted mean HbA1c levels 0.72% higher in patients with severe OSA than in those without sleep-disordered breathing (analysis of covariance, $P < .001$).

Conclusions.—Increasing OSA severity is associated with increased likelihood of concomitant T2DM and worse diabetic control in patients with T2DM (Fig 2).

▶ This is the largest study to date aiming to examine the relationship between obstructive sleep apnea (OSA) severity and type 2 diabetes mellitus (T2DM) prevalence. The study used the European Sleep Apnea Cohort (ESADA)

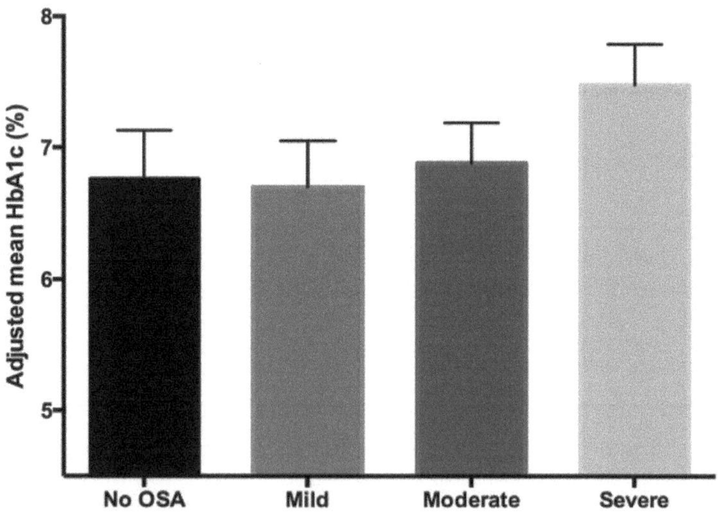

FIGURE 2.—Adjusted mean HbA1c levels among diabetic subjects stratified by OSA severity. Analysis adjusted for age, sex, race, study site, smoking history, alcohol use, average sleep length, BMI, neck circumference, coronary artery disease, congestive heart failure, hyperlipidemia, COPD, psychiatric disease, and medication use. Analysis of covariance, $P < .001$. See Figure 1 legend for expansion of abbreviations. (Reprinted from Kent BD, on behalf of the ESADA collaborators. Diabetes mellitus prevalence and control in sleep-disordered breathing: the European Sleep Apnea Cohort (ESADA) study. *Chest*. 2014;146:982-990, © 2014, American College of Chest Physicians.)

study, which is a prospective multicenter European study. Both full polysomnography or limited cardiopulmonary polygraphy was used in the study population and hemoglobin A1C was used instead of fasting glucose.

The study found a dose-responsive curve between OSA severity and prevalence of T2DM with unadjusted odds ratio ranging from 1.85 to 7.12 for mild to severe OSA. There was still an independent relationship even after adjustment for confounders. Another interesting finding was that increasing severity of OSA predicted increased likelihood of suboptimal glycemic control (higher hemoglobin A1C values) (Fig 2).

One of the major strengths of this study is the sample size of more than 6500 participants. The investigators reported severity of OSA based on the oxygen desaturation index, which is more objective and not subject to bias in the scoring of apneas and hypopneas. This is particularly important because different study types were used (full polysomnography vs cardiopulmonary polygraphy). One of the limitations is the cross-sectional nature of the study, which fails to draw cause-and-effect relationship.

Nevertheless, I find this study an important product from the ESADA collaborators. Being able to conduct large multicenter population-based studies from diverse backgrounds will help us understand impact of OSA on a global level.

S. F. Jones, MD, FCCP, DABSM

Sleep Restriction Therapy for Insomnia is Associated with Reduced Objective Total Sleep Time, Increased Daytime Somnolence, and Objectively Impaired Vigilance: Implications for the Clinical Management of Insomnia Disorder

Kyle SD, Miller CB, Rogers Z, et al (Univ of Manchester, UK; Univ of Sydney, Australia; et al)

Sleep 37:229-237, 2014

Study Objectives.—To investigate whether sleep restriction therapy (SRT) is associated with reduced objective total sleep time (TST), increased daytime somnolence, and impaired vigilance.

Design.—Within-subject, noncontrolled treatment investigation.

Setting.—Sleep research laboratory.

Participants.—Sixteen patients [10 female, mean age = 47.1 (10.8) y] with well-defined psychophysiological insomnia (PI), reporting TST ≤ 6 h.

Interventions.—Patients were treated with single-component SRT over a 4-w protocol, sleeping in the laboratory for 2 nights prior to treatment initiation and for 3 nights (SRT night 1, 8, 22) during the acute interventional phase. The psychomotor vigilance task (PVT) was completed at seven defined time points [day 0 (baseline), day 1,7,8,21,22 (acute treatment) and day 84 (3 mo)]. The Epworth Sleepiness Scale (ESS) was completed at baseline, w 1-4, and 3 mo.

Measurement and Results.—Subjective sleep outcomes and global insomnia severity significantly improved before and after SRT. There was, however, a robust decrease in PSG-defined TST during acute implementation of SRT, by an average of 91 min on night 1, 78 min on night 8, and 69 min on night 22, relative to baseline ($P < 0.001$; effect size range = 1.60-1.80). During SRT, PVT lapses were significantly increased from baseline (at three of five assessment points, all $P < 0.05$; effect size range = 0.69-0.78), returning to baseline levels by 3 mo ($P = 0.43$). A similar pattern was observed for RT, with RTs slowing during acute treatment (at four of five assessment points, all $P < 0.05$; effect size range = 0.57-0.89) and returning to pretreatment levels at 3 mo ($P = 0.78$). ESS scores were increased at w 1, 2, and 3 (relative to baseline; all $P < 0.05$); by 3 mo, sleepiness had returned to baseline (normative) levels ($P = 0.65$).

Conclusion.—For the first time we show that acute sleep restriction therapy is associated with reduced objective total sleep time, increased daytime sleepiness, and objective performance impairment. Our data have important implications for implementation guidelines around the safe and effective delivery of cognitive behavioral therapy for insomnia.

▶ Cognitive behavioral therapy for insomnia (CBTI) is an effective treatment of insomnia with improvements in sleep that are similar to hypnotics but with long-term efficacy. Fundamental in CBTI is the practice of sleep restriction, which includes no napping, and serves to increase the sleep pressure and address the circadian rhythm component of sleep. As the name implies, sleep restriction is less sleep. The minimal amount of sleep prescribed depends on a number of factors but are centered around patient sleep diaries and can vary among practitioners. Using objective measures of polysomnography and psychomotor vigilance testing, the investigators examined the effect of sleep restriction on the early course of CBTI and found increased self-reported sleepiness and impaired performance on the psychomotor vigilance test.

I think this study is interesting with regard to the short-term effects of sleep restriction in CBTI, particularly for the objective approach the authors used. But I also think that their methods may serve as limitations—specifically incongruencies between psychomotor vigilance testing and actual real-life performance. Overall, I think the literature supporting CBTI for insomnia is robust, and CBTI is an effective therapy; I will continue to recommend it to my patients. There may definitely be a "necessary pain to achieve gain" as the authors simply put it, and patients undergoing CBTI need to be aware of this; however, there is also "light at the end of the tunnel," and we need to express that to our patients as well.

S. F. Jones, MD, FCCP, DABSM

A Randomized Controlled Trial of Mindfulness Meditation for Chronic Insomnia

Ong JC, Manber R, Segal Z, et al (Rush Univ Med Ctr, Chicago, IL; Stanford Univ Med Ctr, Palo Alto, CA; Univ of Toronto, Ontario, Canada; et al)
Sleep 37:1553-1563, 2014

Study Objectives.—To evaluate the efficacy of mindfulness meditation for the treatment of chronic insomnia.

Design.—Three-arm, single-site, randomized controlled trial.

Setting.—Academic medical center.

Participants.—Fifty-four adults with chronic insomnia.

Interventions.—Participants were randomized to either mindfulness-based stress reduction (MBSR), mindfulness-based therapy for insomnia (MBTI), or an eight-week self-monitoring (SM) condition.

Measurements and Results.—Patient-reported outcome measures were total wake time (TWT) from sleep diaries, the pre-sleep arousal scale (PSAS), measuring a prominent waking correlate of insomnia, and the Insomnia Severity Index (ISI) to determine remission and response as clinical endpoints. Objective sleep measures were derived from laboratory polysomnography and wrist actigraphy. Linear mixed models showed that those receiving a meditation-based intervention (MBSR or MBTI) had significantly greater reductions on TWT minutes (43.75 vs 1.09), PSAS (7.13 vs 0.16), and ISI (4.56 vs 0.06) from baseline-to-post compared to SM. Post hoc analyses revealed that each intervention was superior to SM on each of the patient-reported measures, but no significant differences were found when comparing MBSR to MBTI from baseline-to-post. From baseline to 6-month follow-up, MBTI had greater reductions in ISI scores than MBSR ($P < 0.05$), with the largest difference occurring at the 3-month follow-up. Remission and response rates in MBTI and MBSR were sustained from post-treatment through follow-up, with MBTI showing the highest rates of treatment remission (50%) and response (78.6%) at the 6-month follow-up.

Conclusions.—Mindfulness meditation appears to be a viable treatment option for adults with chronic insomnia and could provide an alternative to traditional treatments for insomnia.

Trial Registration.—Mindfulness-Based Approaches to Insomnia: clinicaltrials.gov, identifier: NCT00768781 (Fig 2).

▶ Insomnia is a widely prevalent problem in the United States with significant personal health and public impact. Sleeping pills and cognitive behavioral therapy for insomnia are both forms of treatment. Sleeping pills carry significant side effects, as well as the development of tolerance and dependence. Cognitive behavioral therapy for insomnia (CBTI) is not widely available. Many of our patients seek complementary and alternative medicine whether providers know it or not. Techniques that are used in complementary and alternative medicine may be useful in patients with insomnia.

This was a randomized controlled trial to evaluate the efficacy of meditation-based therapies on sleep measures. Two meditation-based therapies were used: mindfulness-based stress reduction (MBSR) and mindfulness-based therapy for insomnia (MBTI), which includes meditation but also principles of sleep restriction. Both of these therapies were compared with self-monitoring of sleep diaries (controls).

Both meditation-based approaches reduced total wake time and presleep arousal scale and improved the insomnia severity index compared with self-monitoring (Fig 2). It is important to note that significant improvements were

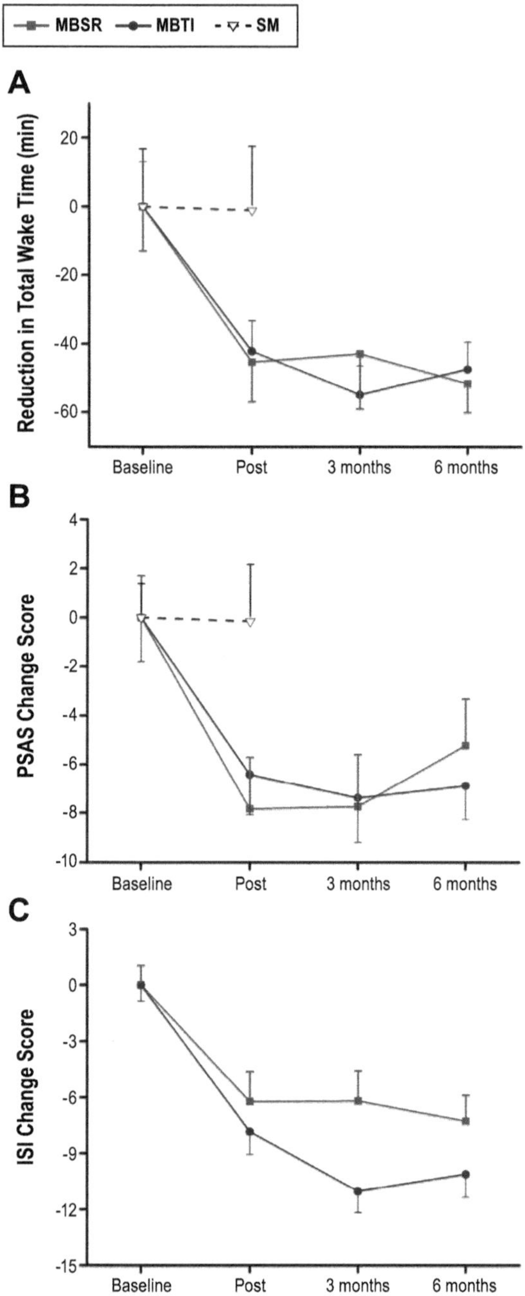

FIGURE 2.—Patient-reported outcomes. (**A**) Total wake time (in minutes; with standard error of the mean) across study arms as reported on sleep diaries. Data presented are change scores from baseline to each assessment point. Raw data (mean, standard deviation, effect sizes) for each arm are reported in Table 2. (**B**) Pre-sleep arousal scale (PSAS) total scores (with standard error of the mean) across study arms. Data presented are change scores from baseline to each assessment point. Raw data (mean, standard deviation, effect sizes) for each arm are reported in Table 2. (**C**) Insomnia Severity Index (ISI) total scores (with standard error of the mean) across the MBSR and MBTI arms. Data presented are change scores from baseline to each assessment point. Raw data (mean, standard deviation, effect sizes) for each arm are reported in Table 2. MBSR, mindfulness-based stress reduction; MBTI, mindfulness-based therapy for insomnia; SM, self-monitoring. (Reprinted from Ong JC, Manber R, Segal Z, et al. A randomized controlled trial of mindfulness meditation for chronic insomnia. *Sleep*. 2014;37:1553-1563, © 2014, American Academy of Sleep Medicine.)

seen only on self-reported measures (sleep diaries) and not on objective measures (PSG and actigraphy). Nevertheless, treatment effects were sustained in the meditation groups with those patients who received MBTI greater that MBSR, which may be due to the addition of the behavioral component of MBTI such as sleep restriction, etc.

Although I am not ready to prescribe mindfulness meditation to all my insomnia patients yet, I do think that this opens the doors to additional research in the field. More questions need to be answered, including applicability, comparative effectiveness research with hypnotics, and with CBTI, for example. Nevertheless, if additional research does show that mindfulness mediation is an effective treatment for chronic insomnia, I think many more patients could be reached and treated.

S. F. Jones, MD, FCCP, DABSM

41 Critical Care Medicine

Catheter-Directed Thrombolytic Intervention Is Effective for Patients with Massive and Submassive Pulmonary Embolism

Akin H, Al-Jubouri M, Assi Z, et al (Jobst Vascular Inst, Toledo, OH)
Ann Vasc Surg 28:1589-1594, 2014

Background.—Massive pulmonary embolism (MPE) is a significant cause of mortality and, with submassive pulmonary embolism (SPE), is associated with chronic thromboembolic pulmonary hypertension, resulting in ongoing patient morbidity. Standard treatment is anticoagulation, although systemic thrombolytic therapy has been shown to reduce early mortality in patients with MPE and improve cardiopulmonary hemodynamics in patients with SPE. However, systemic lysis is associated with significant bleeding risk. Early reports of catheter-directed techniques (CDT) suggest favorable outcomes in patients with MPE and SPE with reduced risk of hemorrhage. The purpose of this study is to evaluate efficacy and safety outcomes in MPE and SPE patients treated with CDT.

Methods.—Seventeen patients treated with CDT for MPE and SPE were clinically and hemodynamically evaluated. Patients were grouped by severity of pulmonary embolism: MPE ($n = 5$) or SPE ($n = 12$). Pre- and post-interventional measures were assessed, including pulmonary artery pressures (PAPs), cardiac biomarkers, tricuspid regurgitation, right ventricular (RV) dilatation, and systolic function. Nine patients had contraindications to systemic thrombolytic therapy.

Results.—PAP was elevated in 94% at presentation. The average dose of recombinant tissue plasminogen activator (rt-PA) was 31 mg; 44 mg in MPE and 26 mg in SPE. Pre- and post-intervention PAPs were recorded in 13 patients. All demonstrated an acute reduction in post-treatment PAP, averaging 37%. At presentation, all MPE and 10 (83%) SPE patients showed both RV dilatation and reduced function on echocardiography, which normalized in 76% (13/ 17) and improved in 24% (4/17) after CDT. Patients who demonstrated left ventricle underfilling before CDT (2 [40%] MPE and 2 [20%] SPE) normalized after CDT. All MPE and 11 (92%) SPE patients had tricuspid regurgitation on echocardiography pretreatment, which resolved in 60% and 58% of MPE and SPE patients, respectively. One delayed mortality occurred in an MPE patient who was hypotensive and hypoxic at presentation. There was one puncture site bleed.

Conclusions.—CDT was successful in the acute management of patients with MPE and SPE. CDT rapidly restores cardiopulmonary hemodynamics using reduced doses of rt-PA. These observations suggest that CDT should be considered in MPE and SPE patients to rapidly restore cardiopulmonary hemodynamics, reduce acute morbidity and mortality, reduce bleeding complications, and potentially avoid long-term morbidity.

▶ This procedure is now commonly performed by interventional radiologists. It is reassuring to know that it is indeed safe and effective for those patients who need it.

J. A. Barker, MD, CPE, FACP, FCCP, FAASM

Early Management of Severe Sepsis: Concepts and Controversies

Marik PE (Eastern Virginia Med School, Norfolk, VA)

Chest 145:1407-1418, 2014

Sepsis is among the most common reasons for admission to ICUs throughout the world, and it is believed to be the third most common cause of death in the United States. The pathogenetic mechanism and physiologic changes associated with sepsis are exceedingly complex, but our understanding is evolving rapidly. The major pathophysiologic changes in patients with septic shock include vasoplegic shock (distributive shock), myocardial depression, altered microvascular flow, and a diffuse endothelial injury. These pathophysiologic changes play a central role in the management of sepsis. The early management of patients with severe sepsis and septic shock centers on the administration of antibiotics, IV fluids, and vasoactive agents, followed by source control. However, the specific approach to the resuscitation of patients with septic shock remains highly controversial. This review provides a practical and physiologic-based approach to the early management of sepsis and explores the controversies surrounding the management of this complex condition.

▶ Dr Marik lays out the current controversies of sepsis management in a thoughtful and clear-cut article. He differs somewhat from the Surviving Sepsis leadership and publications but outlines his rationale and backs it up with literature support. This is a useful read for all intensivists.

J. A. Barker, MD, CPE, FACP, FCCP, FAASM

Difficult Airway Management for Novice Physicians: A Randomized Trial Comparing Direct and Video-Assisted Laryngoscopy

Ambrosio A, Pfannenstiel T, Bach K, et al (Naval Med Ctr San Diego, CA)

Otolaryngol Head Neck Surg 150:775-778, 2014

Objectives.—To detect a difference in (1) intubation success and (2) successful intubation times between novice physicians using a Macintosh-style or video-assisted laryngoscope on a difficult airway manikin.

Study Design.—Prospective randomized trial.

Setting.—Academic, tertiary medical center.

Methods.—Forty first-year residents across a variety of disciplines with fewer than 5 total live intubations were recruited for the study. Testing took place during orientation prior to commencement of clinical duties. The entire group was provided training by faculty otolaryngologists and anesthesiologists using both laryngoscope types on a manikin airway simulator in a standard intubating scenario. Subjects were then randomized into 2 testing groups, using either a Macintosh laryngoscope or video-assisted laryngoscope in a difficult intubation scenario. The difficult airway simulation entailed oral cavity/oropharyngeal obstruction using inflation of the tongue, as well as cervical spine immobilization with a rigid collar preventing extension and elevation of the head and limiting oral cavity opening. Success was defined as a confirmed endotracheal intubation by the testing instructor in 120 seconds or less.

Results.—The Macintosh laryngoscope group ($n = 19$) had an intubation success rate of 47.4% with a mean intubation time of 69.0 seconds (95% confidence interval [CI]: 52.7, 85.2). The video-assisted group ($n = 21$) demonstrated a significantly higher success rate of 100% ($P < .0001$) and a decreased mean intubation time of 23.1 seconds (95% CI: 18.4, 27.8; $P < .0001$). The mean difference in success rate between groups was 52.6% (95% CI: 30.0%, 75.3%).

Conclusions.—Novice physicians with little to no prior intubation experience showed significantly higher intubation success with lower intubation times using a video-assisted laryngoscope in a difficult airway manikin simulator.

► Video laryngoscopy for intubation should now be the standard in teaching hospitals, which this study confirms. One hundred percent success in half the time compared with under 50% success could mean the difference between life and death for a patient. In addition, the mentor can see what the learner is doing both to instruct and to ensure the proper placement of the endotracheal tube.

This simple study is useful as well as elegant.

J. A. Barker, MD, CPE, FACP, FCCP, FAASM

Preparing an ICU room to welcome a critically ill patient with Ebola virus disease

Pasquier P, Ficko C, Mérens A, et al (Bégin Military Teaching Hosp, Saint-Mandé, France)

Intensive Care Med 41:118-119, 2015

Background.—Hospitals are being equipped to manage the care of critically ill patients with Ebola virus disease. The specifics of what is needed for an Ebola virus disease-n-intensive care unit (EVD-ICU) differ from what is available in a regular ICU room.

Patient Equipment.—The EVD-ICU room is entered through an airlock, and negative air pressure is maintained. The pressure gradient increases

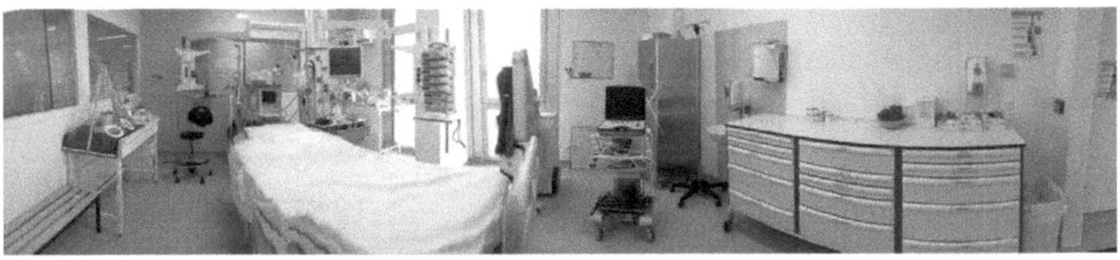

FIGURE 1.—A fully equipped EVD-ICU room. (With kind permission from Springer Science+Business Media. Pasquier P, Ficko C, Mérens A, et al. Preparing an ICU room to welcome a critically ill patient with Ebola virus disease. *Intensive Care Med.* 2015;41:118-119, with permission from Springer-Verlag Berlin Heidelberg and ESICM.)

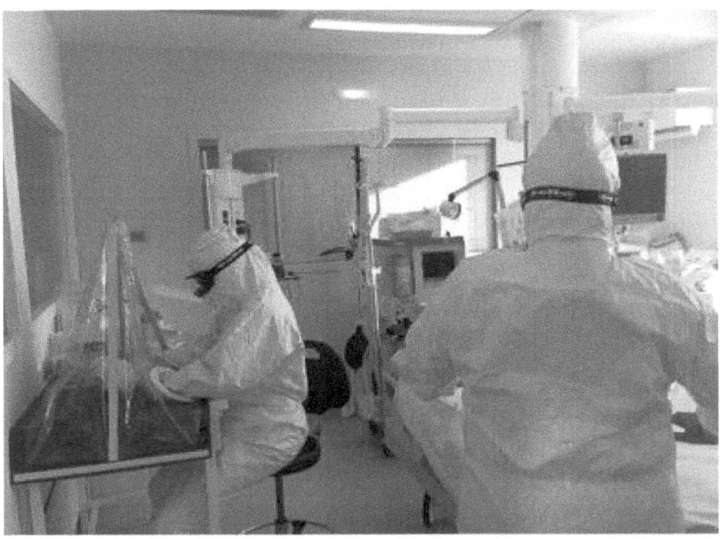

FIGURE 2.—Healthcare providers wearing PPE and training at a field laboratory recovered with a portable glove bag. (With kind permission from Springer Science+Business Media. Pasquier P, Ficko C, Mérens A, et al. Preparing an ICU room to welcome a critically ill patient with Ebola virus disease. *Intensive Care Med.* 2015;41:118-119, with permission from Springer-Verlag Berlin Heidelberg and ESICM.)

from the airlock to the room. The equipment commonly found in an ICU room is present along with a field laboratory recovered with a pyramidal portable glove bag, a mobile system for obtaining radiographs, and a portable ultrasound machine. This equipment is dedicated to the patient throughout his or her stay in the room.

Healthcare Workers.—The safety of healthcare workers requires special equipment for the management of EVD patients. Their personal protective equipment includes a single-use impermeable gown, a hood, a face mask, goggles, two pairs of nitrile gloves, a pair of gloves with extended cuffs, and boots. In addition, specific equipment for the disposal of waste products is also available.

Conclusions.—The safe, appropriate management of EVD patients who require intensive care demands specific equipment in a dedicated ICU room. Both the patient and the healthcare provider must be accommodated (Figs 1 and 2).

▶ This is the reality in which we all now live. If your hospital has not invested the hours of preparation for Ebola or a similarly catastrophic outbreak, this short article will be of great use. Please review Figs 1 and 2, which outline the setup and personal protective equipment that will be needed.

J. A. Barker, MD, CPE, FACP, FCCP, FAASM

PART SIX

HEART AND CARDIOVASCULAR DISEASE

MICHAEL R. GOLD, MD, PhD

Introduction

Reduction in cardiovascular mortality has been one of the major reasons for the prolongation in life expectancy which began in the latter half of the 20th century. Mortality from cardiovascular causes continues to decline with a more than 30% decline in the last 15 years alone. This has been driven by improvements in all facets of cardiovascular care from prevention, to medical therapy and interventional/surgical procedures. The advances in our understanding of cardiovascular disease continued in 2015 and some of the most important studies are highlighted in this edition of the YEAR BOOK OF MEDICINE. Topics include duration of therapy for ischemic heart disease, comparisons of cardiac imaging techniques, the influence of co-morbidities on the prognosis of heart failure, timing of surgery for mitral regurgitation, management of atrial fibrillation, and new device therapy for drug refractory angina pectoris.

Michael R. Gold, MD

42 Arrhythmias

Rivaroxaban vs. vitamin K antagonists for cardioversion in atrial fibrillation

Cappato R, on behalf of the X-VeRT Investigators (Univ of Milan, San Donato Milanese, Italy; et al)

Eur Heart J 35:3346-3355, 2014

Aims.—X-VeRT is the first prospective randomized trial of a novel oral anticoagulant in patients with atrial fibrillation undergoing elective cardioversion.

Methods and Results.—We assigned 1504 patients to rivaroxaban (20 mg once daily, 15 mg if creatinine clearance was between 30 and 49 mL/min) or dose-adjusted vitamin K antagonists (VKAs) in a 2:1 ratio. Investigators selected either an early (target period of 1–5 days after randomization) or delayed (3–8 weeks) cardioversion strategy. The primary efficacy outcome was the composite of stroke, transient ischaemic attack, peripheral embolism, myocardial infarction, and cardiovascular death. The primary safety outcome was major bleeding. The primary efficacy outcome occurred in 5 (two strokes) of 978 patients (0.51%) in the rivaroxaban group and in 5 (two strokes) of 492 patients (1.02%) in the VKA group [risk ratio 0.50; 95% confidence interval (CI) 0.15–1.73]. In the rivaroxaban group, four patients experienced primary efficacy events following early cardioversion (0.71%) and one following delayed cardioversion (0.24%). In the VKA group, three patients had primary efficacy events following early cardioversion (1.08%) and two following delayed cardioversion (0.93%). Rivaroxaban was associated with a significantly shorter time to cardioversion compared with VKAs ($P < 0.001$). Major bleeding occurred in six patients (0.6%) in the rivaroxaban group and four patients (0.8%) in the VKA group (risk ratio 0.76; 95% CI 0.21–2.67).

Conclusion.—Oral rivaroxaban appears to be an effective and safe alternative to VKAs and may allow prompt cardioversion.

Name of the Trial Registry.—Clinicaltrials.gov; Trial registration number: NCT01674647 (Table 2).

▶ Cardioversion is a common therapy for persistent atrial fibrillation (AF). Although it has a high acute success rate, recurrences are frequent, and there are risks of embolic events associated with the termination of this arrhythmia. For this reason, anticoagulation is mandated by guidelines before cardioversion. Traditionally, this entails 3 weeks of therapeutic (international normalized ratio ≥2.0) with vitamin K antagonists (VKA), most commonly warfarin. Surprisingly, this long-standing strategy has not been validated in randomized trials.

TABLE 2.—Number of Patients with Outcome Events

	Total by Treatment			Early		Delayed	
	Rivaroxaban	VKA	RR (95% CI)	Rivaroxaban	VKA	Rivaroxaban	VKA
Efficacy, *n* (%)[a]	*n* = 978	*n* = 492		*n* = 567	*n* = 277	*n* = 411	*n* = 215
Primary end-point	5 (0.51)	5 (1.02)	0.50 (0.15–1.73)	4 (0.71)	3 (1.08)	1 (0.24)	2 (0.93)
Stroke	2 (0.20)	2 (0.41)		2 (0.35)	1 (0.36)	0	1 (0.47)
Haemorrhagic stroke	2 (0.20)	0		2 (0.35)	0	0	0
Ischaemic stroke	0	2 (0.41)		0	1 (0.36)	0	1 (0.47)
TIA	0	0		0	0	0	0
SE	0	1 (0.20)		0	1 (0.36)	0	0
MI	1 (0.10)	1 (0.20)		1 (0.18)	0	0	1 (0.47)
Cardiovascular death	4 (0.41)	2 (0.41)		3 (0.53)	2 (0.72)	1 (0.24)	0
All-cause death	5 (0.51)	3 (0.61)		3 (0.53)	3 (1.08)	2 (0.49)	0
Safety, *n* (%)[b]	*n* = 988	*n* = 499		*n* = 575	*n* = 284	*n* = 413	*n* = 215
Major bleeding	6 (0.61)	4 (0.80)	0.76 (0.21–2.67)	3 (0.52)	3 (1.06)	3 (0.73)	1 (0.47)
Fatal	1 (0.10)	2 (0.40)		1 (0.17)	2 (0.70)	0	0
Critical site	2 (0.20)	3 (0.60)		2 (0.35)	2 (0.70)	0	1 (0.47)
ICH	2 (0.20)	1 (0.20)		2 (0.35)	0	0	1 (0.47)
Hb decrease ≥2 g/dL	4 (0.40)	1 (0.20)		1 (0.17)	1 (0.35)	3 (0.73)	0
Transfusion ≥2 units RBCs or whole blood	3 (0.30)	1 (0.20)		1 (0.17)	1 (0.35)	2 (0.48)	0

Cumulative incidence risk for adjudicated outcomes from randomization up to the date of last study medication plus 2 days. Per protocol, study treatment was to be continued up to 42 days after cardioversion.

CI, confidence interval; CV, cardiovascular; Hb, haemoglobin; ICH, intracranial haemorrhage; MI, myocardial infarction; N/A, not applicable; RBC, red blood cells; RR, risk ratio; SE, systemic embolism; TIA, transient ischaemic attack; VKA, vitamin K antagonist.

[a]mITT population.

[b]Safety population.

Reprinted from Cappato R; on behalf of the X-VeRT Investigators. Rivaroxaban vs. vitamin K antagonists for cardioversion in atrial fibrillation. *Eur Heart J*. 2014;35:3346-3355, by permission of The European Society of Cardiology.

The novel oral anticoagulants (NOAC) have the potential to allow for more rapid anticoagulation and avoid the need for frequent monitoring of anticoagulation status or heparin bridging strategies. The X-VeRT study was a prospective randomized trial of rivaroxaban, a NOAC, with VKA for cardioversion. Either an early cardioversion strategy primarily with transesophageal echo guidance or a delayed strategy after at least 3 weeks of therapeutic anticoagulation. Both the rates of embolic events, including stroke and major bleeding, were lower with rivaroxaban (Table 2), although these differences were not statistically significant. Moreover, the time to cardioversion was shorter with rivaroxaban, presumably because of delays achieving therapeutic anticoagulation with VKA. These are important findings and establish the safety and efficacy of rivaroxaban for rapid and safe cardioversion, with a observed stroke rate <0.5%. This adds to the accumulating evidence that NOACs have significant advantages for the early treatment of AF.

M. Gold, MD

43 Cardiomyopathy

Angiotensin–Neprilysin Inhibition versus Enalapril in Heart Failure

McMurray JJ, for the PARADIGM-HF Investigators and Committees (Univ of Glasgow, UK; et al)

N Engl J Med 371:993-1004, 2014

Background.—We compared the angiotensin receptor–neprilysin inhibitor LCZ696 with enalapril in patients who had heart failure with a reduced ejection fraction. In previous studies, enalapril improved survival in such patients.

Methods.—In this double-blind trial, we randomly assigned 8442 patients with class II, III, or IV heart failure and an ejection fraction of 40% or less to receive either LCZ696 (at a dose of 200 mg twice daily) or enalapril (at a dose of 10 mg twice daily), in addition to recommended therapy. The primary outcome was a composite of death from cardiovascular causes or hospitalization for heart failure, but the trial was designed to detect a difference in the rates of death from cardiovascular causes.

Results.—The trial was stopped early, according to prespecified rules, after a median follow-up of 27 months, because the boundary for an overwhelming benefit with LCZ696 had been crossed. At the time of study closure, the primary outcome had occurred in 914 patients (21.8%) in the LCZ696 group and 1117 patients (26.5%) in the enalapril group (hazard ratio in the LCZ696 group, 0.80; 95% confidence interval [CI], 0.73 to 0.87; $P < 0.001$). A total of 711 patients (17.0%) receiving LCZ696 and 835 patients (19.8%) receiving enalapril died (hazard ratio for death from any cause, 0.84; 95% CI, 0.76 to 0.93; $P < 0.001$); of these patients, 558 (13.3%) and 693 (16.5%), respectively, died from cardiovascular causes (hazard ratio, 0.80; 95% CI, 0.71 to 0.89; $P < 0.001$). As compared with enalapril, LCZ696 also reduced the risk of hospitalization for heart failure by 21% ($P < 0.001$) and decreased the symptoms and physical limitations of heart failure ($P = 0.001$). The LCZ696 group had higher proportions of patients with hypotension and nonserious angioedema but lower proportions with renal impairment, hyperkalemia, and cough than the enalapril group.

Conclusions.—LCZ696 was superior to enalapril in reducing the risks of death and of hospitalization for heart failure. (Funded by Novartis; PARADIGM-HF ClinicalTrials.gov number, NCT01035255.)

► The authors examined the effects of LCZ696, an angiotensin receptor neprilysin inhibitor, versus the gold standard therapy of angiotensin-converting enzyme inhibitor, enalapril, on cardiovascular outcomes, including death from cardiovascular causes and hospitalization for heart failure (HF). The morbidity and mortality gains in those randomly assigned to LCZ696 in addition to optimal medical management led to this randomized trial being stopped early. In fact, the number of HF patients needed to treat to prevent 1 death of only 35 is similar to that of other landmark trials in HF with reduced ejection fraction (EF; Fig 1 in the original article). The angiotensin receptor neprilysin inhibitors represent the first new and beneficial class of drugs for HF treatment in more than a decade. Neprilysin is a neutral endopeptidase that inhibits natriuretic peptides and degrades bradykinin.[1] It is, therefore, not surprising that neprilysin inhibition has added benefits over inhibition of angiotensin-converting enzyme alone. Additionally, LCZ696 was extremely well tolerated, with a primary side effect of increased symptomatic hypotension compared with enalapril (14.0% vs 9.2%; $P < .001$) but significantly less hyperkalemia, cough, and worsening renal function. Importantly, nearly 75% of the patients enrolled in the trial had either New York Heart Association class I or II symptoms, and this subgroup experienced a more pronounced reduction in the primary endpoint than those with more severe symptoms ($P = .03$). Although the future replacement of angiotensin-converting inhibitors and angiotensin receptor blockers with LCZ696 in the treatment of less sick HF patients is likely given the results of this study, further research is necessary to determine the benefits of a similar strategy for the more symptomatic HF patient with a reduced EF.

M. A. Brisco, MD, MSCE

Reference

1. Jessup M. Neprilysin inhibition—a novel therapy for heart failure. *N Engl J Med.* 2014;371:1062-1064.

Cardiac Remodeling in Response to 1 Year of Intensive Endurance Training

Arbab-Zadeh A, Perhonen M, Howden E, et al (Texas Health Presbyterian Hosp, Dallas; et al)

Circulation 130:2152-2161, 2014

Background.—It is unclear whether, and to what extent, the striking cardiac morphological manifestations of endurance athletes are a result of exercise training or a genetically determined characteristic of talented athletes. We hypothesized that prolonged and intensive endurance training in previously sedentary healthy young individuals could induce cardiac remodeling similar to that observed cross-sectionally in elite endurance athletes.

Methods and Results.—Twelve previously sedentary subjects (aged 29 ± 6 years; 7 men and 5 women) trained progressively and intensively for 12 months such that they could compete in a marathon. Magnetic resonance images for assessment of right and left ventricular mass and volumes were obtained at baseline and after 3, 6, 9, and 12 months of training. Maximum oxygen uptake (*Vȯ2max*) and cardiac output at rest and during exercise (C_2H_2 rebreathing) were measured at the same time periods. Pulmonary artery catheterization was performed before and after 1 year of training, and pressure-volume and Starling curves were constructed during decreases (lower body negative pressure) and increases (saline infusion) in cardiac volume. Mean *V̇o2max* rose from 40.3 ± 1.6 to 48.7 ± 2.5 mL/kg per minute after 1 year ($P < 0.00001$), associated with an increase in both maximal cardiac output and stroke volume. Left and right ventricular mass increased progressively with training duration and intensity and reached levels similar to those observed in elite endurance athletes. In contrast, left ventricular volume did not change significantly until 6 months of training, although right ventricular volume increased progressively from the outset; Starling and pressure-volume curves approached but did not match those of elite athletes.

Conclusions.—One year of prolonged and intensive endurance training leads to cardiac morphological adaptations in previously sedentary young subjects similar to those observed in elite endurance athletes; however, it is not sufficient to achieve similar levels of cardiac compliance and performance. Contrary to conventional thinking, the left ventricle responds to exercise with initial concentric but not eccentric remodeling during the first 6 to 9 months after commencement of endurance training depending on the duration and intensity of exercise. Thereafter, the left ventricle dilates and restores the baseline mass-to-volume ratio. In contrast, the right ventricle responds to endurance training with eccentric remodeling at all levels of training.

► Cross-sectional studies and autopsy examinations have previously revealed the distinctive pathophysiologic characteristics of endurance athletes, particularly the presence of eccentric left ventricular hypertrophy. However, given the prior lack of prospective clinical data, the question remained as to whether these observed cardiac changes were the result of endurance training or merely a preexisting and essential requirement for endurance development. Arbab-Zadeh and colleagues sought to answer this "chicken-or-egg" question of exercise physiology in a prospective study of 12 previously sedentary subjects who had never engaged in endurance training. At the conclusion of a 12-month endurance exercise program, myocardial compliance improved such that at any filling pressure, the end-diastolic volume achieved in the left ventricle was larger compared with baseline. Although eccentric hypertrophy did ensue after 9 months of training, the initial left ventricular response was actually concentric hypertrophy for the first 6 months. Interestingly, the right ventricular wall thickness and volume increased to a greater degree than the left ventricle. Despite these improvements in cardiac mass and compliance, the *V̇o2max* achieved after 12 months did not approach what has been reported in endurance athletes. The authors speculate that it may take more time and training to achieve the cardiac performance of an elite athlete. Regardless, this elegant study is the first to reveal that with the appropriate exercise intensity and duration, improvements in cardiac compliance are possible in previously sedentary individuals. These results demonstrate the remarkable plasticity of the human heart and suggest the endurance athlete's heart is not born, but created.

M. A. Brisco, MD, MSCE

Association between renal function and cardiovascular structure and function in heart failure with preserved ejection fraction

Gori M, for the PARAMOUNT Investigators (Brigham and Women's Hosp, Boston, MA; et al)

Eur Heart J 35:3442-3451, 2014

Aim.—Renal dysfunction is a common comorbidity in patients with heart failure and preserved ejection fraction (HFpEF). We sought to determine whether renal dysfunction was associated with measures of cardiovascular structure/function in patients with HFpEF.

Methods.—We studied 217 participants from the PARAMOUNT study with HFpEF who had echocardiography and measures of kidney function. We evaluated the relationships between renal dysfunction [estimated glomerular filtration rate (eGFR) >30 and <60 mL/min/1.73 m^2 and/or albuminuria] and cardiovascular structure/function.

Results.—The mean age of the study population was 71 years, 55% were women, 94% hypertensive, and 40% diabetic. Impairment of at least one parameter of kidney function was present in 62% of patients (16% only albuminuria, 23% only low eGFR, 23% both). Renal dysfunction was associated with abnormal LV geometry (defined as concentric hypertrophy, or eccentric hypertrophy, or concentric remodelling) (adjusted $P = 0.048$), lower midwall fractional shortening (MWFS) ($P = 0.009$), and higher NT-proBNP ($P = 0.006$). Compared with patients without renal dysfunction, those with low eGFR and no albuminuria had a higher prevalence of abnormal LV geometry ($P = 0.032$) and lower MWFS ($P < 0.01$), as opposed to those with only albuminuria. Conversely, albuminuria alone was associated with greater LV dimensions ($P < 0.05$). Patients with combined renal impairment had mixed abnormalities (higher LV wall thicknesses, NT-proBNP; lower MWFS).

Conclusion.—Renal dysfunction, as determined by both eGFR and albuminuria, is highly prevalent in HFpEF, and associated with cardiac remodelling and subtle systolic dysfunction. The observed differences in cardiac structure/function between each type of renal damage suggest that both parameters of kidney function might play a distinct role in HFpEF.

► The PARAMOUNT study randomized 301 patients with New York Heart Association class II or III heart failure (HF), left ventricular ejection fraction (EF) of 45% or higher, and N-terminal pro-brain natriuretic peptide (NT-proBNP) greater than 400 pg/mL to the angiotensin receptor neprilysin inhibitor LCZ696 at 200 mg twice daily or the angiotensin receptor blocker valsartan at 160 mg twice daily. Patients with estimated glomerular filtration rate (eGFR) less than 30 mL/min/1.73m^2 were excluded. At 12 weeks, LCZ696 achieved a greater statistically significant reduction in NT-proBNP compared with valsartan, the primary end point of the trial.

The prognostic and mechanistic value of albuminuria independent of a reduced eGFR has been repeatedly demonstrated in HF with reduced EF;

however, only recently evidence has emerged as it relates to HF with preserved EF (HFpEF). In this cross-sectional subanalysis of the PARAMOUNT trial, the authors explore the relationships between 2 metrics of renal dysfunction (eGFR reduction and albuminuria) and markers of cardiac structure and function as measured with echocardiography in enrolled patients. Using both domains of kidney function revealed that nearly two-third of HFpEF patients experience significant renal dysfunction. Importantly, 16% of patients had albuminuria (defined as a urine albumin to creatinine ratio greater than 17 mg/g for men and 25 mg/g for women) in the presence of an eGFR greater than 60 mL/min/m^2, demonstrating that there is likely more than 1 mechanism responsible for renal dysfunction in HFpEF. In further support of this argument, those patients with eGFR reduction without albuminuria exhibited greater concentric hypertrophy and remodeling, whereas those with albuminuria in the setting of a more normal eGFR displayed more eccentric hypertrophy and chamber dilation. There are a variety of processes including endothelial dysfunction, venous congestion, and activation of the renin-angiotensin-aldosterone system that have been implicated in HFpEF and both eGFR reduction and albuminuria and could account for some of the observed relationships.

Although the authors highlighted some interesting cardiac structural differences between patients without a low eGFR or albuminuria and those with at least 1 metric of renal dysfunction, small sample size limited more extensive comparisons between those with at least 1 metric of renal dysfunction (i.e., patients with albuminuria and normal eGFR vs patients with no albuminuria and low eGFR etc.). The exclusion of patients with eGFR less than 30 likely led to an underestimation of renal functional impairment in HFpEF and is a limitation. Furthermore, the authors did not explore the potential involvement of right ventricular dysfunction and pulmonary hypertension, both of which have been linked to albuminuria in a previous HFpEF population. Given the aforementioned associations between cardiac structure in HFpEF and renal dysfunction were evaluated at baseline, the results of this study offer no prognostic information and instead serve to highlight the pathophysiologic complexities of HFpEF and concomitant renal disease. Further research is required to better understand the mechanisms involved in renal dysfunction in HFpEF and, in turn, suggest potential therapeutic targets in these patients.

M. A. Brisco, MD, MSCE

Cardiac Positron Emission Tomography Enhances Prognostic Assessments of Patients With Suspected Cardiac Sarcoidosis

Blankstein R, Osborne M, Naya M, et al (Brigham and Women's Hosp, Boston, MA)

J Am Coll Cardiol 63:329-336, 2014

Objectives.—This study sought to relate imaging findings on positron emission tomography (PET) to adverse cardiac events in patients referred for evaluation of known or suspected cardiac sarcoidosis.

Background.—Although cardiac PET is commonly used to evaluate patients with suspected cardiac sarcoidosis, the relationship between PET findings and clinical outcomes has not been reported.

Methods.—We studied 118 consecutive patients with no history of coronary artery disease, who were referred for PET, using [^{18}F]fluorodeoxyglucose (FDG) to assess for inflammation and rubidium-82 to evaluate for perfusion defects (PD), following a high-fat/low-carbohydrate diet to suppress normal myocardial glucose uptake. Blind readings of PET data categorized cardiac findings as normal, positive PD or FDG, positive PD and FDG. Images were also used to identify whether findings of extracardiac sarcoidosis were present. Adverse events (AE)—death or sustained ventricular tachycardia (VT)—were ascertained by electronic medical records, defibrillator interrogation, patient questionnaires, and telephone interviews.

Results.—Among the 118 patients (age 52 ± 11 years; 57% males; mean ejection fraction: 47 ± 16%), 47 (40%) had normal and 71 (60%) had abnormal cardiac PET findings. Over a median follow-up of 1.5 years, there were 31 (26%) adverse events (27 VT and 8 deaths). Cardiac PET findings were predictive of AE, and the presence of both a PD and abnormal FDG (29% of patients) was associated with hazard ratio

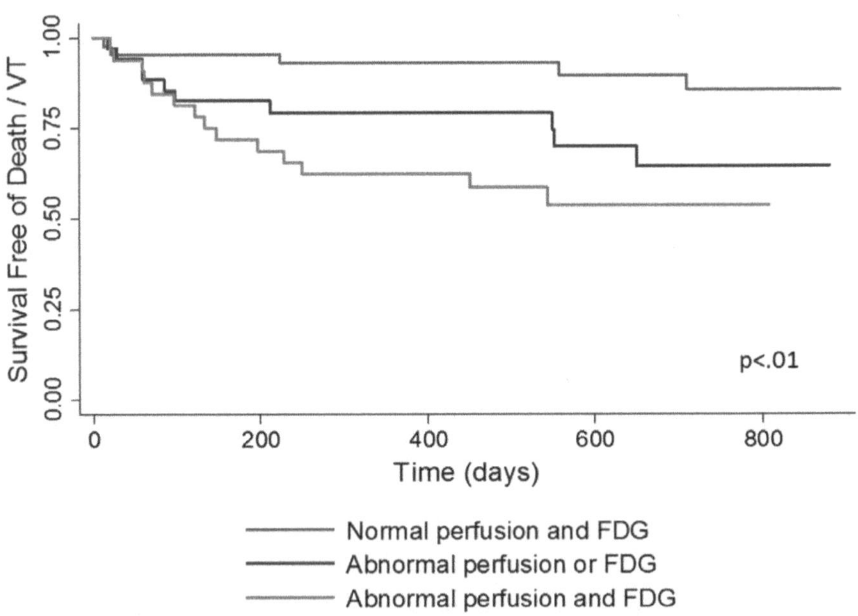

FIGURE 3.—Survival free of death or VT stratified by cardiac PET examination results. Survival free of death or VT stratified by cardiac PET examination results. VT = ventricular tachycardia; other abbreviations as in Figures 1 and 2. (Reprinted from Blankstein R, Osborne M, Naya M, et al. Cardiac positron emission tomography enhances prognostic assessments of patients with suspected cardiac sarcoidosis. *J Am Coll Cardiol.* 2014;63:329-336, with permission from the American College of Cardiology Foundation.)

of 3.9 ($p < 0.01$) and remained significant after adjusting for left ventricular ejection fraction (LVEF) and clinical criteria. Extra-cardiac FDG uptake (26% of patients) was not associated with AE.

Conclusions.—The presence of focal PD and FDG uptake on cardiac PET identifies patients at higher risk of death or VT. These findings offer prognostic value beyond Japanese Ministry of Health and Welfare clinical criteria, the presence of extra-cardiac sarcoidosis and LVEF (Figs 3 and 4).

▶ Definitive diagnosis of cardiac sarcoidosis has long been an elusive proposition. Owing to the diffuse patchy patterns of involvement, the sensitivity of endomyocardial biopsies remains low (20%-30%). More recently, advanced imaging techniques have been used to assist in diagnosis; these include cardiac MRI and cardiac position emission tomography (PET). However, the findings of these imaging modalities have not been used consistently in an attempt to risk stratify patients with suspected disease. This prospective, single-center, observational trial studied 118 consecutive patients referred for cardiac PET for evaluation of known or suspected cardiac sarcoidosis. All patients underwent perfusion imaging using rubidium-82 and metabolic imaging with 18F-

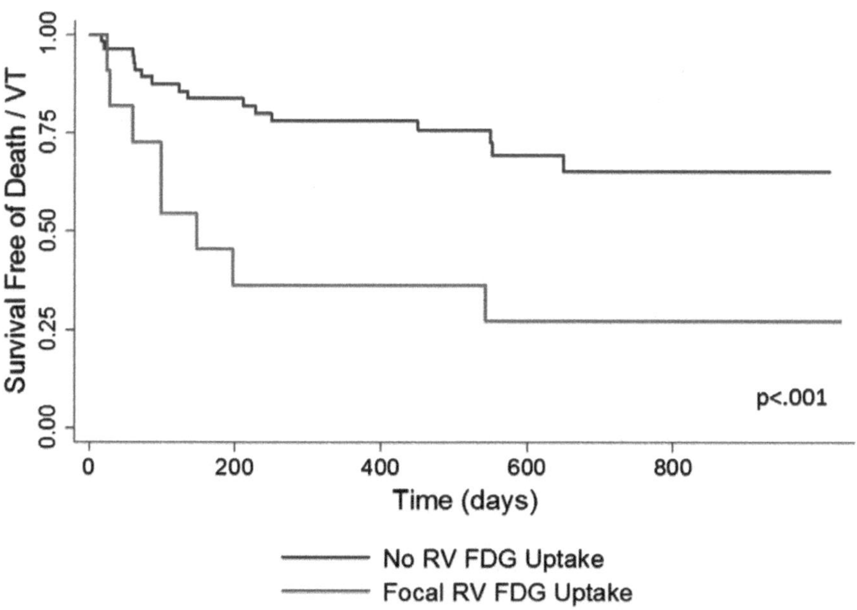

FIGURE 4.—Survival free of death or VT stratified by focal RV inflammation. Survival free of death or VT stratified by the presence or absence of focal right ventricular FDG uptake among individuals with abnormal cardiac PET examination findings. RV = right ventricular; other abbreviations as in Figure 1 to 3. (Reprinted from Blankstein R, Osborne M, Naya M, et al. Cardiac positron emission tomography enhances prognostic assessments of patients with suspected cardiac sarcoidosis. *J Am Coll Cardiol.* 2014;63:329-336, with permission from the American College of Cardiology Foundation.)

labeled fluorodeoxyglucose (FDG). Findings were classified as normal (both perfusion and metabolic), abnormal (perfusion or metabolic), and abnormal (perfusion and metabolic). Over a median follow-up time of 1.5 years, the patients were monitored for a primary endpoint of death from any cause or sustained ventricular tachycardia (VT) and a secondary endpoint of cardiac death or sustained VT. Over that follow-up period, the primary endpoint was observed in 31 patients, 6 of whom had normal PET images. In the 25 patients with abnormal PET images, 11 had abnormal perfusion or metabolism, and 14 had abnormal perfusion and metabolism (Fig 3). Of note, 8 patients with abnormal metabolic imaging showed focal right ventricular uptake of FDG (Fig 4). In a univariate analysis of the imaging findings, the presence of abnormal myocardial perfusion and metabolism (hazard ratio [HR] of 3.94) and focal right ventricular (RV) uptake of FDG (HR, 4.22) was strongly associated with adverse events. Additional factors such as a depressed left ventricular ejection fraction (LVEF) and positive criteria via the Japanese Ministry of Health and Welfare (JMHW) were also associated with adverse events. In a multivariate analysis, addition of abnormal perfusion and metabolism to LVEF and JMHW was associated to death or VT, whereas focal RV uptake of FDG in combination with LVEF and JMHW also remained associated with adverse events. This association was also noted for the secondary endpoint of cardiac death or VT. These results suggest that patients with suspected or confirmed cardiac sarcoidosis in whom cardiac PET shows abnormal perfusion and metabolism or focal RV FDG uptake are at the highest risk of death or VT. Although this finding may indicate a patient population that is more likely to benefit from intervention (treatment with systemic anti-inflammatory medications or implantable cardiac defibrillators), it does not identify low-risk populations. This is evidenced by the 7% event rate that occurred within the group of patients with normal cardiac PET images. Thus, although this is a step forward in risk stratification of cardiac sarcoid, there is still the need for further refinement of the strategy of assessing these patients.

R. Bayer II, MD

Association Between Frequency of Atrial and Ventricular Ectopic Beats and Biventricular Pacing Percentage and Outcomes in Patients With Cardiac Resynchronization Therapy

Ruwald MH, Mittal S, Ruwald A-C, et al (Univ of Rochester Med Ctr, NY; Valley Health System of New York; et al)
J Am Coll Cardiol 64:971-981, 2014

Background.—A high percentage of biventricular pacing is required for optimal outcome in patients treated with cardiac resynchronization therapy (CRT), but the influence of ectopic beats on the success of biventricular pacing has not been well established.

Objectives.—This study sought to determine if increased ectopic beats reduce the chance of high biventricular pacing percentage and are associated with subsequent adverse outcomes.

Methods.—From the MADIT-CRT (Multicenter Automatic Defibrillator Implantation Trial With Cardiac Resynchronization Therapy), 801 patients with an implanted CRT-defibrillator device with data available on biventricular pacing percentage and pre-implantation 24-h Holter recordings were included. Using logistic regression, we estimated the influence of ectopic beats on the percentage of biventricular pacing. Reverse remodeling was measured as reductions in atrial and left ventricular end-systolic volumes (LVESV) at 1 year. Cox models were used to assess the influence of ectopic beats on the outcomes of heart failure (HF) or death, ventricular tachyarrhythmias (VTAs), and death.

Results.—In the pre-implantation Holter recording, ectopic beats accounted for a mean 3.2 ± 5.5% of all beats. The probability of subsequent low biventricular pacing percentage (<97%) was increased 3-fold (odds ratio: 3.37; 95% confidence interval: 1.74 to 6.50; $p < 0.001$) in patients with 0.1% to 1.5% ectopic beats and 13-fold (odds ratio: 13.42; 95% confidence interval: 7.02 to 25.66; $p < 0.001$) in patients with >1.5% ectopic beats compared with those with <0.1% ectopic beats. Patients with ≥0.1% ectopic beats had significantly less reverse remodeling (percent reduction in LVESV 31 ± 15%) than patients

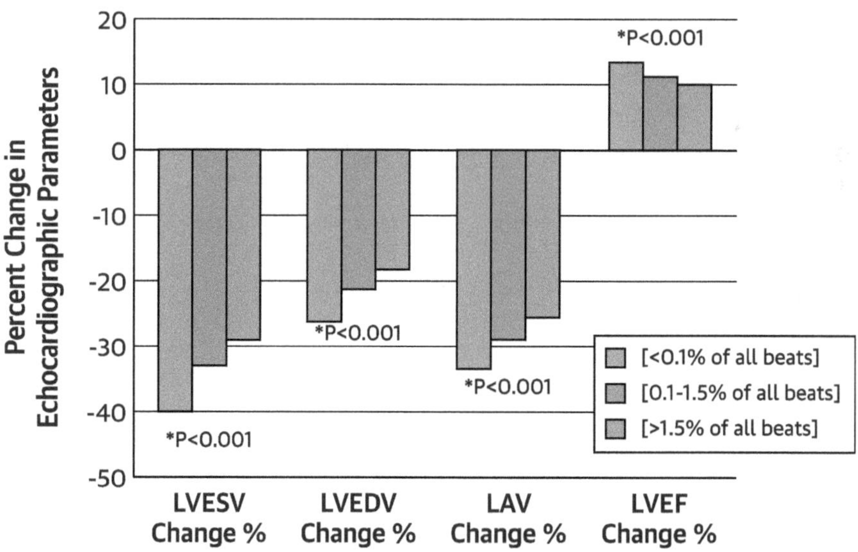

FIGURE 4.—Echocardiography-Measured Changes at 1-Year Follow-Up by Ectopic Burden During Pre-Implantation 24-h Holter Monitoring in Cardiac Resynchronization Therapy Patients. Increasing baseline ectopic burden resulted in less reverse remodeling as measured by 1-year changes in left ventricular end-systolic volume (LVESV), left ventricular end-diastolic volume (LVEDV), left atrial volume (LAV), and left ventricular ejection fraction (LVEF). (Reprinted from the Journal of American College of Cardiology. Ruwald MH, Mittal S, Ruwald A-C, et al. Association between frequency of atrial and ventricular ectopic beats and biventricular pacing percentage and outcomes in patients with cardiac resynchronization therapy. *J Am Coll Cardiol.* 2014;64:971-981, Copyright 2014, with permission from The American College of Cardiology.)

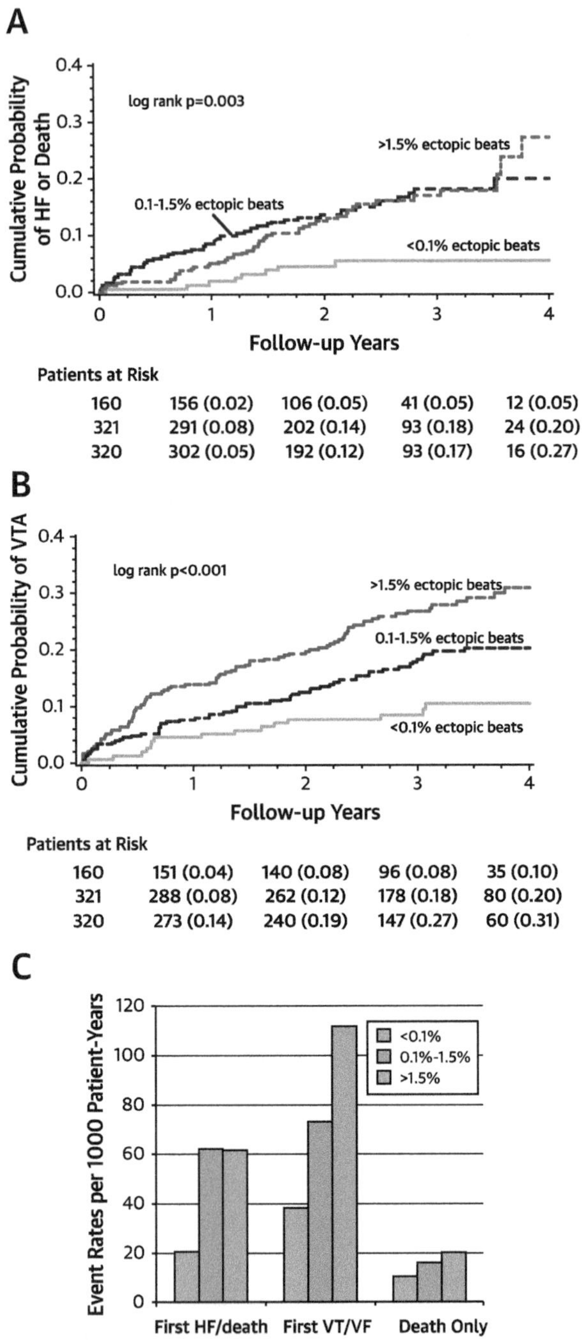
A
Cumulative Probability of HF or Death
0.4
0.3
0.2
0.1
0.0
log rank p=0.003
>1.5% ectopic beats
0.1-1.5% ectopic beats
<0.1% ectopic beats
0
1
2
3
4
Follow-up Years
Patients at Risk
160 156 (0.02) 106 (0.05) 41 (0.05) 12 (0.05)
321 291 (0.08) 202 (0.14) 93 (0.18) 24 (0.20)
320 302 (0.05) 192 (0.12) 93 (0.17) 16 (0.27)
B
Cumulative Probability of VTA
0.4
0.3
0.2
0.1
0.0
log rank p<0.001
>1.5% ectopic beats
0.1-1.5% ectopic beats
<0.1% ectopic beats
0
1
2
3
4
Follow-up Years
Patients at Risk
160 151 (0.04) 140 (0.08) 96 (0.08) 35 (0.10)
321 288 (0.08) 262 (0.12) 178 (0.18) 80 (0.20)
320 273 (0.14) 240 (0.19) 147 (0.27) 60 (0.31)
C
Event Rates per 1000 Patient-Years
120
100
80
60
40
20
0
<0.1%
0.1%-1.5%
>1.5%
First HF/death
First VT/VF
Death Only

with <0.1% ectopic beats (percent reduction in LVESV 39 ± 14%; $p < 0.001$). The risk of HF/death and VTA was increased significantly in those with 0.1% to 1.5% ectopic beats (hazard ratio: 3.13 and 1.84, respectively) and for >1.5% ectopic beats (hazard ratio: 2.38 and 2.74, respectively).

Conclusions.—Relatively low frequencies of ectopic beats (≥0.1%) dramatically increase the probability of low biventricular pacing (<97%), with reduced CRT efficacy by less reverse remodeling and higher risk of HF/death and VTA. This supports pre-implantation Holter monitoring of patients selected for CRT for optimal outcome. (MADIT-CRT: Multicenter Automatic Defibrillator Implantation With Cardiac Resynchronization Therapy; NCT00180271) (Figs 4 and 5).

▶ Cardiac resynchronization therapy (CRT) is well established in the treatment of patients with left ventricular systolic dysfunction, heart failure, and QRS prolongation, primarily left bundle branch block. Many previous studies showed that a surprisingly high percentage of biventricular (BiV) pacing is needed to maximize the benefit of CRT. Early studies suggested at least 90% BiV pacing was needed, but this threshold has been revised upward with subsequent larger studies. Large data analyses from registries now suggest that 99% BiV pacing may be required. In contrast, studies of the deleterious effect of right ventricular pacing suggest that at least 40% percent pacing is needed before systolic function declines. The mechanism for the impact of even small decreases in BiV pacing on CRT is not clear. One explanation is that PVCs and other causes of reduced pacing are a marker of sicker patients so that the BiV pacing percentage is not a primary cause. Interestingly, in the present study, a careful analysis of MADIT-CRT was performed. These investigators again show that small reductions in pacing result in less reverse remodeling (Fig 4) and worse clinical outcomes (Fig 5). Moreover, the effect appears independent of the etiology of ectopic beats because similar responses were noted for atrial and ventricular premature complexes. Thus, a reduction in pacing appears to be deleterious to CRT independent of cause. This provides further

FIGURE 5.—Kaplan-Meier Estimates of Primary Endpoint of Hospitalization for HF or Death and Secondary Endpoint of Hospitalization for VTAs, and Event Rates of Total HF or Death Events and Total VTAs, by Ectopic Burden at Pre-Implantation 24-h Holter Monitoring. (**A**) An increasing ectopic burden (>0.1%) resulted in a significantly increased risk of heart failure (HF)/death compared with <0.1% ectopic beats. No significant difference was found between groups with 0.1% to 1.5% ectopic beats and those with >1.5% ectopic beats for risk of HF/death. (**B**) An increase in the number of ectopic beats was significantly associated with increased risk of ventricular tachyarrhythmia (VTA). (**C**) An increase in the amount of ectopic beats resulted in an increased risk of HF/death with no further increase in event rates for >1.5% ectopic beats compared with 0.1% to 1.5% ectopic beats. VF = ventricular fibrillation; VT = ventricular tachycardia. (Reprinted from the Journal of American College of Cardiology. Ruwald MH, Mittal S, Ruwald A-C, et al. Association between frequency of atrial and ventricular ectopic beats and biventricular pacing percentage and outcomes in patients with cardiac resynchronization therapy. *J Am Coll Cardiol.* 2014;64:971-981, Copyright 2014, with permission from The American College of Cardiology.)

evidence in support of aggressive strategies to maximize pacing, particularly in nonresponders.

M. Gold, MD

44 Chronic Coronary Artery Disease

Association of NSAID Use With Risk of Bleeding and Cardiovascular Events in Patients Receiving Antithrombotic Therapy After Myocardial Infarction

Schjerning Olsen A-M, Gislason GH, McGettigan P, et al (Copenhagen Univ Hosp Gentofte, Hellerup, Denmark; William Harvey Research Inst (WHRI), London, UK; et al)

JAMA 313:805-814, 2015

Importance.—Antithrombotic treatment is indicated for use in patients after myocardial infarction (MI); however, concomitant use of nonsteroidal anti-inflammatory drugs (NSAIDs) could pose safety concerns.

Objective.—To examine the risk of bleeding and cardiovascular events among patients with prior MI taking antithrombotic drugs and for whom NSAID therapy was then prescribed.

Design, Setting, and Participants.—Using nationwide administrative registries in Denmark (2002-2011), we studied patients 30 years or older admitted with first-time MI and alive 30 days after discharge. Subsequent treatment with aspirin, clopidogrel, or oral anticoagulants and their combinations, as well as ongoing concomitant NSAID use, was determined.

Exposures.—Use of NSAIDs with ongoing antithrombotic treatment after first-time MI.

Main Outcomes and Measures.—Risk of bleeding (requiring hospitalization) or a composite cardiovascular outcome (cardiovascular death, nonfatal recurrent MI, and stroke) according to ongoing NSAID and antithrombotic therapy, calculated using adjusted time-dependent Cox regression models.

Results.—We included 61 971 patients (mean age, 67.7 [SD, 13.6] years; 63% men); of these, 34% filled at least 1 NSAID prescription. The number of deaths during a median follow-up of 3.5 years was 18 105 (29.2%). A total of 5288 bleeding events (8.5%) and 18 568 cardiovascular events (30.0%) occurred. The crude incidence rates of bleeding (events per 100 person-years) were 4.2 (95% CI, 3.8-4.6) with concomitant NSAID treatment and 2.2 (95% CI, 2.1-2.3) without NSAID treatment, whereas the rates of cardiovascular events were 11.2 (95% CI, 10.5-11.9) and 8.3 (95% CI, 8.2-8.4). The multivariate-adjusted Cox regression analysis found increased risk of bleeding with NSAID treatment compared with no NSAID treatment (hazard ratio, 2.02 [95% CI, 1.81-2.26]), and the cardiovascular risk was also increased (hazard ratio, 1.40 [95% CI, 1.30-1.49]). An increased risk of bleeding and cardiovascular events was evident with concomitant use of NSAIDs, regardless of antithrombotic treatment, types of NSAIDs, or duration of use.

Conclusions and Relevance.—Among patients receiving antithrombotic therapy after MI, the use of NSAIDs was associated with increased risk of bleeding and excess thrombotic events, even after short-term treatment. More research is needed to confirm these findings; however, physicians should exercise appropriate caution when prescribing NSAIDs for patients who have recently experienced MI.

▶ Patients with ischemic heart disease often have other medical conditions that are typically treated with anti-inflammatory drugs. Nonsteroidal anti-inflammatory drugs (NSAIDs) are readily available over the counter and have become ubiquitous for the treatment of many conditions such as arthritis, headaches, and general musculoskeletal pain. These drugs increase the risk of bleeding, which may be additive to other agents. There is also concern that they may increase the risk of ischemic events. In this study, the national Danish database was used to evaluate the effect of NSAIDs on bleeding and cardiovascular events in more than 60 000 subjects. Such big data analyses allow assessment of drug interactions that often cannot be adequately studied with traditional randomized trials. NSAID use was associated with a 2-fold increased risk of significant bleeding events and 40% increase in cardiovascular events (Fig 1 in the original article). This finding was observed whether antiplatelet therapy or anticoagulants were used. Importantly, the increased risk was observed independent of the duration of NSAID therapy. These findings support the recommendation that NSAIDs should be avoided whenever possible in the presence of antiplatelet drugs, including aspirin and anticoagulants, among patients with known ischemic heart disease.

M. Gold, MD

Ivabradine in Stable Coronary Artery Disease without Clinical Heart Failure

Fox K, for the SIGNIFY Investigators (Royal Brompton Hosp, London, UK; et al)

N Engl J Med 371:1091-1099, 2014

Background.—An elevated heart rate is an established marker of cardiovascular risk. Previous analyses have suggested that ivabradine, a heart-rate–reducing agent, may improve outcomes in patients with stable coronary artery disease, left ventricular dysfunction, and a heart rate of 70 beats per minute or more.

Methods.—We conducted a randomized, double-blind, placebo-controlled trial of ivabradine, added to standard background therapy, in 19,102 patients who had both stable coronary artery disease without clinical heart failure and a heart rate of 70 beats per minute or more (including 12,049 patients with activity-limiting angina [class ≥II on the Canadian Cardiovascular Society scale, which ranges from I to IV, with higher classes indicating greater limitations on physical activity owing to angina]). We randomly assigned patients to placebo or ivabradine, at a dose of up to 10 mg twice daily, with the dose adjusted to achieve a target heart rate of 55 to 60 beats per minute. The primary end point was a composite of death from cardiovascular causes or nonfatal myocardial infarction.

Results.—At 3 months, the mean (±SD) heart rate of the patients was 60.7 ± 9.0 beats per minute in the ivabradine group versus 70.6 ± 10.1 beats per minute in the placebo group. After a median follow-up of 27.8 months, there was no significant difference between the ivabradine group and the placebo group in the incidence of the primary end point (6.8% and 6.4%, respectively; hazard ratio, 1.08; 95% confidence interval, 0.96 to 1.20; $P = 0.20$), nor were there significant differences in the incidences of death from cardiovascular causes and nonfatal myocardial infarction. Ivabradine was associated with an increase in the incidence of the primary end point among patients with activity-limiting angina but not among those without activity-limiting angina ($P = 0.02$ for interaction). The incidence of bradycardia was higher with ivabradine than with placebo (18.0% vs. 2.3%, $P < 0.001$).

Conclusions.—Among patients who had stable coronary artery disease without clinical heart failure, the addition of ivabradine to standard background therapy to reduce the heart rate did not improve outcomes. (Funded by Servier; SIGNIFY Current Controlled Trials number, ISRCTN61576291.)

▶ Ivabradine is a specific blocker of the If current in sinoatrial cells, leading to heart rate slowing. It has been shown to be effective in the treatment of heart failure with an elevated heart rate, as well as inappropriate sinus tachycardia. The SIGNIFY study was a large randomized, multicenter trial of ivabradine among subjects with stable coronary artery disease and no risk factors. No benefit of this drug was noted despite a heart rate decease of about 10 beats per minute (Fig 1 in the original article). This is in clear contrast to the data for cohorts with heart failure. However, it is consistent with older literature showing no benefit of other classes of drugs that decrease heart rate, such as non-dihydropyridine calcium channel blockers and digoxin. The authors postulate that the lack of benefit of ivabradine in this study was due to the lack of neurohormonal activation, which is a reasonable hypothesis. Importantly, this study reinforces that treating risk factors for cardiovascular events may not reduce risk, and in some cases may even increase risk (eg, antiarrhythmic drugs for premature ventricular contractions after myocardial infarction). This study clearly shows that ivabradine should not be used to treat stable coronary artery disease in the absence of heart failure.

M. Gold, MD

Long-Term Use of Ticagrelor in Patients with Prior Myocardial Infarction

Bonaca MP, for the PEGASUS-TIMI 54 Steering Committee and Investigators
(Brigham and Women's Hosp and Harvard Med School, Boston, MA; et al)

N Engl J Med 372:1791-1800, 2015

Background.—The potential benefit of dual antiplatelet therapy beyond 1 year after a myocardial infarction has not been established. We investigated the efficacy and safety of ticagrelor, a $P2Y_{12}$ receptor antagonist with established efficacy after an acute coronary syndrome, in this context.

Methods.—We randomly assigned, in a double-blind 1:1:1 fashion, 21,162 patients who had had a myocardial infarction 1 to 3 years earlier to ticagrelor at a dose of 90 mg twice daily, ticagrelor at a dose of 60 mg twice daily, or placebo. All the patients were to receive low-dose aspirin and were followed for a median of 33 months. The primary efficacy end point was the composite of cardiovascular death, myocardial infarction, or stroke. The primary safety end point was Thrombolysis in Myocardial Infarction (TIMI) major bleeding.

Results.—The two ticagrelor doses each reduced, as compared with placebo, the rate of the primary efficacy end point, with Kaplan–Meier rates at 3 years of 7.85% in the group that received 90 mg of ticagrelor twice daily, 7.77% in the group that received 60 mg of ticagrelor twice daily, and 9.04% in the placebo group (hazard ratio for 90 mg of ticagrelor vs. placebo, 0.85; 95% confidence interval [CI], 0.75 to 0.96; $P = 0.008$; hazard ratio for 60 mg of ticagrelor vs. placebo, 0.84; 95% CI, 0.74 to 0.95; $P = 0.004$). Rates of TIMI major bleeding were higher with ticagrelor (2.60% with 90 mg and 2.30% with 60 mg) than with placebo (1.06%) ($P < 0.001$ for each dose vs. placebo); the rates of intracranial hemorrhage or fatal bleeding in the three groups were 0.63%, 0.71%, and 0.60%, respectively.

Conclusions.—In patients with a myocardial infarction more than 1 year previously, treatment with ticagrelor significantly reduced the risk of cardiovascular death, myocardial infarction, or stroke and increased the risk of major bleeding. (Funded by AstraZeneca; PEGASUS-TIMI 54 ClinicalTrials.gov number, NCT01225562.)

▶ Platelet activation is an integral component in the development of ischemic coronary artery events. In patients who have suffered a myocardial infarction (MI), the addition of a P2Y12 receptor antagonist to aspirin therapy significantly reduced the risk of recurrent ischemic events in the first year after their MI. However, the benefit of continued aggressive long-term secondary prevention with the use of P2Y12 receptor antagonists is not well defined. Prior studies evaluating long-term use of clopidogrel in a broad population failed to show benefit. This multinational, randomized, double-blind, placebo-controlled trial sought to investigate the benefit of ticagrelor in addition to baseline aspirin use in patients who had an MI 1 to 3 years earlier. A group of 21 162 patients were randomly assigned to placebo, ticagrelor 60 mg twice a day, or ticagrelor 90 mg twice a day, in addition to low-dose aspirin (75-150 mg daily). The primary efficacy endpoint was a composite of cardiovascular death, MI, or stroke. The primary safety endpoint was thrombolysis in myocardial infarction (TIMI) major bleeding. After a mean follow-up period of 33 months, there was a significant reduction in the primary endpoint in both of the ticagrelor groups. The primary endpoint occurred in 7.85% of patients receiving 90 mg of ticagrelor twice a day, 7.77% in the group receiving 60 mg of ticagrelor twice a day, and in 9.04% of the placebo group. In a subgroup analysis, including age, sex, race, weight, type of MI, time from qualifying MI, history of percutaneous coronary intervention, presence of multivessel coronary artery disease, presence of chronic kidney disease, and aspirin dose, this benefit was observed across all groups. Although exploratory, a posthoc analysis found a significant reduction in the rates of myocardial infarction in both ticagrelor treatment groups when compared with placebo (Fig 1 in the original article). Despite these promising findings, there was an increase in primary safety endpoints. The rates of TIMI major bleeding were higher in both ticagrelor groups (2.60% with 90 mg twice a day and 2.3% with 60 mg twice a day) when compared with placebo (1.06%). In addition, rates on TIMI minor bleeding, rates of transfusion, and bleeding leading to drug discontinuation were also significantly higher in both ticagrelor groups (Table 3 in the original article). In addition, all cause mortality was the same among all groups. The use of the P2Y12 receptor antagonist ticagrelor more than 1 year after an MI reduces the rate of combined cardiovascular death, MI, and stroke but does so at the expense of increased rates of TIMI major bleeding. Given these increased risks and the lack of mortality reduction, it remains unclear if prolonging the recommended duration of dual antiplatelet therapy will become standard.

R. Bayer II, MD

Efficacy of a Device to Narrow the Coronary Sinus in Refractory Angina

Verheye S, Jolicœur EM, Behan MW, et al (Antwerp Cardiovascular Ctr, Belgium; Montreal Heart Inst, Quebec, Canada; Royal Infirmary of Edinburgh, UK; et al)

N Engl J Med 372:519-527, 2015

Background.—Many patients with coronary artery disease who are not candidates for revascularization have refractory angina despite standard medical therapy. The balloon-expandable, stainless steel, hourglass-shaped, coronary-sinus reducing device creates a focal narrowing and increases pressure in the coronary sinus, thus redistributing blood into ischemic myocardium.

Methods.—We randomly assigned 104 patients with Canadian Cardiovascular Society (CCS) class III or IV angina (on a scale from I to IV, with higher classes indicating greater limitations on physical activity owing to angina) and myocardial ischemia, who were not candidates for revascularization, to implantation of the device (treatment group) or to a sham procedure (control group). The primary end point was the proportion of patients with an improvement of at least two CCS angina classes at 6 months.

Results.—A total of 35% of the patients in the treatment group (18 of 52 patients), as compared with 15% of those in the control group (8 of 52), had an improvement of at least two CCS angina classes at 6 months ($P = 0.02$). The device was also associated with improvement of at least one CCS angina class in 71% of the patients in the treatment group (37 of 52 patients), as compared with 42% of those in the control group (22 of 52) ($P = 0.003$). Quality of life as assessed with the use of the Seattle Angina Questionnaire was significantly improved in the treatment group, as compared with the control group (improvement on a 100-point scale, 17.6 vs. 7.6 points; $P = 0.03$). There were no significant between-group differences in improvement in exercise time or in the mean change in the wall-motion index as assessed by means of dobutamine echocardiography. At 6 months, 1 patient in the treatment group had had a myocardial infarction; in the control group, 1 patient had died and 3 had had a myocardial infarction.

Conclusions.—In this small clinical trial, implantation of the coronary-sinus reducing device was associated with significant improvement in symptoms and quality of life in patients with refractory angina who were not candidates for revascularization. (Funded by Neovasc; COSIRA ClinicalTrials.gov number, NCT01205893.)

▶ Many patients with refractory angina, despite maximal medical therapy, are not candidates for coronary artery revascularization. As the prevalence of debilitating refractory angina increases, so does the need for novel therapies. Preliminary first-in-human data of using a novel coronary sinus-reducing device has shown significant improvement in angina class in 15 patients with refractory angina. The coronary sinus reducer device is a balloon-expandable, stainless steel, hourglass-shaped designed for percutaneous insertion into the coronary sinus (Reducer, Neovasc; Fig 1 in the original article). It is hypothesized to redistribute blood into ischemic myocardium by creating a focal narrowing and increasing the pressure in the coronary sinus. The aim of the Coronary Sinus Reducer for Treatment of Refractory Angina (COISTRA) trial is to examine whether implantation of the coronary sinus-reducing device can effectively improve angina in patients with advanced coronary artery disease and evidence of reversible myocardial ischemia who are not candidates for coronary artery revascularization. A total of 104 patients (mean age 67.8 ± 9.4 y and 81% males) with Canadian Cardiovascular Society (CCS) class III or IV angina and myocardial ischemia were randomly assigned to implantation of the device (treatment group, $n = 52$) or to sham procedure (control group, $n = 52$). The prespecified primary endpoint was the proportion of patients with an improvement of 2 or more CCS angina classes from baseline to 6 months after the procedure. The device was successfully placed in 50 of 52 (96%) patients assigned to treatment group. A total of 18 of 52 (35%) patients in the treatment group and 8 of 52 (15%) patients in the control group had an improvement of at least 2 CCS classes ($P = .02$; Fig 2A in the original article). The mean CCS class was reduced from 3.2 ± 0.4 at baseline to 2.1 ± 1.0 at 6 months in the treatment group compared with a reduction from 3.1 ± 0.3 to 2.6 ± 0.9 in the control group (*P* < .001; Fig 2B in the original article). Overall, there were no differences in adverse events between the groups. Although the number of enrolled patients was small, this trial found that a coronary sinus-reducing device was associated with improvement in CCS angina class and is a promising new therapy for treatment of patients with refractory angina. Further studies are needed to determine safety and clinical benefit.

T. Todoran, MD

45 Coronary Intervention Procedures

Cardioverter defibrillator implantation without induction of ventricular fibrillation: a single-blind, non-inferiority, randomised controlled trial (SIMPLE)

Healey JS, on behalf of the Shockless IMPLant Evaluation [SIMPLE] investigators (McMaster Univ, Hamilton, Ontario, Canada; et al)

Lancet 385:785-791, 2015

Background.—Defibrillation testing by induction and termination of ventricular fibrillation is widely done at the time of implantation of implantable cardioverter defibrillators (ICDs). We aimed to compare the efficacy and safety of ICD implantation without defibrillation testing versus the standard of ICD implantation with defibrillation testing.

Methods.—In this single-blind, randomised, multicentre, non-inferiority trial (Shockless IMPLant Evaluation [SIMPLE]), we recruited patients aged older than 18 years receiving their first ICD for standard indications at 85 hospitals in 18 countries worldwide. Exclusion criteria included pregnancy, awaiting transplantation, particpation in another randomised trial, unavailability for follow-up, or if it was expected that the ICD would have to be implanted on the right-hand side of the chest. Patients undergoing initial implantation of a Boston Scientific ICD were randomly assigned (1:1) using a computer-generated sequence to have either defibrillation testing (testing group) or not (no-testing group). We used random block sizes to conceal treatment allocation from the patients, and randomisation was stratified by clinical centre. Our primary efficacy analysis tested the intention-to-treat population for non-inferiority of no-testing versus testing by use of a composite outcome of arrhythmic death or failed appropriate shock (ie, a shock that did not terminate a spontaneous episode of ventricular tachycardia or fibrillation). The non-inferiority margin was a hazard ratio (HR) of 1·5 calculated from a proportional hazards model with no-testing versus testing as the only covariate; if the upper bound of the 95% CI was less than 1·5, we concluded that ICD insertion without testing was non-inferior to ICD with testing. We examined safety with two, 30 day, adverse event outcome clusters. The trial is registered with ClinicalTrials.gov, number NCT00800384.

Findings.—Between Jan 13, 2009, and April 4, 2011, of 2500 eligible patients, 1253 were randomly assigned to defibrillation testing and 1247 to no-testing, and followed up for a mean of 3·1 years (SD 1·0). The primary outcome of arrhythmic death or failed appropriate shock occurred in fewer patients (90 [7% per year]) in the no-testing group than patients who did receive it (104 [8% per year]; HR 0·86, 95% CI 0·65–1·14; $P_{non\text{-}inferiority}$ <0·0001). The first safety composite outcome occurred in 69 (5·6%) of 1236 patients with no-testing and in 81 (6·5%) of 1242 patients with defibrillation testing, $p = 0{\cdot}33$. The second, pre-specified safety composite outcome, which included only events most likely to be directly caused by testing, occurred in 3·2% of patients with no-testing and in 4·5% with defibrillation testing, $p = 0{\cdot}08$. Heart failure needing intravenous treatment with inotropes or diuretics was the most common adverse event (in 20 [2%] of 1236 patients in the no-testing group vs 28 [2%] of 1242 patients in the testing group, $p = 0{\cdot}25$).

Interpretation.—Routine defibrillation testing at the time of ICD implantation is generally well tolerated, but does not improve shock efficacy or reduce arrhythmic death (Figs 2 and 3).

▶ The implantable cardioverter defibrillator (ICD) is found to reduce mortality in high-risk cohorts for sudden cardiac death. A standard practice at the time

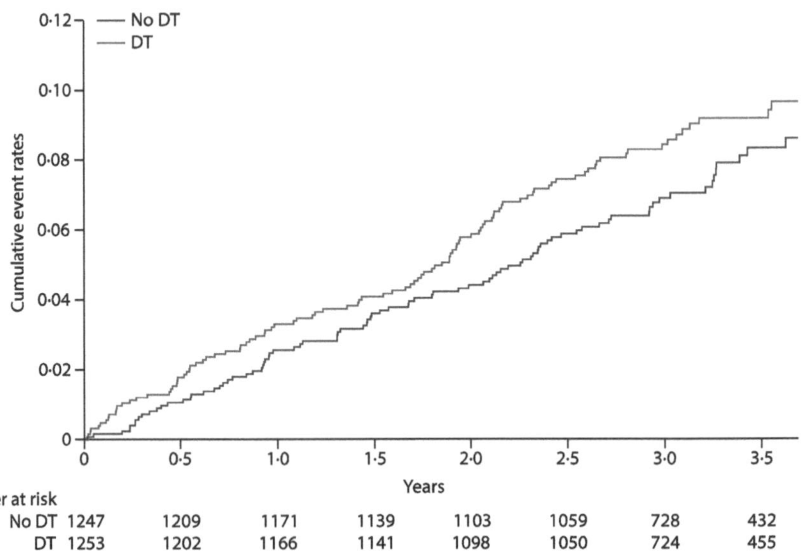

FIGURE 2.—Failed appropriate shock or arrhythmic death. DT = defibrillation testing. Mortality curve was constructed with the Kaplan-Meier method. (Reprinted from The Lancet. Healey JS, on behalf of the Shockless IMPLant Evaluation [SIMPLE] investigators. Cardioverter defibrillator implantation without induction of ventricular fibrillation: a single-blind, non-inferiority, randomised controlled trial (SIMPLE). *Lancet*. 2015;385:785-791, Copyright 2015, with permission from Elsevier.)

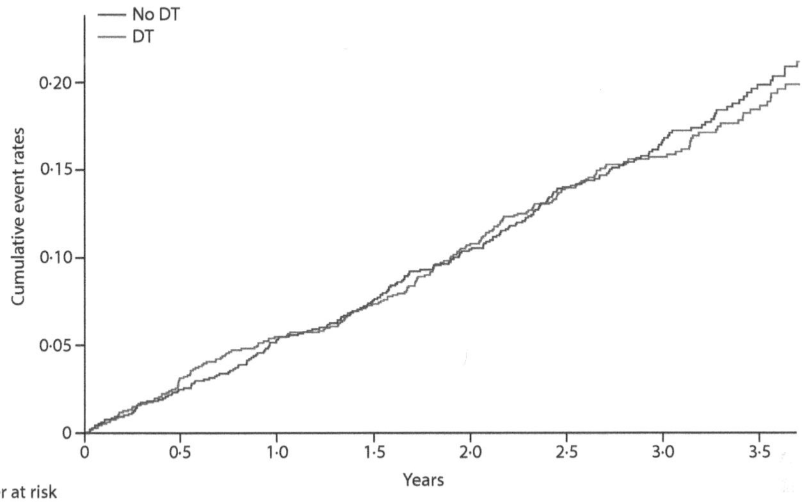

Number at risk

	0	0·5	1·0	1·5	2·0	2·5	3·0	3·5
No DT	1247	1215	1180	1154	1121	1078	742	441
DT	1253	1211	1182	1159	1118	1071	742	463

FIGURE 3.—Total mortality. DT = defibrillation testing. Mortality curve was constructed with the Kaplan-Meier method. (Reprinted from The Lancet. Healey JS, on behalf of the Shockless IMPLant Evaluation [SIMPLE] investigators. Cardioverter defibrillator implantation without induction of ventricular fibrillation: a single-blind, non-inferiority, randomised controlled trial (SIMPLE). *Lancet*. 2015; 385:785-791, Copyright 2015, with permission from Elsevier.)

of ICD placement is to perform testing of the system to ensure adequate sensing of ventricular tachyarrhythmias and termination with shock. Such defibrillation threshold (DFT) testing was used in all the pivotal studies leading to current guidelines for ICD use. However, with advances in shocking leads, waveforms, and detection algorithms, the need for testing at implantation has been questioned. More worrisome is that analysis of several trials shows that ICD shocks are associated with increased mortality. Whether this is a direct cause of such shocks, or more likely a marker of high-risk patients more prone to arrhythmias, is actively debated and further heightens the controversy regarding the need to perform DFT testing. The Shockless IMPLant Evaluation study was the first multicenter, randomized trial to address this issue. A total of 2500 patients were randomly assigned to testing or no testing. The no-testing arm was noninferior for the primary endpoint of arrhythmic death and failed shock (Fig 2). Moreover, mortality did not differ between groups either (Fig 3). In general, testing was well tolerated. This study showed that a no-testing strategy is safe and reasonable in many patients undergoing ICD implantation. Further subgroup analyses will be useful to determine if there are patients more likely to benefit from testing or others in whom testing should clearly be avoided.

M. Gold, MD

A Randomized Comparison of Drug-Eluting Balloon Versus Everolimus-Eluting Stent in Patients With Bare-Metal Stent–In-Stent Restenosis: The RIBS V Clinical Trial (Restenosis Intra-Stent of Bare Metal Stents: Paclitaxel-eluting Balloon vs. Everolimus-eluting Stent)

Alfonso F, RIBS V Study Investigators, Under the Auspices of the Working Group on Interventional Cardiology of the Spanish Society of Cardiology (Hospital Universitario de La Princesa, Madrid, Spain; et al)

J Am Coll Cardiol 63:1378-1386, 2014

Objectives.—This study sought to compare the efficacy of drug-eluting balloons (DEB) with that of everolimus-eluting stents (EES) in patients with bare-metal stents (BMS) in-stent restenosis (ISR).

Background.—Treatment of patients with ISR remains a challenge.

Methods.—This was a prospective, multicenter, randomized trial comparing DEB with EES in patients with bare-metal stents (BMS) in-stent restenosis (ISR). The primary endpoint was the minimal lumen diameter at 9 months' follow-up.

Results.—A total of 189 patients with BMS-ISR from 25 Spanish sites were included (95 were allocated to DEB and 94 to EES). Procedural success was achieved in all patients. At late angiography (median 249 days; 92% of eligible patients), patients in the EES arm had a significantly larger minimal lumen diameter (2.36 ± 0.6 mm vs. 2.01 ± 0.6 mm, $p < 0.001$; absolute mean difference: 0.35 mm; 95% confidence interval [CI]: 0.16 to 0.53) and a lower percent of diameter stenosis (13 ± 17% vs. 25 ± 20%, $p < 0.001$). However, late loss (0.04 ± 0.5 mm vs. 0.14 ± 0.5 mm, $p = 0.14$) and binary restenosis rate (4.7% vs. 9.5%, $p = 0.22$) were very low and similar in both groups. Clinical follow-up (median 365 days) was obtained in all (100%) patients. Occurrences of the combined clinical outcome measure (cardiac death, myocardial infarction, and target vessel revascularization; 6% vs. 8%; hazard ratio [HR]: 0.76; 95% CI: 0.26 to 2.18, $p = 0.6$) and the need for target vessel revascularization (2% vs. 6%; HR: 0.32: 95% CI: 0.07 to 1.59, $p = 0.17$) were similar in the 2 groups.

Conclusions.—In patients with BMS-ISR, both DEB and EES provided excellent clinical results with a very low rate of clinical and angiographic recurrences. However, compared with DEB, EES provide superior late angiographic findings. (Restenosis Intra-stent of Bare Metal Stents: Paclitaxel-eluting Balloon vs. Everolimus-eluting Stent [RIBS V]; NCT01239953).

▶ Despite the associated risk of in-stent restenosis (ISR), bare-metal stents (BMS) are still used in coronary artery interventions. Treatment of BMS ISR is challenging and until recently has been limited to either balloon angioplasty or placement of a drug-eluting stent (DES). The advent of drug-eluting balloon (DEB) has provided an alternative to treatment of ISR. Although second-generation DES such as everolimus-eluting stents (EES) have demonstrated efficacy in subsets of patients with BMS ISR, the relative efficacy to that of DEB is unknown.

The aim of this study was to compare the results of DEB to EES in patients with BMS ISR. There were 189 patients with BMS ISR presenting with either angina or objective evidence of ischemia randomized to receive DEB ($n = 95$) or EES ($n = 94$). Primary end point was in-stent minimal luminal diameter at 9-month follow-up. On acute quantitative angiography, patients treated with EES obtained had larger minimal lumen diameter (2.38 ± 0.5 mm vs 2.16 ± 0.5 mm, respectively), a lower residual stenosis (11 ± 11% vs 19 ± 11%, respectively), and a larger acute gain (1.45 ± 0.5 mm vs 1.14 ± 0.6 mm, respectively; $P < .01$ for all). At late follow-up, minimal luminal diameter was significantly larger (2.36 ± 0.6 mm vs 2.01 ± 0.6 mm, respectively, $P < .001$) and net lumen gain (1.41 ± 0.6 mm vs 0.99 ± 0.6 mm, respectively, $P < .001$) in patients treated with EES compared with DEB. Angiographic late loss and binary restenosis were similar between both groups. The rates of major cardiac events, major adverse events, and target vessel revascularization were also similar between both groups. This study demonstrates that EES provides better late angiographic results compared to DEB in patients with ISR BMS. However, these late angiographic findings do not translate into improved long-term clinical outcomes, so the decision to use a DES rather than simply a novel balloon for dilation is less clear.

T. Todoran, MD

Everolimus-Eluting Stents or Bypass Surgery for Multivessel Coronary Disease

Bangalore S, Guo Y, Samadashvili Z, et al (New York Univ School of Medicine; State Univ of New York at Albany)

N Engl J Med 372:1213-1222, 2015

Background.—Results of trials and registry studies have shown lower long-term mortality after coronary-artery bypass grafting (CABG) than after percutaneous coronary intervention (PCI) among patients with multivessel disease. These previous analyses did not evaluate PCI with second-generation drug-eluting stents.

Methods.—In an observational registry study, we compared the outcomes in patients with multivessel disease who underwent CABG with the outcomes in those who underwent PCI with the use of everolimus-eluting stents. The primary outcome was all-cause mortality. Secondary outcomes were the rates of myocardial infarction, stroke, and repeat revascularization. Propensity-score matching was used to assemble a cohort of patients with similar baseline characteristics.

Results.—Among 34,819 eligible patients, 9223 patients who underwent PCI with everolimus-eluting stents and 9223 who underwent CABG had similar propensity scores and were included in the analyses. At a mean follow-up of 2.9 years, PCI with everolimus-eluting stents, as compared with CABG, was associated with a similar risk of death (3.1% per year and 2.9% per year, respectively; hazard ratio, 1.04; 95% confidence interval [CI], 0.93 to 1.17; $P = 0.50$), higher risks of myocardial infarction (1.9% per year vs. 1.1% per year; hazard ratio, 1.51;

95% CI, 1.29 to 1.77; $P < 0.001$) and repeat revascularization (7.2% per year vs. 3.1% per year; hazard ratio, 2.35; 95% CI, 2.14 to 2.58; $P < 0.001$), and a lower risk of stroke (0.7% per year vs. 1.0% per year; hazard ratio, 0.62; 95% CI, 0.50 to 0.76; $P < 0.001$). The higher risk of myocardial infarction with PCI than with CABG was not significant among patients with complete revascularization but was significant among those with incomplete revascularization ($P = 0.02$ for interaction).

Conclusions.—In a contemporary clinical-practice registry study, the risk of death associated with PCI with everolimus-eluting stents was similar to that associated with CABG. PCI was associated with a higher risk of myocardial infarction (among patients with incomplete revascularization) and repeat revascularization but a lower risk of stroke. (Funded by Abbott Vascular.)

▶ Previous studies found a mortality benefit in coronary artery bypass grafting (CABG) surgery for treatment of patients with multivessel coronary artery disease (CAD) compared with percutaneous coronary artery intervention (PCI). However, these studies did not compare CABG with PCI using second-generation drug-eluting stents. The aim of this study was to evaluate the outcomes with CABG compared with PCI with everolimus-eluting stents (EES) in patients identified from the Cardiac Surgery Reporting System and Percutaneous Coronary Intervention Reporting System registries of New York State Department of Health. The primary outcome was all-cause mortality. A total of 34 819 patients with multivessel CAD were identified and 16 876 (48.5%) underwent PCI with EES and 17 943 (51.5%) underwent CABG. After propensity score matching there were 9223 patients in each group (C-statistic 0.814 with <10% differences for all variables). In-hospital or ≤30-day outcomes favored PCI with EES over CABG. PCI was associated with significantly lower risk of death (0.6% vs 1.1%; hazard ratio [HR], 0.49; $P < .0001$) and stroke (0.2% vs 1.2%; HR, 0.18; $P < .001$), but there was no difference in risk of myocardial infarction between the groups (0.5% vs 0.4%; HR, 1.37; $P = .16$). After a mean follow-up of 2.9 years, PCI with EES and CABG had similar risk of death (3.1% vs 2.9% per year), a higher risk of myocardial infarction (1.9% vs 1.1% per year), a higher rate of repeat revascularization (7.2% vs 3.1% per year), and lower risk of stroke (0.7% vs 1.0% per year; Fig 2 in the original article). In this cohort of patients with multivessel CAD from a contemporary clinical practice registry, risk of death associated with PCI using EES is similar to that of CABG. Short-term outcomes favored PCI with lower risk of death and stroke. Although PCI was associated with increased risk of myocardial infarction in both short- and long-term follow-up, this difference was primarily among patients with incomplete revascularization. This study suggests that PCI using EES is comparable to CABG in treatment of patients with multivessel CAD.

T. Todoran, MD

46 Non-Invasive Testing

T1 mapping and survival in systemic light-chain amyloidosis

Banypersad SM, Fontana M, Maestrini V, et al (The Heart Hosp, London, UK; et al)

Eur Heart J 36:244-251, 2015

Aims.—To assess the prognostic value of myocardial pre-contrast T1 and extracellular volume (ECV) in systemic amyloid light-chain (AL) amyloidosis using cardiovascular magnetic resonance (CMR) T1 mapping.

Methods and Results.—One hundred patients underwent CMR and T1 mapping pre- and post-contrast. Myocardial ECV was calculated at contrast equilibrium (ECV_i) and 15 min post-bolus (ECV_b). Fifty-four healthy volunteers served as controls. Patients were followed up for a median duration of 23 months and survival analyses were performed. Mean ECV_i was raised in amyloid (0.44 ± 0.12) as was ECV_b (mean 0.44 ± 0.12) compared with healthy volunteers (0.25 ± 0.02), $P < 0.001$. Native pre-contrast T1 was raised in amyloid (mean 1080 ± 87 ms vs. 954 ± 34 ms, $P < 0.001$). All three correlated with pre-test probability of cardiac involvement, cardiac biomarkers, and systolic and diastolic dysfunction. During follow-up, 25 deaths occurred. An ECV_i of >0.45 carried a hazard ratio (HR) for death of 3.84 [95% confidence interval (CI): 1.53–9.61], $P = 0.004$ and pre-contrast T1 of >1044 ms = HR 5.39 (95% CI: 1.24–23.4), $P = 0.02$. Extracellular volume after primed infusion and ECV_b performed similarly. Isolated post-contrast T1 was non-predictive. In Cox regression models, ECV_i was independently predictive of mortality (HR = 4.41, 95% CI: 1.35–14.4) after adjusting for E:E′, ejection fraction, diastolic dysfunction grade, and NT-proBNP.

Conclusion.—Myocardial ECV (bolus or infusion technique) and pre-contrast T1 are biomarkers for cardiac AL amyloid and they predict mortality in systemic amyloidosis (Fig 3).

► The presence of cardiac involvement in systemic light-chain amyloidosis (AL) has important prognostic implications. Cardiac involvement can be present in up to 50% of patients at the time of their initial presentation. To date, predictive models use surrogate markers of cardiac involvement, such as serum biomarkers (NT-proBNP and troponin), electrocardiogram criteria (low limb lead voltages, fragmented QRS complexes), and echocardiographic findings (left and right ventricular hypertrophy and diastolic dysfunction). Newer techniques in myocardial T1 mapping using cardiovascular magnetic resonance (CMR) imaging allow for the quantification of the myocardial extracellular volume (ECV). Because this

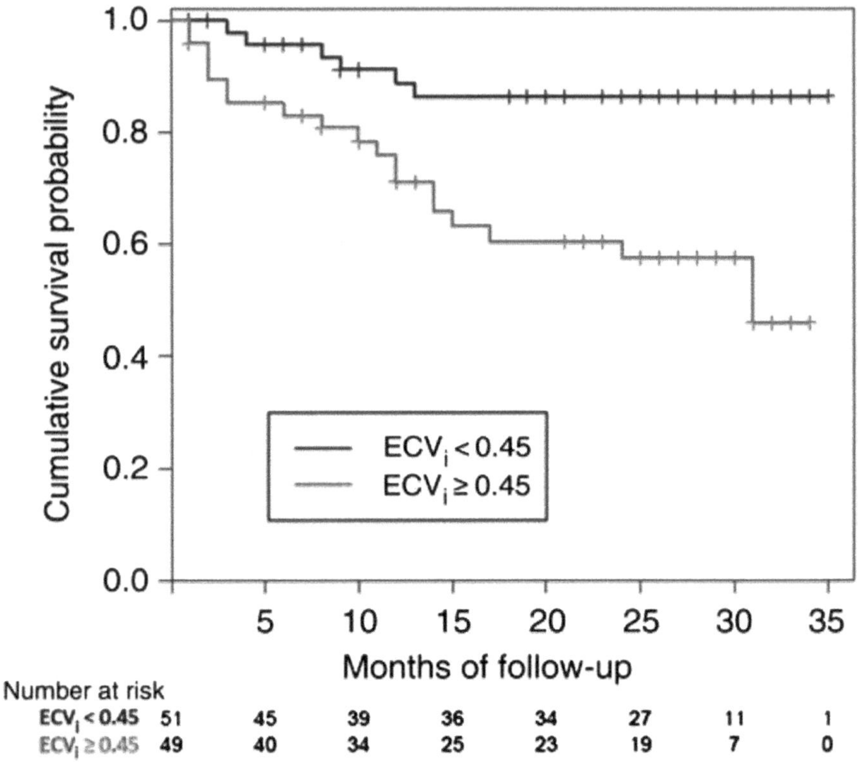

FIGURE 3.—Kaplan–Meier survival curves for extracellular volume after primed infusion. (Reprinted from Banypersad SM, Fontana M, Maestrini V, et al. T1 mapping and survival in systemic light-chain amyloidosis. *Eur Heart J*. 2015;36:244-251, by permission of The European Society of Cardiology.)

represents a measurement of the myocardial interstitium, it has the potential to be used as a marker for amyloid burden within the myocardium and as a marker for outcomes. This prospective, single-center, observational study studied 100 consecutive patients presenting to the National Amyloidosis Center for evaluation, in whom no contraindication to CMR existed and 50 healthy volunteers. All patients underwent precontrast T1 mapping, ECV measurement following primed infusion (ECV$_i$) and bolus-only (ECV$_b$), and postcontrast T1 mapping. In patients with known AL, the mean cardiac ECV was elevated (0.44 ± 0.12) compared with healthy volunteers (0.25 ± 0.02). Similarly, the precontrast myocardial T1 values were also increased in AL patients (1080 ± 87 ms) compared with healthy volunteers (954 ± 34 ms). At a median 23-month follow-up, 25 patients had died. A ECV$_i$ value of ≥0.45 predicted a 40% chance of mortality, compared with only a 15% risk with a value less than 0.45. Precontrast T1 (>1044 ms) and ECV$_b$ (>0.44) also predicted mortality with hazard ratios of 5.39 and 5.09, respectively. Postcontrast T1 mapping did not correlate with survival. In addition, at least modest increases in ECV were noted in AL patients without other criteria to indicate cardiac involvement, which may suggest the presence of low-level disease. These findings indicate that precontrast T1 mapping and ECV measurements detect cardiac involvement of systemic light chain amyloidosis and predict mortality in this patient population. Prospective validation of this finding is warranted, but it may represent an important new diagnostic criteria for amyloid heart disease.

R. Bayer II, MD

Outcomes of Anatomical versus Functional Testing for Coronary Artery Disease

Douglas PS, for the PROMISE Investigators (Duke Univ School of Medicine, Durham, NC; et al)

N Engl J Med 372:1291-1300, 2015

Background.—Many patients have symptoms suggestive of coronary artery disease (CAD) and are often evaluated with the use of diagnostic testing, although there are limited data from randomized trials to guide care.

Methods.—We randomly assigned 10,003 symptomatic patients to a strategy of initial anatomical testing with the use of coronary computed tomographic angiography (CTA) or to functional testing (exercise electrocardiography, nuclear stress testing, or stress echocardiography). The composite primary end point was death, myocardial infarction, hospitalization for unstable angina, or major procedural complication. Secondary end points included invasive cardiac catheterization that did not show obstructive CAD and radiation exposure.

Results.—The mean age of the patients was 60.8 ± 8.3 years, 52.7% were women, and 87.7% had chest pain or dyspnea on exertion. The mean pretest likelihood of obstructive CAD was 53.3 ± 21.4%. Over a median follow-up period of 25 months, a primary end-point event occurred in 164 of 4996 patients in the CTA group (3.3%) and in 151 of 5007 (3.0%) in the functional-testing group (adjusted hazard ratio, 1.04; 95% confidence interval, 0.83 to 1.29; $P = 0.75$). CTA was associated with fewer catheterizations showing no obstructive CAD than was functional testing (3.4% vs. 4.3%, $P = 0.02$), although more patients in the CTA group underwent catheterization within 90 days after randomization (12.2% vs. 8.1%). The median cumulative radiation exposure per patient was lower in the CTA group than in the functional-testing group (10.0 mSv vs. 11.3 mSv), but 32.6% of the patients in the functional-testing group had no exposure, so the overall exposure was higher in the CTA group (mean, 12.0 mSv vs. 10.1 mSv; $P < 0.001$).

Conclusions.—In symptomatic patients with suspected CAD who required noninvasive testing, a strategy of initial CTA, as compared with functional testing, did not improve clinical outcomes over a median follow-up of 2 years. (Funded by the National Heart, Lung, and Blood Institute; PROMISE ClinicalTrials.gov number, NCT01174550.)

▶ The evaluation of chest pain is a common scenario in ambulatory patients. Typically, this evaluation focuses on the diagnosis of significant coronary artery disease (CAD) as the cause of symptoms. With growing technologic advances, there are multiple modalities for the evaluation of CAD. These modalities fall into 2 overarching strategies: functional versus anatomic testing. This prospective, multicenter study evaluated clinical endpoints of patients, without a known history of CAD, who were referred for evaluation of symptoms concerning for were CAD. Just more than 10 000 patients were enrolled and subsequently randomly assigned to an initial evaluation using function testing (stress electrocardiogram [EKG], stress echocardiography, or exercise/pharmacologic nuclear imaging) or anatomic testing (cardiac computed tomography angiography [CCTA]). After randomization, 4686 patients underwent CCTA, and 4692 patients underwent functional testing with a breakdown of 3159 patients undergoing nuclear imaging, 1056 stress echocardiography, and 477 stress EKG. The primary endpoint was a composite of major adverse cardiac events (death, myocardial infarction, hospitalization for unstable angina, or major procedural complication) with secondary endpoint of invasive coronary angiography demonstrating nonobstructive CAD to the primary endpoint. At the end of 2-year follow-up period, there was no statistical difference between the 2 testing strategies with the primary endpoint occurring in 3.3% in the CTA group and 3.0% in the functional testing group (Fig 2 in the original article). In addition, there was no significant difference in the secondary endpoint (6.6% vs 7.1% in the CTA and functional testing groups, respectively). Additionally, median radiation dose was lower in the CCTA arm (10 mSv vs 11.3 mSv), whereas mean exposure was higher (12 mSv vs 10.1 mSv). This difference is explained by the fact that 2 of the 3 functional modalities had no radiation exposure. However, when compared with only patients undergoing nuclear imaging, both the median and mean radiation exposure were lower in the CCTA group. These data would suggest that in symptomatic patients referred for evaluation of CAD, there is no difference in hard clinical endpoints between functional and anatomic testing.

R. Bayer II, MD

47 Risk Factors

Blood pressure and incidence of twelve cardiovascular diseases: lifetime risks, healthy life-years lost, and age-specific associations in 1·25 million people

Rapsomaniki E, Timmis A, George J, et al (The Farr Inst of Health Informatics Res, London, UK; et al)

Lancet 383:1899-1911, 2014

Background.—The associations of blood pressure with the different manifestations of incident cardiovascular disease in a contemporary population have not been compared. In this study, we aimed to analyse the associations of blood pressure with 12 different presentations of cardiovascular disease.

Methods.—We used linked electronic health records from 1997 to 2010 in the CALIBER (CArdiovascular research using LInked Bespoke studies and Electronic health Records) programme to assemble a cohort of 1·25 million patients, 30 years of age or older and initially free from cardiovascular disease, a fifth of whom received blood pressure-lowering treatments. We studied the heterogeneity in the age-specific associations of clinically measured blood pressure with 12 acute and chronic cardiovascular diseases, and estimated the lifetime risks (up to 95 years of age) and cardiovascular disease-free life-years lost adjusted for other risk factors at index ages 30, 60, and 80 years. This study is registered at ClinicalTrials.gov, number NCT01164371.

Findings.—During 5·2 years median follow-up, we recorded 83 098 initial cardiovascular disease presentations. In each age group, the lowest risk for cardiovascular disease was in people with systolic blood pressure of 90—114 mm Hg and diastolic blood pressure of 60—74 mm Hg, with no evidence of a J-shaped increased risk at lower blood pressures. The effect of high blood pressure varied by cardiovascular disease endpoint, from strongly positive to no effect. Associations with high systolic blood pressure were strongest for intracerebral haemorrhage (hazard ratio 1·44 [95% CI 1·32—1·58]), subarachnoid haemorrhage (1·43 [1·25—1·63]), and stable angina (1·41 [1·36—1·46]), and weakest for abdominal aortic aneurysm (1·08 [1·00—1·17]). Compared with diastolic blood pressure, raised systolic blood pressure had a greater effect on angina, myocardial infarction, and peripheral arterial disease, whereas raised diastolic blood pressure had a greater effect on abdominal aortic aneurysm than did raised systolic pressure. Pulse pressure associations were inverse for abdominal aortic aneurysm (HR per 10 mm Hg 0·91 [95% CI 0·86—0·98]) and strongest for peripheral arterial disease (1·23 [1·20–1·27]). People with hypertension (blood pressure ≥140/90 mm Hg or those receiving blood pressure-lowering drugs) had a lifetime risk of overall cardiovascular disease at 30 years of age of 63·3% (95% CI 62·9–63·8) compared with 46·1% (45·5–46·8) for those with normal blood pressure, and developed cardiovascular disease 5·0 years earlier (95% CI 4·8–5·2). Stable and unstable angina accounted for most (43%) of the cardiovascular disease-free years of life lost associated with hypertension from index age 30 years, whereas heart failure and stable angina accounted for the largest proportion (19% each) of years of life lost from index age 80 years.

Interpretation.—The widely held assumptions that blood pressure has strong associations with the occurrence of all cardiovascular diseases across a wide age range, and that diastolic and systolic associations are concordant, are not supported by the findings of this high-resolution study. Despite modern treatments, the lifetime burden of hypertension is substantial. These findings emphasise the need for new blood pressure-lowering strategies, and will help to inform the design of randomised trials to assess them.

▶ In 2010, the Institute for Health Metrics and Evaluation identified hypertension (HTN) as the single largest contributor to overall mortality and global burden of disease. Although the role of HTN as a primary risk factor for cardiovascular disease is well known, the relationships between HTN and multiple forms of incident cardiovascular diseases across age and sex groups in a contemporary population are less clear. Rapsomaniki and colleagues provide in this report the most detailed examination of HTN as a major risk factor to date harnessing the power of the electronic medical record across the United Kingdom. In addition to exploring the effect of HTN on the development of 12 incident cardiovascular conditions, including heart failure and peripheral arterial disease, the authors studied the effect of elevations in systolic blood pressure alone (140 mm Hg or greater), diastolic blood pressure alone (90 mm Hg or greater), mean arterial pressure, pulse pressure, and mid-blood pressure on these outcomes. Interestingly, systolic blood pressure appears to significantly impact stable angina, myocardial infarction, and peripheral arterial disease, whereas diastolic blood pressure may play more of a role in abdominal aortic aneurysm development. These varied associations suggest different pathophysiology of these forms of cardiovascular disease and will likely inform prevention strategies accordingly. Still, the most sobering statistic from this analysis is the 63.3% lifetime risk of cardiovascular disease development and subsequent 5 years of life lost in a 30-year-old patient with HTN in the modern era. This is of particular importance given the increasing incidence of HTN in children (likely secondary to childhood obesity).

As the authors state in their report, one of the most beneficial applications of these data will occur at the bedside, serving as powerful evidence during discussions of cardiovascular risk with patients. The extensive analyses of age- and sex-related differences in risk as well as years lost to particular cardiovascular diseases will allow for further personalization of these discussions for the individual patient. Additionally, these results will support the continued efforts to both diagnose and treat HTN, particularly in younger patients who suffer the greatest amount of years of life lost to this highly prevalent and powerful risk factor.

M. A. Brisco, MD, MSCE

Percutaneous closure of patent foramen ovale in patients with cryptogenic embolism: a network meta-analysis

Stortecky S, da Costa BR, Mattle HP, et al (Bern Univ Hosp, Bern, Switzerland; Clinical Trials Unit, Bern, Switzerland; et al)

Eur Heart J 36:120-128, 2015

Background.—Up to 40% of ischaemic strokes are cryptogenic. A strong association between cryptogenic stroke and the prevalence of patent foramen ovale (PFO) suggests paradoxical embolism via PFO as a potential cause. Randomized trials failed to demonstrate superiority of PFO closure over medical therapy.

Methods and Results.—Randomized trials comparing percutaneous PFO closure against medical therapy or devices head-to-head published or presented by March 2013 were identified through a systematic search. We performed a network meta-analysis to determine the effectiveness and safety of PFO closure with different devices when compared with medical therapy. We included four randomized trials (2963 patients with 9309 patient-years). Investigated devices were Amplatzer (AMP), STARFlex (STF), and HELEX (HLX). Patients allocated to PFO closure with AMP were less likely to experience a stroke than patients allocated to medical therapy [rate ratio (RR) 0.39; 95% CI: 0.17–0.84]. No significant differences were found for STF (RR 1.01; 95% CI: 0.44–2.41), and HLX (RR, 0.71; 95% CI: 0.17–2.78) when compared with medical therapy. The probability to be best in preventing strokes was 77.1% for AMP, 20.9% for HLX, 1.7% for STF, and 0.4% for medical therapy. No significant differences were found for transient ischaemic attack and death. The risk of new-onset atrial fibrillation was more pronounced for STF (RR 7.67; 95% CI: 3.25–19.63), than AMP (RR 2.14; 95% CI: 1.00–4.62) and HLX (RR 1.33; 95%-CI 0.33–4.50), when compared with medical therapy.

Conclusions.—The effectiveness of PFO closure depends on the device used. PFO closure with AMP appears superior to medical therapy in preventing strokes in patients with cryptogenic embolism (Fig 2).

► Stroke is one of the leading causes of death and disability in most western civilizations. It is growing in incidence as the population ages. Although the cause of stroke is often apparent, more than one-third of the time no etiology is identified. Such cryptogenic strokes have been the subject of much study. The association of a patent foramen ovale (PFO) with such strokes has led to the hypothesis that paradoxical emboli are the cause in such cases. To test this hypothesis, multiple randomized trials have been performed evaluating the role of PFO closure in patients with cryptogenic strokes. This study is a

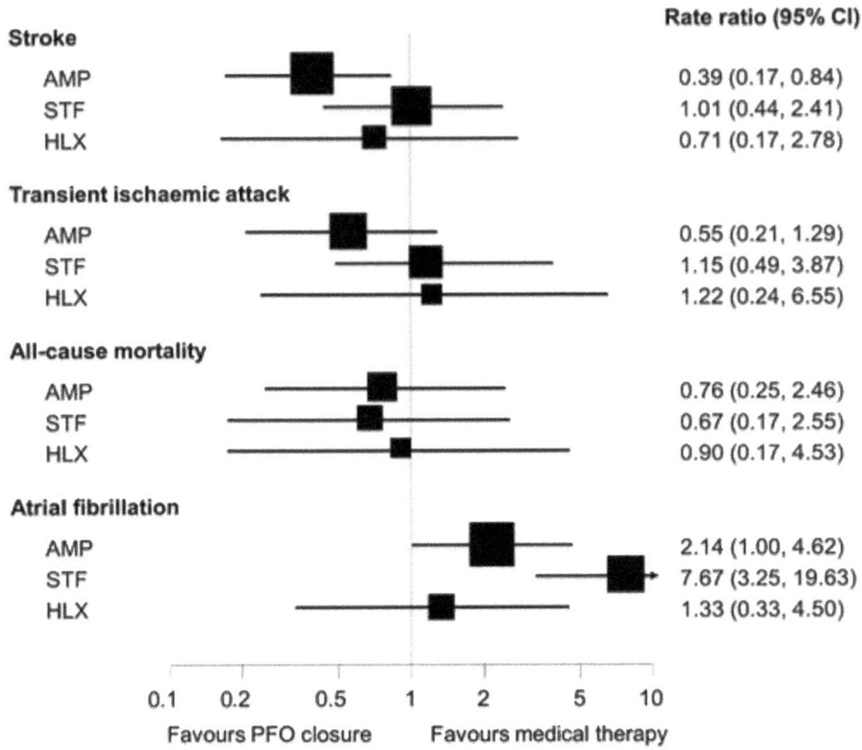

FIGURE 2.—Primary and secondary clinical outcomes with medical therapy as a reference compound. AMP, Amplatzer; STF, STARFlex; HLX, HELEX; CI, credibility interval. (Reprinted from Stortecky S, da Costa BR, Mattle HP, et al. Percutaneous closure of patent foramen ovale in patients with cryptogenic embolism: a network meta-analysis. *Eur Heart J*. 2015;36:120-128, by permission of The European Society of Cardiology.)

meta-analysis of such trials. The authors show that the effectiveness of PFO closure is strongly dependent on the device used (Fig 2) with the best results for prevention of recurrent stroke noted with the Amplatzer device. However, PFO closure is associated with increased atrial fibrillation, an independent cause of stroke, indicating that close monitoring is needed to determine which patients will need long-term anticoagulation. Importantly, no mortality benefit was noted with PFO closure even by pooling multiple studies in a meta-analysis. These results indicate that PFO closure may have a role in certain patients with cryptogenic stroke but there are likely other processes contributing to these episodes.

M. Gold, MD

Efficacy and Safety of Alirocumab in Reducing Lipids and Cardiovascular Events

Robinson JG, for the ODYSSEY LONG TERM Investigators (Centre Hospitalier Universitaire de Nantes—Hôpital Nord Laennec, Saint-Herblain, France; et al)

N Engl J Med 372:1489-1499, 2015

Background.—Alirocumab, a monoclonal antibody that inhibits proprotein convertase subtilisin—kexin type 9 (PCSK9), has been shown to reduce low-density lipoprotein (LDL) cholesterol levels in patients who are receiving statin therapy. Larger and longer-term studies are needed to establish safety and efficacy.

Methods.—We conducted a randomized trial involving 2341 patients at high risk for cardiovascular events who had LDL cholesterol levels of 70 mg per deciliter (1.8 mmol per liter) or more and were receiving treatment with statins at the maximum tolerated dose (the highest dose associated with an acceptable side-effect profile), with or without other lipid-lowering therapy. Patients were randomly assigned in a 2:1 ratio to receive alirocumab (150 mg) or placebo as a 1-ml subcutaneous injection every 2 weeks for 78 weeks. The primary efficacy end point was the percentage change in calculated LDL cholesterol level from baseline to week 24.

Results.—At week 24, the difference between the alirocumab and placebo groups in the mean percentage change from baseline in calculated LDL cholesterol level was −62 percentage points ($P < 0.001$); the treatment effect remained consistent over a period of 78 weeks. The alirocumab group, as compared with the placebo group, had higher rates of injection-site reactions (5.9% vs. 4.2%), myalgia (5.4% vs. 2.9%), neurocognitive events (1.2% vs. 0.5%), and ophthalmologic events (2.9% vs. 1.9%). In a post hoc analysis, the rate of major adverse cardiovascular events (death from coronary heart disease, nonfatal myocardial infarction, fatal or nonfatal ischemic stroke, or unstable angina requiring hospitalization) was lower with alirocumab than with placebo (1.7% vs. 3.3%; hazard ratio, 0.52; 95% confidence interval, 0.31 to 0.90; nominal $P = 0.02$).

Conclusions.—Over a period of 78 weeks, alirocumab, when added to statin therapy at the maximum tolerated dose, significantly reduced LDL cholesterol levels. In a post hoc analysis, there was evidence of a reduction in the rate of cardiovascular events with alirocumab. (Funded by Sanofi and Regeneron Pharmaceuticals; ODYSSEY LONG TERM ClinicalTrials.gov number, NCT01507831.)

► In patients at high risk of cardiovascular events, lowering of cholesterol, specifically low-density lipoprotein (LDL), is a major treatment goal. Despite high-intensity or maximal tolerated statin therapy, many patients may not reach a targeted LDL level of less than 70 mg/dL. Monoclonal antibodies targeted at proprotein convertase subtilisin-kexin type 9 (PCSK9) have been shown previously to lower LDL levels in patients who are already on high-intensity or maximally tolerated statin therapy. However, these studies were short in duration, and longer term follow-up was needed for additional assessment of safety and efficacy. This multinational, randomized, double-blind, placebo-controlled study followed 2341 patients at high risk of cardiovascular events over a 78-week period. Patients who were already being treated with high-intensity or maximally tolerated statin therapy were randomly selected in a 2:1 fashion to the PCSK9 inhibitor alirocumab (150 mg every 2 weeks) or placebo. The primary efficacy endpoint was percentage change of LDL from baseline to week 24. Safety endpoints included symptoms; laboratory, vital sign, and electrocardiographic abnormalities; and adjudicated major adverse cardiac events. At baseline, the mean calculated LDL level for both groups was 122 mg/dL. At week 24, the mean LDL level in the alirocumab group was 48 mg/dL, a reduction of 61%, compared with the placebo group with a mean LDL of 119 mg/dL, a reduction of only 0.8%. The goal LDL level of less than 70 mg/dL was achieved in 79.3% of patients in the alirocumab group compared with only 8.0% of patients in the placebo group. At week 78, the LDL reduction remained, although slightly less robust, with a reduction of 52.4%. This difference was thought to be related to the population of patients for whom there was premature discontinuation of the drug prior to the 78-week analysis. With regard to the safety endpoints, patients who received alirocumab were more likely to have injection site reactions (5.9% vs 4.2%), myalgias (5.4% vs 2.9%), neurocognitive events (1.2% vs 0.5%), and ophthalmologic events (2.9% vs 1.9%). In a posthoc analysis using prespecified cardiovascular endpoints (composite of death from coronary artery disease, nonfatal myocardial infarction, fatal or nonfatal ischemic stroke, or unstable angina requiring hospitalization), patients receiving alirocumab experienced fewer events (1.7% vs 3.3%) when compared with placebo. However, when congestive heart failure requiring hospitalization and ischemia-driven coronary revascularization were added, the difference between the 2 treatment groups was no longer observed. The study clearly shows that the PCSK9 inhibitor alirocumab significantly reduces LDL cholesterol levels in patients at high risk for cardiovascular events who are already on high-intensity or maximally tolerated statin therapy. The impact on cardiovascular events is less clear. The follow-up period of 78 weeks may not have been sufficient to detect changes in hard clinical endpoints, and a longer trial with 5-yr follow-up is currently underway.

R. Bayer II, MD

48 Valvular Heart Disease

Survival and Outcomes Following Bioprosthetic vs Mechanical Mitral Valve Replacement in Patients Aged 50 to 69 Years

Chikwe J, Chiang YP, Egorova NN, et al (Icahn School of Medicine at Mount Sinai, NY)

JAMA 313:1435-1442, 2015

Importance.—In nonelderly patients with mitral disease requiring valve replacement, deciding between bioprosthetic and mechanical prosthetic valves is challenging because long-term survival and morbidity are not well defined.

Objective.—To quantify survival and major morbidity after mitral valve replacement in patients aged 50 to 69 years.

Design, Setting, and Participants.—Retrospective cohort analysis of 3433 patients (aged 50-69 years) who underwent primary, isolated mitral valve replacement in New York State hospitals from 1997-2007. Follow-up ended November 30, 2013; median duration was 8.2 years (range, 0-16.8 years). Propensity score matching for 19 baseline characteristics yielded 664 patient pairs.

Exposures.—Bioprosthetic vs mechanical prosthetic mitral valve replacement.

Main Outcomes and Measures.—All-cause mortality, stroke, reoperation, and major bleeding events.

Results.—No survival difference was observed between use of mechanical prosthetic and bioprosthetic mitral valves in patients aged 50 to 69 years matched by propensity score or in a subgroup analysis of age by decade. Among patients matched by propensity score, the incidences of stroke and bleeding events were both significantly higher in those who received mechanical prosthetic mitral valves compared with those who received bioprosthetic mitral valves; however, the incidence of reoperation was lower in the mechanical prosthesis group compared with the bioprosthesis group.

Outcome at 15 Years	No. (%) [95% CI] by Type of Mitral Valve Replacement Mechanical Prosthetic (n = 664)	Bioprosthetic (n = 664)	Hazard Ratio (95% CI)
Death	209	221	
Actuarial 15-year survival, % (95% CI)	57.5 (50.5-64.4)	59.9 (54.8-65.0)	0.95 (0.79-1.15)
Stroke	65 (14.0) [9.5-18.6]	41 (6.8) [4.5-8.8]	1.62 (1.10-2.39)
Reoperation	28 (5.0) [3.1-6.9]	47 (11.1) [7.6-14.6]	0.59 (0.37-0.94)
Bleeding events	72 (14.9) [11.0-18.7]	49 (9.0) [6.4-11.5]	1.50 (1.05-2.16)

Conclusions and Relevance.—Among patients aged 50 to 69 years undergoing mitral valve replacement in New York State, there was no significant survival difference at 15 years in patients matched by propensity score who underwent mechanical prosthetic vs bioprosthetic mitral valve replacement. Mechanical prosthetic valves were associated with lower risk of reoperation but greater risk of bleeding and stroke. Even though these findings suggest bioprosthetic mitral valve replacement may be a reasonable alternative to mechanical prosthetic valve replacement in patients aged 50 to 69 years, the 15-year follow-up was insufficient to fully assess lifetime risks, particularly of reoperation.

▶ Age is one of the major determinants in the selection of prosthetic valve type (mechanical vs bioprosthetic) to be used when performing mitral valve replacement. Consensus guidelines recommend bioprosthetic valves for patients older than 70 years. This guideline is related to the relative low change of reoperation secondary to valve degeneration. Similarly, in very young patients, owing to the accelerated rate of bioprosthetic valve degeneration, mechanical valves are more appropriate. However, the optimal prosthesis in an intermediate-age patient (age 50-70 years) is less well defined. This retrospective cohort analysis compared patients undergoing mitral valve replacement with patients receiving both mechanical and bioprosthetic prostheses in the state of New York between 1997 and 2007. Owing to the differing baseline characteristics of the 2 populations, propensity score matching was used to identify 664 patient pairs for the analysis. The primary endpoint was all-cause mortality with secondary endpoints of stroke, reoperation, and major bleeding events. At 15 years, there was no difference in survival rates between the mechanical prosthetic group and the bioprosthetic group (57.5% and 59.9%, respectively). However, there were several differences between the 2 groups with regard to the secondary endpoints. Specifically, there was a significantly higher risk of stroke in the mechanical valve group (14% vs 6.8%). In addition, rates of bleeding events were also significantly higher in the mechanical group (14.9% vs 9.0%). Conversely, there were higher rates of reoperation in the bioprosthetic valve group (11.1% vs 5.0%). The data indicate that there is no difference with respect to long-term survival in patients aged 50 to 69 undergoing mechanical or bioprosthetic mitral valve replacement. However, the implantation of a mechanical valve, although offering lower rates of reoperation, comes with a trade off of higher stroke and bleeding events.

R. Bayer II, MD

Surgical Treatment of Moderate Ischemic Mitral Regurgitation

Smith PK, for the Cardiothoracic Surgical Trials Network Investigators (Duke Univ Med Ctr, Durham, NC; et al)

N Engl J Med 371:2178-2188, 2014

Background.—Ischemic mitral regurgitation is associated with increased mortality and morbidity. For surgical patients with moderate regurgitation, the benefits of adding mitral-valve repair to coronary-artery bypass grafting (CABG) are uncertain.

Methods.—We randomly assigned 301 patients with moderate ischemic mitral regurgitation to CABG alone or CABG plus mitral-valve repair (combined procedure). The primary end point was the left ventricular end-systolic volume index (LVESVI), a measure of left ventricular remodeling, at 1 year. This end point was assessed with the use of a Wilcoxon rank-sum test in which deaths were categorized as the lowest LVESVI rank.

Results.—At 1 year, the mean LVESVI among surviving patients was 46.1 ± 22.4 ml per square meter of body-surface area in the CABG-alone group and 49.6 ± 31.5 ml per square meter in the combined-procedure group (mean change from baseline, −9.4 and −9.3 ml per square meter, respectively). The rate of death was 6.7% in the combined-procedure group and 7.3% in the CABG-alone group (hazard ratio with mitral-valve repair, 0.90; 95% confidence interval, 0.38 to 2.12; $P = 0.81$). The rank-based assessment of LVESVI at 1 year (incorporating deaths) showed no significant between-group difference (z score, 0.50; $P = 0.61$). The addition of mitral-valve repair was associated with a longer bypass time ($P < 0.001$), a longer hospital stay after surgery ($P = 0.002$), and more neurologic events ($P = 0.03$). Moderate or severe mitral regurgitation was less common in the combined-procedure group than in the CABG-alone group (11.2% vs. 31.0%, $P < 0.001$). There were no significant between-group differences in major adverse cardiac or cerebrovascular events, deaths, readmissions, functional status, or quality of life at 1 year.

Conclusions.—In patients with moderate ischemic mitral regurgitation, the addition of mitral-valve repair to CABG did not result in a higher degree of left ventricular reverse remodeling. Mitral-valve repair was associated with a reduced prevalence of moderate or severe mitral regurgitation but an increased number of untoward events. Thus, at 1 year, this trial did not show a clinically meaningful advantage of adding mitral-valve repair to CABG. Longer-term follow-up may determine whether the lower prevalence of mitral regurgitation translates into a net clinical benefit. (Funded by the National Institutes of Health and the Canadian Institutes of Health Research; ClinicalTrials.gov number, NCT00806988.)

▶ Ischemic mitral valve regurgitation (MR) occurs in up to 50% of patients following a myocardial infarction. The presence of any degree of ischemic mitral regurgitation results in excess mortality. In patients who are to undergo coronary artery bypass graft surgery (CABG), there is uncertainty of the benefit of concomitant of mitral valve repair (MVR) in the presence of moderate ischemic MR. It has been proposed that the addition of MVR and subsequent reduction of ischemic MR may prevent further adverse remodeling and subsequently improve left ventricular function. In this prospective, multicenter, randomized clinical trial, 301 patients with moderate ischemic mitral valve regurgitation were randomly assigned to CABG alone or combined CABG with MVR. The primary endpoint at 1 year was the left ventricular end systolic volume index (LVESVI) with secondary endpoints of major adverse cardiac or cerebrovascular events, mortality, residual MR, New York Heart Association functional class, and quality of assessment. There was no statistical difference in the groups with regard to the primary endpoint. In the CABG-alone group, the LVESI decreased from 54.8 ± 24.9 mL/m^2 to 46.1 ± 22.4 mL/m^2 (mean change of 9.4 mL/m^2), whereas in the combined CABG MVR group it decreased from 59.6 ± 25.7 mL/m^2 to 49.6 ± 31.5 mL/m^2 (mean change of 9.3 mL/m^2). In addition, there was no difference in secondary endpoints of mortality, composite major adverse cardiac or cerebrovascular events, or quality-of-life scores. However, there were differences between the 2 groups with regard to serious neurologic events (CABG alone 3.1% vs combined CABG MVR 9.6%), mean length of stay (CABG alone 9.4 ± 5.9 days vs combined CABG MVR 11.3 ± 8.3 days), and intensive care unit length of stay (CABG alone 4.0 ± 5.7 days vs combined CABG MVR 4.8 ± 6.1 days) in favoring CABG alone. With regard to residual mitral valve regurgitation, 30% of patients in the CABG-alone group had moderate-to-severe MR compared with only 11.2% in the combined CABG MVR group. Although this study found that addition of MVR to CABG in patients with moderate mitral regurgitation results in less residual mitral regurgitation at 1 year, this did not translate into a clinical benefit and occurred at the cost of an increased rate of serious neurologic events and longer hospital stay. Accordingly, routine repair of moderate MR cannot be advocated at the time of CABG unless the longer-term (2 years) planned follow-up of this cohort shows clinical improvement.

R. Bayer II, MD

49 Acute Coronary Syndromes

Outcomes 1 Year after Thrombus Aspiration for Myocardial Infarction

Lagerqvist B, Fröbert O, Olivecrona GK, et al (Uppsala Univ, Sweden; Lund Univ, Sweden; et al)

N Engl J Med 371:1111-1120, 2014

Background.—Routine intracoronary thrombus aspiration before primary percutaneous coronary intervention (PCI) in patients with ST-segment elevation myocardial infarction (STEMI) has not been proved to reduce short-term mortality. We evaluated clinical outcomes at 1 year after thrombus aspiration.

Methods.—We randomly assigned 7244 patients with STEMI to undergo manual thrombus aspiration followed by PCI or to undergo PCI alone, in a registry-based, randomized clinical trial. The primary end point of all-cause mortality at 30 days has been reported previously. Death from any cause at 1 year was a prespecified secondary end point of the trial.

Results.—No patients were lost to follow-up. Death from any cause occurred in 5.3% of the patients (191 of 3621 patients) in the thrombus-aspiration group, as compared with 5.6% (202 of 3623) in the PCI-only group (hazard ratio, 0.94; 95% confidence interval [CI], 0.78 to 1.15; $P = 0.57$). Rehospitalization for myocardial infarction at 1 year occurred in 2.7% and 2.7% of the patients, respectively (hazard ratio, 0.97; 95% CI, 0.73 to 1.28; $P = 0.81$), and stent thrombosis in 0.7% and 0.9%, respectively (hazard ratio, 0.84; 95% CI, 0.50 to 1.40; $P = 0.51$). The composite of death from any cause, rehospitalization for myocardial infarction, or stent thrombosis occurred in 8.0% and 8.5% of the patients, respectively (hazard ratio, 0.94; 95% CI, 0.80 to 1.11; $P = 0.48$). The results were consistent across all the major subgroups, including grade of thrombus burden and coronary flow before PCI.

Conclusions.—Routine thrombus aspiration before PCI in patients with STEMI did not reduce the rate of death from any cause or the composite of death from any cause, rehospitalization for myocardial infarction, or stent thrombosis at 1 year. (Funded by the Swedish Research Council and others; TASTE ClinicalTrials.gov number, NCT01093404.)

▶ The utility of intracoronary thrombus aspiration in the setting of ST-segment myocardial infarction remains controversial. Two randomized clinical trials found no reduction in mortality at 30 days. To date, there are no adequately powered randomized data showing a reduction in mortality at 1 year. The aim of the Thrombus Aspiration in ST-Elevation in Myocardial Infarction in Scandinavia (TASTE) trial was to determine clinical outcomes 1 year after thrombus aspiration. A total of 7244 patients were randomly assigned in a 1:1 ratio either to thrombus aspiration followed by percutaneous coronary intervention (PCI) or to PCI alone. The primary endpoint was all-cause mortality at 30 days and prespecified secondary endpoints at 1 year: death from any cause, myocardial infarction, stent thrombosis, target-vessel revascularization, and target-lesion revascularization. Data on clinical endpoints were obtained from national health registries. These endpoint events were not adjudicated. There were no study-specific follow-up studies done. Data regarding deaths were obtained from national population registries and other clinical endpoints from the Swedish Web System for Enhancement and Development of Evidence-based Care in Heart Disease Evaluated According to Recommended Therapies registry. One year after the PCI, there was no difference in death (hazard ratio [HR], 0.94; 95% confidence interval [CI], 0.78-1.15; $P = .57$), myocardial infarction (HR, 0.97; 95% CI, 0.73-1.28; $P = .81$), or stent thrombosis (HR, 0.84; 95% CI, 0.50-1.40; $P = .51$) between the thrombus aspiration and PCI groups (Fig 1 in the original article). Additionally, there was no difference in composite endpoint of death from any cause, myocardial infarction or stent thrombosis (HR, 0.94; 95% CI, 0.80-1.11; $P = .48$) at 1 year between the groups (Fig 2 in the original article). These data strongly suggest that routine thrombus aspiration before PCI does not result in lower all-cause mortality or composite all-cause mortality, myocardial infarction, and stent thrombosis when compared with PCI alone. One limitation of this study was that the outcome events were obtained from registry data and were not adjudicated. However, such a multicenter, randomized, registry-based clinical trial design is a novel alternative to traditional clinical trials and allows more cost effective and rapid trials to be completed.

T. Todoran, MD

PART SEVEN

THE DIGESTIVE SYSTEM

KENNETH R. DEVAULT, MD

Introduction

There have been numerous advances in the field of gastroenterology and hepatology over the past year. Reviewing studies for this publication gives me an excellent opportunity to view the major trends, which this year include advances in our understanding of how food and psychological factors influence functional gastrointestinal disorders, additional data on how to best prevent colon cancer, data on the treatment and significance of liver disease such as hepatitis C and fatty liver disease, improved understanding of pancreatic lesions, and many others.

It was very hard to put together the best articles in this very productive year, but hopefully this collection will both inform the reader and encourage a deeper examination of each of these important topics.

Kenneth R. DeVault, MD

50 Esophagus

Hospital and surgeon volume in relation to long-term survival after oesophagectomy: systematic review and meta-analysis

Brusselaers N, Mattsson F, Lagergren J (Karolinska Institutet, Stockholm, Sweden)

Gut 63:1393-1400, 2014

Background.—Centralisation of healthcare, especially for advanced cancer surgery, has been a matter of debate. Clear short-term mortality benefits have been described for oesophageal cancer surgery conducted at high-volume hospitals and by high-volume surgeons.

Objective.—To clarify the association between hospital volume, surgeon volume and hospital type in relation to long-term survival after oesophagectomy for cancer, by a meta-analysis.

Design.—The systematic literature search included PubMed, Web of Science, Cochrane library, EMBASE and Science Citation Index, for the period 1990–2013. Eligible articles were those which reported survival (time to death) as HRs after oesophagectomy for cancer by hospital volume, surgeon volume or hospital type. Fully adjusted HRs for the longest follow-up were the main outcomes. Results were pooled by a meta-analysis, and reported as HRs and 95% CIs.

Results.—Sixteen studies from seven countries met the inclusion criteria. These studies reported hospital volume (N = 13), surgeon volume (N = 4) or hospital type (N = 4). A survival benefit was found for high-volume hospitals (HR = 0.82, 95% CI 0.75 to 0.90), and possibly also, for high-volume surgeons (HR = 0.87, 95% CI 0.74 to 1.02) compared with their low-volume counterparts. No association with survival remained for hospital volume after adjustment for surgeon volume (HR = 1.01, 95% CI 0.97 to 1.06; N = 2), while a survival benefit was found in favour of high-volume surgeons after adjustment for hospital volume (HR = 0.91, 95% CI 0.85 to 0.98; N = 2).

Conclusions.—This meta-analysis demonstrated better long-term survival (even after excluding early deaths) after oesophagectomy with high-volume surgery, and surgeon volume might be more important than hospital volume. These findings support centralisation with fewer surgeons working at large centres.

▶ Esophagectomy is a radical procedure associated with high rates of both morbidity and mortality. Previous studies have suggested that having surgery in high-volume centers leads to better outcomes. This systematic review and meta-analysis of many of those studies confirms the assertion of better outcomes in high-volume centers and with high-volume surgeons. In fact, in contrast to some prior data, the surgeon volume may be more important than the center volume.

These and other data support the centralization of esophagectomy to high-volume centers and surgeons. What is the downside, if any of that approach? It would be reasonable to believe that removing these elective cases might lead to poor outcomes in emergent cases presenting to low-volume centers. That is a rare enough occurrence that it can likely be discounted. Another possible concern would be that removing complex cases might produce poorer skills in more routine operations, but there are also no data to support that. The studies used in this analysis had a wide variation in what they considered high volume (ranging from >9 per year to >40 per year) and low volume (ranging form 1.2 per year to <10 per year). The correct cutoff is probably somewhere between 10 and 20 per year. The bottom line is that it is clearly in the esophagectomy patient's best interest to have surgery performed in a sufficiently experienced environment by an experienced surgeon.

K. R. DeVault, MD

Efficacy of Transoral Fundoplication vs Omeprazole for Treatment of Regurgitation in a Randomized Controlled Trial

Hunter JG, Kahrilas PJ, Bell RCW, et al (Oregon Health & Science Univ, Portland; Northwestern Univ, Chicago, IL; SurgOne Foregut Inst, Englewood, CO; et al)

Gastroenterology 148:324-333, 2015

Background & Aims.—Transoral esophagogastric fundoplication (TF) can decrease or eliminate features of gastroesophageal reflux disease (GERD) in some patients whose symptoms persist despite proton pump inhibitor (PPI) therapy. We performed a prospective, sham-controlled trial to determine if TF reduced troublesome regurgitation to a greater extent than PPIs in patients with GERD.

Methods.—We screened 696 patients with troublesome regurgitation despite daily PPI use with 3 validated GERD-specific symptom scales, on and off PPIs. Those with at least troublesome regurgitation (based on the Montreal definition) on PPIs underwent barium swallow, esophagogastroduodenoscopy, 48-hour esophageal pH monitoring (off PPIs), and high-resolution esophageal manometry analyses. Patients with GERD and hiatal hernias ≤2 cm were randomly assigned to groups that underwent TF and then received 6 months of placebo (n = 87), or sham surgery and 6 months of once- or twice-daily omeprazole (controls, n = 42). Patients were blinded to therapy during follow-up period and reassessed at 2, 12, and 26 weeks. At 6 months, patients underwent 48-hour esophageal pH monitoring and esophagogastroduodenoscopy.

Results.—By intention-to-treat analysis, TF eliminated troublesome regurgitation in a larger proportion of patients (67%) than PPIs (45%)

($P = .023$). A larger proportion of controls had no response at 3 months (36%) than subjects that received TF (11%; $P = .004$). Control of esophageal pH improved after TF (mean 9.3% before and 6.3% after; $P < .001$), but not after sham surgery (mean 8.6% before and 8.9% after). Subjects from both groups who completed the protocol had similar reductions in GERD symptom scores. Severe complications were rare (3 subjects receiving TF and 1 receiving the sham surgery).

Conclusions.—TF was an effective treatment for patients with GERD symptoms, particularly in those with persistent regurgitation despite PPI therapy, based on evaluation 6 months after the procedure. Clinicaltrials.gov no: NCT01136980.

► This report examined the latest endoscopic procedure designed to control reflux. Transoral fundoplication (TF) uses a series of pledgets placed endoscopically to hopefully control reflux. This study compared TF with omeprazole therapy and concluded that it was a helpful treatment in patients with regurgitation refractory to proton pump inhibitor therapy. Indeed, patients who had TF had less troublesome regurgitation when compared with those with a sham TF. Overall quality of life was not different between the 2 groups. Similarly, the study from the *American Journal of Gastroenterology* (AJG) showed an improvement in symptoms with TF.

Why then would we not apply this broadly? The problem with this and all endoscopic treatments of gastroesophageal reflux disease to date is that although symptoms often improve, acid exposure does not. The report presented here found an improvement in reflux measures, but less than 50% of patients had normalization at 6 months. In addition, the AJG trial found acid control in only 29% of subjects at 12 months, and 61% were back on proton pump inhibitors. Traditional surgery (fundoplication and, more recently, magnetic augmentation) controls both symptoms and acid exposure.

It is possible that some endoscopic intervention in the future may take the place of traditional surgery, but nothing to date (including TF) meets that standard. Recent guidelines from the American College of Gastroenterology did not advocate endoscopic approaches at this time, and data from these 2 studies are unlikely to change that opinion.

K. R. DeVault, MD

Long-term recurrence of neoplasia and Barrett's epithelium after complete endoscopic resection

Anders M, Bähr C, El-Masry MA, et al (Univ Hosp Hamburg-Eppendorf, Germany; et al)
Gut 63:1535-1543, 2014

Background.—Current endoscopic therapy for neoplastic Barrett's oesophagus (BO) consists of complete resection/ablation of all Barrett's tissue including neoplastic lesions. Recurrence seems to be frequent after thermal therapy, such as radiofrequency ablation.

Objective.—To analyse long-term recurrence of neoplasia and BO after successful widespread endoscopic mucosal resection (EMR).

Design.—In a retrospective analysis, all patients undergoing widespread EMR of neoplastic BO between 2002 and 2007 at two referral centres were followed for at least 3 years after completion of endotherapy. Recurrence was diagnosed if neoplasia and/or BO were detected following previous successful complete removal, defined as at least two negative endoscopies and biopsies.

Results.—Ninety patients undergoing widespread EMR were included (mean age 63 years; 82 male), 58% of whom underwent additional thermal ablation for minor residual disease. Complete eradication of neoplasia and Barrett's tissue was achieved in 90% of patients. On further follow-up (mean 64.8 months), recurrence of neoplastic and non-neoplastic BO was found in 6.2% and 39.5%, respectively. Recurring neoplasia (3 adenocarcinomas, 1 low-grade and 1 high-grade dysplasia) were found after a median of 44 months (range 38–85) and could be retreated endoscopically. In a multivariate analysis, Barrett's length was the only factor significantly associated with recurrence (OR 2.73).

Conclusions.—Even after seemingly complete endoscopic resection, recurrence of BO is frequent and independent of additional thermal therapy. Due to the possibility of neoplasia recurrence even after long disease-free intervals, follow-up should be extended beyond 5 years.

▶ Barrett's esophagus (BE) is a common complication of gastroesophageal reflux disease. Current guidelines suggest eradication of BE when either low- or high-grade dysplasia is diagnosed. Methods for that eradication include thermal ablation, endoscopic mucosal resection (EMR), or a combination of both. This study followed patients after complete EMR of BE, which usually had high-grade dysplasia or limited carcinoma before resection. More than half also required thermal ablation. They were able to achieve complete eradication in 90% of patients, yet the recurrence of nondysplastic and dysplastic BE (39.5 and 6.2%, respectively) were relatively common. Among the 5 patients with recurrence of neoplastic BE, there were 3 cancers and 1 high-grade and 1 low-grade dysplasia with recurrences happening as far out as 85 months. All were treated successfully with additional endoscopy and brought back into remission.

What can we take from this study? First, it is clear that patients with BE that has been eradicated are not necessarily "cured" of their disease. It is possible that the use of argon plasma coagulation in this study could be inferior to radiofrequency ablation (RFA), but the numbers were too small to make any conclusion. The initial grade of dysplasia or presence of cancer did not predict recurrence, but recurrence was more likely in those with longer segments of BE. The lag between eradication and recurrence suggests that patients with eradicated BE may need to stay in lifelong surveillance programs. This may call into question the practice of eradicating low-grade dysplasia and nondysplastic BE (particularly the cost-effectiveness of that practice), although again, this was not directly evaluated in this study. On a more positive note, the fact that they could be brought back into remission is important and suggests that if we do appropriate surveillance, we can control cancer even if the ablations are not permanent.

K. R. DeVault, MD

51 Stomach

Peptic Ulcer Bleeding Risk. The Role of *Helicobacter Pylori* Infection in NSAID/Low-Dose Aspirin Users

Sostres C, Carrera-Lasfuentes P, Benito R, et al (Universitary Hosp Lozano Blesa, Zaragoza, Spain; CIBERehd, Madrid, Spain; et al)

Am J Gastroenterol 110:684-689, 2015

Objectives.—*Helicobacter pylori* (*H. pylori*) infection and NSAID/low-dose aspirin (ASA) use are associated with peptic ulcer disease. The risk of peptic ulcer bleeding (PUB) associated with the interaction of these factors remains unclear. The objective of this study was to determine the risk of PUB associated with the interaction between *H. pylori* infection and current nonsteroidal anti-inflammatory drugs (NSAIDs) or low-dose ASA use.

Methods.—This was a case-control study of consecutive patients hospitalized because of PUB. Controls were matched by age, sex, and month of admission. *H. pylori* infection status was determined in all cases and controls by serology. Drug use was determined by structured questionnaire. Adjusted relative risk (RR) associated with different factors, and the interaction between NSAID/ASA and *H. pylori* infection was estimated by logistic regression analysis.

Results.—The study included 666 cases of PUB and 666 controls; 74.3% cases and 54.8% controls (RR: 2.6; 95% confidence interval (CI): 2.0–3.3) tested positive for *H. pylori* infection; 34.5% of cases had current NSAID use compared with 13.4% of controls (RR: 4.0; 95% CI: 3.0–5.4). Respective proportions for low-dose ASA use were 15.8 and 12%, respectively (RR: 1.9; 95% CI: 1.3–2.7). The RR of PUB for concomitant NSAID use and *H. pylori* infection suggested an additive effect (RR: 8.0; 95% CI: 5.0–12.8), whereas no interaction was observed with ASA use (RR: 3.5; 95% CI: 2.0–6.1).

Conclusions.—NSAID, low-dose ASA use, and *H. pylori* infection are three independent risk factors for the development of PUB, but there were differences in the interaction effect between low-dose ASA (no interaction) or NSAID (addition) use and *H. pylori* infection, which may have implications for clinical practice in prevention strategies.

► Peptic ulcer disease (PUD) is associated with *Helicobacter pylori* (HP) infection, nonsteroidal anti-inflammatory drugs (NSAID)/low-dose aspirin (ASA) use or a combination in a majority of patients. Interactions between these risk factors are incompletely defined. Some guidelines advocate eradication of HP in all patients at risk of developing PUD. This case-control study confirmed an interaction between HP infection and NSAID use but found no such interaction between low-dose ASA use and PUD.

How can we use the data from this study? First, the authors demonstrated that the risk of PUD was greatest in NSAID users, followed by HP, and less so with low-dose ASA. It confirms that added care should be taken in patients with HP and NSAID, and in fact, it may be reasonable to test for and eradicate HP in a patient taking NSAIDs with other risk factors for bleeding. The same cannot be said for HP and low-dose ASA. It is important to remember that this is not a randomized trial and thus could be affected by several potential biases.

K. R. DeVault, MD

52 Small Bowel

Small Amounts of Gluten in Subjects With Suspected Nonceliac Gluten Sensitivity: A Randomized, Double-Blind, Placebo-controlled, Cross-Over Trial

Di Sabatino A, Volta U, Salvatore C, et al (Univ of Pavia, Italy; Univ of Bologna, Italy)

Clin Gastroenterol Hepatol 2015 [Epub ahead of print]

Background & Aims.—There is debate over the existence of nonceliac gluten sensitivity (NCGS) intestinal and extraintestinal symptoms in response to ingestion of gluten-containing foods by people without celiac disease or wheat allergy. We performed a randomized, double-blind, placebo-controlled, cross-over trial to determine the effects of administration of low doses of gluten to subjects with suspected NCGS.

Methods.—We enrolled 61 adults without celiac disease or a wheat allergy who believed ingestion of gluten-containing food to be the cause of their intestinal and extraintestinal symptoms. Participants were assigned randomly to groups given either 4.375 g/day gluten or rice starch (placebo) for 1 week, each via gastrosoluble capsules. After a 1-week gluten-free diet, participants crossed over to the other group. The primary outcome was the change in overall (intestinal and extraintestinal) symptoms, determined by established scoring systems, between gluten and placebo intake. A secondary outcome was the change in individual symptom scores between gluten vs placebo.

Results.—According to the per-protocol analysis of data from the 59 patients who completed the trial, intake of gluten significantly increased overall symptoms compared with placebo ($P = .034$). Abdominal bloating ($P = .040$) and pain ($P = .047$), among the intestinal symptoms, and foggy mind ($P = .019$), depression ($P = .020$), and aphthous stomatitis ($P = .025$), among the extraintestinal symptoms, were significantly more severe when subjects received gluten than placebo.

Conclusions.—In a cross-over trial of subjects with suspected NCGS, the severity of overall symptoms increased significantly during 1 week of intake of small amounts of gluten, compared with placebo. Clinical trial no: ISRCTN72857280.

▶ The concept of gluten sensitivity in patients without serological or histological evidence of celiac disease has received increased attention in the recent past. Many practitioners are more accepting of the diagnosis and agree with patients following a gluten-free diet if their symptoms are improved by that diet. We know that even small exposures to gluten can result in mucosal changes and increased symptoms in patients with celiac disease, but whether similar exposures result in symptom changes in nonceliac, gluten sensitivity is not known.

The patients in this study were exposed to a daily dose of just over 4 g of gluten compared with placebo while they maintained an otherwise gluten-free diet. Overall symptoms as well as specific symptoms such as abdominal bloating and pain were significantly worse when exposed to gluten. Interestingly, there were a few nonspecific symptoms that also improved, including "foggy mind," depression, and aphthous stomatitis. This important study provides guidance to physicians treating these patients. It is still reasonable to make the diagnosis based on response to diet. Although small amounts of gluten exposure are unlikely to produce sustained damage as they does in celiac disease, patients need to understand that poor adherence to their diet may well result in an increase in symptoms. Because gluten is ubiquitous in our environment, a visit with a dietician may be needed to help educate these patients on what constitutes a truly gluten-free diet.

K. R. DeVault, MD

Effect of Antidepressants and Psychological Therapies, Including Hypnotherapy, in Irritable Bowel Syndrome: Systematic Review and Meta-Analysis

Ford AC, Quigley EMM, Lacy BE, et al (St James's Univ Hosp, Leeds, UK; Houston Methodist Hospital, TX; Dartmouth-Hitchcock Medical Center, Lebanon, NH; et al)

Am J Gastroenterol 109:1350-1365, 2014

Objectives.—Irritable bowel syndrome (IBS) is a chronic functional gastrointestinal disorder. Evidence relating to the treatment of this condition with antidepressants and psychological therapies continues to accumulate.

Methods.—We performed an updated systematic review and meta-analysis of randomized controlled trials (RCTs). MEDLINE, EMBASE, and the Cochrane Controlled Trials Register were searched (up to December 2013). Trials recruiting adults with IBS, which compared antidepressants with placebo, or psychological therapies with control therapy or "usual management," were eligible. Dichotomous symptom data were pooled to obtain a relative risk (RR) of remaining symptomatic after therapy, with a 95% confidence interval (CI).

Results.—The search strategy identified 3,788 citations. Forty-eight RCTs were eligible for inclusion: thirty-one compared psychological therapies with control therapy or "usual management," sixteen compared antidepressants with placebo, and one compared both psychological therapy and antidepressants with placebo. Ten of the trials of psychological therapies, and four of the RCTs of antidepressants, had been published since our previous meta-analysis. The RR of IBS symptom not improving with antidepressants vs. placebo was 0.67 (95% CI = 0.58–0.77), with similar treatment effects for both tricyclic antidepressants and selective serotonin reuptake inhibitors. The RR of symptoms not improving with psychological therapies was 0.68 (95% CI = 0.61–0.76). Cognitive behavioral therapy, hypnotherapy, multicomponent psychological therapy, and dynamic psychotherapy were all beneficial.

Conclusions.—Antidepressants and some psychological therapies are effective treatments for IBS. Despite the considerable number of studies published in the intervening 5 years since we last examined this issue, the overall summary estimates of treatment effect have remained remarkably stable.

▶ Irritable bowel syndrome (IBS) is one of the most commonly diagnosed conditions in both gastroenterology and primary care. Effective therapies for the common and life-altering condition are limited. Because IBS is considered a "functional" disorder with a neuroenteric etiology, several therapies designed to lower sensitivity have been proposed and widely used. This analysis looked at the published efficacy of several of these therapies when grouped together included the following:

1. Antidepressants: in pooled analysis of several agents, there was an improvement over placebo (35% improvement with placebo and 56% with active treatment). Agents with a positive and similar effects included tricyclic antidepressants and selective serotonin reuptake inhibitors.
2. Psychological therapies were also superior to control groups (48.1% improvement vs 23.9%). Forms of therapy included cognitive behavioral therapy, relaxation therapy, and hypnotherapy, among several others.

These data provide support for this type of intervention in IBS. The treating physician should counsel patients of that efficacy and ensure them that the effect is not dependent on underlying, non-IBS related, psychological issues. After structural disease has been excluded, these therapies should be considered early in IBS management and likely are as effective as more commonly used therapies such as fiber and antispasmodics. Given the common nature of the problem, mental health providers should be open to seeing and treating this group of patients.

K. R. DeVault, MD

Lack of Utility of Symptoms and Signs at First Presentation as Predictors of Inflammatory Bowel Disease in Secondary Care

Ford AC, Moayyedi P, Bercik P, et al (St James's Univ Hosp, Leeds, UK; McMaster Univ, Hamilton, Ontario, Canada; et al)

Am J Gastroenterol 110:716-724, 2015

Objectives.—There are few data concerning the utility of symptoms and signs at first presentation in predicting a diagnosis of ulcerative colitis (UC) or Crohn's disease (CD). We conducted a study to examine this issue in secondary care.

Methods.—We collected complete symptom, colonoscopy, and histology data prospectively from 1,981 consecutive adult patients with lower gastrointestinal symptoms at two hospitals in Hamilton, Ontario. Assessors were blinded to symptom status. The reference standard used to define the presence of UC or CD was according to accepted histological criteria. Patients without UC or CD served as controls. Sensitivity, specificity, and positive and negative likelihood ratios (LRs) were calculated for individual items from the clinical history, as well as combinations of these.

Results.—In identifying 302 patients with inflammatory bowel diseases (IBD), positive LRs for individual items ranged from 1.18 (incomplete emptying) to 2.30 (passage of stools more than four times per day at least most of the time) and negative LRs from 0.70 (bloody stools) to 0.96 (incomplete emptying). Combinations of items had a high specificity, but at the expense of sensitivity. Items that were independent predictors of IBD after logistic regression analysis were family history of IBD, younger age, passage of stools more than four times per day ≥75% of the time, urgency most of the time, and anemia.

Conclusions.—Individual items from the clinical history are not helpful in predicting a diagnosis of UC or CD. However, this may be because some items lacked sufficient detail. Combinations of symptoms and computer models had a high specificity, but overall were only modestly useful diagnostically. Future studies should evaluate biological markers in combination with symptoms to improve accuracy.

▶ When patients present with gastrointestinal symptoms such as abdominal pain and diarrhea, the diagnosis of inflammatory bowel disease (IBD) is often considered. This consideration frequently leads to expensive endoscopic tests, the results of which are normal in most patients. This report looked at clinical data from a group of 1981 patients, of which, 302 had IBD. There was no attempt at matching, so the IBD patients were predictably younger by more than 10 years, but the other demographic factors were for the most part similar.

Individual symptoms did not clearly distinguish those with IBD, although the most suggestive factors were family history of IBD, urgency, and more than 4 bowel movements per day. No single factor had sensitivity greater than 53%. The best prediction was a combination of anemia, greater than 5 kg weight loss in the last year, and passage of stools more than 4 times per day. The symptoms also did not perform better when the controls were limited to those with a normal colonoscopy. Prior results from the same group suggest that symptoms also were not really effective in distinguishing between irritable bowel syndrome (IBS) and other nonfunctional findings such as colorectal cancer.

Where does this leave us? It is disappointing that we cannot exclude IBD based on historical factors, leading many patients to continue to need investigation. Future studies may be able to combine symptoms with simple blood tests looking at inflammation to yield better performance. It is important to follow up with patients for some time before investigation, as symptoms may remit spontaneously or with an IBS approach, allowing one to avoid colonoscopy. It is also important to understand that patients with IBD often also suffer from IBS.

K. R. DeVault, MD

53 Colon

The Effect of Fiber Supplementation on Irritable Bowel Syndrome: A Systematic Review and Meta-analysis

Moayyedi P, Quigley EMM, Lacy BE, et al (McMaster Univ, Hamilton, Ontario, Canada; Houston Methodist Hosp, TX; Dartmouth-Hitchcock Medical Ctr, Lebanon, NH; et al)

Am J Gastroenterol 109:1367-1374, 2014

Objectives.—Fiber has been used for many years to treat irritable bowel syndrome (IBS). This approach had fallen out of favor until a recent resurgence, which was based on new randomized controlled trial (RCT) data that suggested it might be effective. We have previously conducted a systematic review of fiber in IBS, but new RCT data for fiber therapy necessitate a new analysis; thus, we have conducted a systematic review of this intervention.

Methods.—MEDLINE, EMBASE, and the Cochrane Controlled Trials Register were searched up to December 2013. Trials recruiting adults with IBS, which compared fiber supplements with placebo, control therapy, or "usual management", were eligible. Dichotomous symptom data were pooled to obtain a relative risk (RR) of remaining symptomatic after therapy as well as number needed to treat (NNT) with a 95% confidence interval (CI).

Results.—We identified 14 RCTs involving 906 patients that had evaluated fiber in IBS. There was a significant benefit of fiber in IBS (RR = 0.86; 95% CI 0.80–0.94 with an NNT = 10; 95% CI = 6–33). There was no significant heterogeneity between results ($I^2 = 0\%$, Cochran $Q = 13.85$ (d.f. = 14), $P = 0.46$). The benefit was only seen in RCTs on soluble fiber (RR = 0.83; 95% CI 0.73–0.94 with an NNT = 7; 95% CI 4–25) with no effect seen with bran (RR = 0.90; 95% CI 0.79–1.03).

Conclusions.—Soluble fiber is effective in treating IBS. Bran did not appear to be of benefit, although we did not uncover any evidence of harm from this intervention, as others have speculated from uncontrolled data.

▶ Fiber supplementation is considered first-line therapy for irritable bowel syndrome (IBS). This review and analysis confirmed soluble fiber but not bran as beneficial. It is interesting that the majority of trials did not distinguish between various subtypes of IBS (constipation, diarrhea, and pain predominant). The types of fiber were quite variable. As above in the article, no benefit was noted with bran. Positive effects were seen with ispaghula husk, concentrated fiber, and linseeds. Importantly, there were no adverse events. This analysis was more supportive of fiber than previous reviews by the same group and also more supportive than a Cochrane review. The authors attributed that change to the inclusion of recent, positive studies.

Should fiber be tried in all patients with IBS? I think that given the potential efficacy and low side effect profile, the answer is likely yes. Use of soluble fiber, not bran, should be emphasized. That having been said, additional studies should focus on the 3 subtypes of IBS and attempt to define which patients are more likely to respond. Those with bloating and distention may actually be made worse, although it would be good to have better data to support that statement. Finally, it is interesting that despite our long use of these agents and their efficacy, the mechanism of action is mostly unknown and likely involves more than simply increasing the bulk of stools.

K. R. DeVault, MD

Efficacy of Prebiotics, Probiotics, and Synbiotics in Irritable Bowel Syndrome and Chronic Idiopathic Constipation: Systematic Review and Meta-analysis

Ford AC, Quigley EMM, Lacy BE, et al (St James's Univ Hosp, Leeds, UK; Houston Methodist Hosp, TX; Dartmouth-Hitchcock Med Ctr, Lebanon, NH; et al)

Am J Gastroenterol 109:1547-1561, 2014

Objectives.—Irritable bowel syndrome (IBS) and chronic idiopathic constipation (CIC) are functional bowel disorders. Evidence suggests that disturbance in the gastrointestinal microbiota may be implicated in both conditions. We performed a systematic review and meta-analysis to examine the efficacy of prebiotics, probiotics, and synbiotics in IBS and CIC.

Methods.—MEDLINE, EMBASE, and the Cochrane Controlled Trials Register were searched (up to December 2013). Randomized controlled trials (RCTs) recruiting adults with IBS or CIC, which compared prebiotics, probiotics, or synbiotics with placebo or no therapy, were eligible. Dichotomous symptom data were pooled to obtain a relative risk (RR) of remaining symptomatic after therapy, with a 95% confidence interval (CI). Continuous data were pooled using a standardized or weighted mean difference with a 95% CI.

Results.—The search strategy identified 3,216 citations. Forty-three RCTs were eligible for inclusion. The RR of IBS symptoms persisting with probiotics vs. placebo was 0.79 (95% CI 0.70–0.89). Probiotics had beneficial effects on global IBS, abdominal pain, bloating, and flatulence scores. Data for prebiotics and synbiotics in IBS were sparse. Probiotics appeared to have beneficial effects in CIC (mean increase in number of stools per week = 1.49; 95% CI = 1.02–1.96), but there were only two RCTs. Synbiotics also appeared beneficial (RR of failure to respond to therapy = 0.78; 95% CI 0.67—0.92). Again, trials for prebiotics were few in number, and no definite conclusions could be drawn.

Conclusions.—Probiotics are effective treatments for IBS, although which individual species and strains are the most beneficial remains unclear. Further evidence is required before the role of prebiotics or synbiotics in IBS is known. The efficacy of all three therapies in CIC is also uncertain.

▶ Probiotics, prebiotics, and synbiotics are commonly used in patients with gastrointestinal symptoms, yet the efficacy, dose, and duration are incompletely defined. This systematic review and meta-analysis adds to our understanding of this area. Most of the data were on probiotics, which showed improvement in the global irritable bowel syndrome (IBS) symptom as well as in several specific symptoms of IBS (abdominal pain, bloating, and flatulence). In addition, they increased the number of stools per week in chronic idiopathic constipation (CIC).

Although this analysis once again confirmed the efficacy of these agents, we are still left with a great deal of uncertainty in regard to which agent to give and the dose and duration of that agent. It appears the greatest efficacy was found with combination probiotics containing various agents and perhaps monotherapy with *Lactobacillus plantarum*. When compared with other, traditional pharmacologic agents, probiotics have similar efficacy and lower side effects. They therefore should have an early and prominent role in IBS. The improvement in CIC was a little more unexpected, but a trial in that disorder may also be reasonable.

K. R. DeVault, MD

Incidence, Prevalence, and Temporal Trends of Microscopic Colitis: A Systematic Review and Meta-Analysis

Tong J, Zheng Q, Zhang C, et al (Shanghai Jiao Tong Univ, China; et al)
Am J Gastroenterol 110:265-276, 2015

Objectives.—A systematic review and meta-analysis was conducted to provide an accurate estimate of the incidence rate of microscopic colitis (MC) and to assess the association between medication use and the risk of MC.

Methods.—We searched Medline, Embase, and Institute for Scientific Information (ISI) Web of Science up to 26 September 2014 to identify published epidemiological studies of MC. The pooled incidence rate, female-to-male incidence rate ratio, age at diagnosis, prevalence, as well as odds ratios (ORs) of MC in association with medication use were calculated using a fixed-effects model or a random-effects model.

Results.—Of the 1,972 citations retrieved, 25 studies were included. Pooled incidence rate of collagenous colitis (CC) was 4.14 (95% confidence interval (CI) 2.89—5.40) per 100,000 person-years and 4.85 (95% CI, 3.45—6.25) for lymphocytic colitis (LC). The female-to-male incidence rate ratios were 3.05 (95% CI 2.92–3.19) for CC and 1.92 (95% CI 1.53–2.31) for LC. The median age at diagnosis for CC was 64.9 (range, 57.03–72.78) years, similar to LC (median 62.18, range 53.99–70.38). Furthermore, the incidence rate of MC increased with rising age. A steadily increasing trend of incidence rate for both CC and LC was observed before 2000; however, the incidence rate since then has become stable in the United States, Sweden, and Spain. An increased risk of MC was associated with the use of proton pump inhibitors (PPIs) and selective serotonin reuptake inhibitors (SSRIs) (OR 2.68, 95% CI 1.73–4.17 and OR 2.41, 95% CI 1.64–3.53, respectively).

Conclusions.—MC is a common disease process. Female gender, increased age, and the use of PPIs and SSRIs are associated with a significantly increased risk of developing MC. Further work is needed to evaluate reported data from developing countries and to elucidate the biologic mechanisms behind the risk factors for MC.

▶ When patients, particularly older patients, present with diarrhea, microscopic colitis (MC) should be in the differential diagnosis. MC has 2 subtypes: lymphocytic and collagenous colitis. Patients with MC are often first diagnosed with irritable bowel syndrome and may suffer for a prolonged period before the appropriate diagnosis. Because the disease is more common in older, female patients, increased morbidity often occurs when there is coexistent fecal incontinence.

There was a gradual increase in the incidence of MC before 2000, but that has recently stabilized. In this study, there was also an association with the use of proton pump inhibitors and selective serotonin reuptake inhibitors. Unlike previous studies, there was only a slight association with nonsteroidal antiinflammatory drugs use. There is also no clear explanation for the increase in incidence of this disorder, nor do we understand the age and gender associations.

The bottom line is that MC should be considered in any patient with chronic, watery diarrhea, especially in older females. It is best diagnosed with mucosal biopsies taken at colonoscopy. Because the mucosa is grossly normal appearing, random biopsies should be obtained on any colonoscopy or sigmoidoscopy performed for diarrhea.

K. R. DeVault, MD

Burden of *Clostridium difficile* Infection in the United States

Lessa FC, Mu Y, Bamberg WM, et al (Emory Univ School of Medicine, Atlanta, GA; Colorado Dept of Public Health and Environment, Denver; et al)

N Engl J Med 372:825-834, 2015

Background.—The magnitude and scope of *Clostridium difficile* infection in the United States continue to evolve.

Methods.—In 2011, we performed active population- and laboratory-based surveillance across 10 geographic areas in the United States to identify cases of *C. difficile* infection (stool specimens positive for *C. difficile* on either toxin or molecular assay in residents ≥1 year of age). Cases were classified as community-associated or health care-associated. In a sample of cases of *C. difficile* infection, specimens were cultured and isolates underwent molecular typing. We used regression models to calculate estimates of national incidence and total number of infections, first recurrences, and deaths within 30 days after the diagnosis of *C. difficile* infection.

Results.—A total of 15,461 cases of *C. difficile* infection were identified in the 10 geographic areas; 65.8% were health care-associated, but only 24.2% had onset during hospitalization. After adjustment for predictors of disease incidence, the estimated number of incident *C. difficile* infections in the United States was 453,000 (95% confidence interval [CI], 397,100 to 508,500). The incidence was estimated to be higher among females (rate ratio, 1.26; 95% CI, 1.25 to 1.27), whites (rate ratio, 1.72; 95% CI, 1.56 to 2.0), and persons 65 years of age or older (rate ratio, 8.65; 95% CI, 8.16 to 9.31). The estimated number of first recurrences of *C. difficile* infection was 83,000 (95% CI, 57,000 to 108,900), and the estimated number of deaths was 29,300 (95% CI, 16,500 to 42,100). The North American pulsed-field gel electrophoresis type 1 (NAP1) strain was more prevalent among health care—associated infections than among community-associated infections (30.7% vs. 18.8%, $P < 0.001$).

Conclusions.—*C. difficile* was responsible for almost half a million infections and was associated with approximately 29,000 deaths in 2011.

► *Clostridium difficile* infection is a major health hazard and is now one of the reportable nosocomial infections by which hospital quality is judged. This study reports the burden that this illness is inflicting on the health care system in the United States. Data were obtained by examination of a well-constructed reporting system, then extrapolating to the US population. Major and important findings included estimated yearly mortality of almost 30 000. The number of cases are estimated at 453 000 and first recurrences of 83 000. The risk for a first recurrence was 14% in community and 21% in health care-associated infection. Although the majority of cases were health care-associated (65.8%), almost two-thirds of those were identified outside the hospital.

The take-home message from this study is that we have to respect both the widespread nature of *C. difficile* infection as well as the high mortality and morbidity associated with this infection. Any patient with substantial diarrhea should probably be tested for this agent regardless of their exposure to antibiotics or to a health care environment. The study also confirmed the high rate of recurrence (or perhaps lack of clearance) of infection after initial treatment. Because we know refractory cases are expensive and difficult to treat, added research is needed on optimization of initial therapy. Hospitals also must make sure known and suspected *C. difficile* patients have appropriate isolation. In addition, decontamination processes need to be tailored to the unique challenges of this infection.

K. R. DeVault, MD

A Randomized, Placebo-Controlled Trial of Lubiprostone for Opioid-Induced Constipation in Chronic Noncancer Pain

Jamal MM, Adams AB, Jansen J-P, et al (Long Beach VA Med Ctr, CA; AB Clinical Trials, Las Vegas, NV; SZ Schmerzzentrum Berlin GmbH, Germany; et al)

Am J Gastroenterol 110:725-732, 2015

Objectives.—This multicenter, phase 3 trial evaluated oral lubiprostone for constipation associated with non-methadone opioids in patients with chronic noncancer-related pain.

Methods.—Adults with opioid-induced constipation (OIC; <3 spontaneous bowel movements [SBMs] per week) were randomized 1:1 to double-blind lubiprostone 24 μg or placebo twice daily for 12 weeks. The primary end point was the overall SBM response rate. Responders had at least moderate response (≥1 SBM improvement over baseline frequency) in all treatment weeks with available observed data, as well as full response (≥3 SBMs per week) for at least 9 of the 12 treatment weeks.

Results.—In total, 431 patients were randomized; 212 each received lubiprostone and placebo, and 7 were not treated. Overall, the SBM response rate was significantly higher for patients treated with lubiprostone vs. placebo (27.1 vs. 18.9%, respectively; $P = 0.030$). Overall mean change from baseline in SBM frequency was significantly greater with lubiprostone vs. placebo (3.2 vs. 2.4, respectively; $P = 0.001$). The median time to first SBM was significantly shorter with lubiprostone vs. placebo (23.5 vs. 37.7 h, respectively; $P = 0.004$). Compared with placebo, the patients treated with lubiprostone exhibited significant improvements in straining ($P = 0.004$), stool consistency ($P < 0.001$), and constipation severity ($P = 0.010$). No significant differences were observed in quality-of-life measures or the use of rescue medication; however, the percentage of patients who used rescue medication was consistently lower in the lubiprostone group than in the placebo group at months 1 (34.9 vs. 37.7%), 2 (23.4 vs. 26.6%), and 3 (20.5 vs. 22.0%). Adverse events (AEs) >5% were diarrhea, nausea, vomiting, and abdominal pain (lubiprostone: 11.3, 9.9, 4.2, and 7.1%, respectively; placebo, 3.8, 4.7, 5.2, and 0%, respectively). None of the serious AEs (lubiprostone, 3.3%; placebo, 2.8%) were related to lubiprostone.

Conclusions.—Lubiprostone significantly improved symptoms of OIC and was well tolerated in patients with chronic noncancer pain.

▶ Opioid use is constantly increasing around the world. An unavoidable consequence of opioid use is constipation, which is reported in 15% to 80% of patients. This constipation can be difficult to deal with and at times produces increased pain, resulting in a downward spiral of increased opioid use and constipation. In addition, some patients will stop their opioids because of constipation and then suffer from worsening pain. This study evaluated an agent previously approved for constipation-predominant irritable bowel syndrome and chronic idiopathic constipation.

Lubiprostone (24 mcg twice daily) produced a modest but statistically significant improvement in number of spontaneous bowel movements in a week. There was also improvement in associated symptoms such as straining, stool consistency, and self-reported constipation severity. This drug is now approved in the United States for this indication. Because narcotics affect motility of the entire gastrointestinal tract, it is not surprising that high-volume agents like polyethylene glycol-containing laxatives could produce more bloating and increased discomfort. A pill-based therapy such as lubiprostone is therefore advantageous. Given cost concerns, it remains reasonable to start these patients on simple, over-the-counter measures, but if they do not respond or have agent-specific side effects, lubiprostone should be considered.

K. R. DeVault, MD

Optimizing Adequacy of Bowel Cleansing for Colonoscopy: Recommendations From the US Multi-Society Task Force on Colorectal Cancer

Johnson DA, Barkun AN, Cohen LB, et al (Eastern VA Med School, Norfolk; McGill Univ, Montreal, Canada; Icahn School of Medicine at Mount Sinai, NY; et al)
Am J Gastroenterol 109:1528-1545, 2014

Background.—Colonoscopy can prevent colorectal cancer (CRC) by detecting and removing precancerous lesions, but inadequate bowel preparation can compromise the process. Bowel preparation formulations are designed to be efficacious, safe, and tolerable for patients, but for the best results, efficacy must be given precedence over tolerability. The US Multi-Society Task Force on Colorectal Cancer formulated recommendations regarding the best way to optimize colonoscopy preparation and patient safety using the Grades of Recommendation Assessment, Development and Evaluation (GRADE) scoring system to evaluate current literature.

Method.—The medical literature in MEDLINE, PubMed EMBASE, Scopus, CENTRAL, and ISI Web of knowledge was searched between 1980 and 2013. The published articles and abstracts given at national meetings were also reviewed systematically to yield the recommendations.

Recommendations.—Beginning with the rectosigmoid colon, the preparation quality should be assessed. If polyps measuring more than 5 mm cannot be detected, the procedure should be terminated or additional cleansing done. A repeat examination within 1 year is required if the preparation is inadequate past the cecum. If advanced neoplasia is detected, the procedure should be repeated sooner. Adequate preparation should be achieved in 85% or more of all examinations.

Preparation for elective colonoscopy should ideally use a split-dose bowel cleansing regimen, but a same-day regimen can be substituted, especially for patients having an afternoon procedure. In all cases, the second dose of the split preparation is ideally begun 4 to 6 hours before procedure time and completed at least 2 hours before colonoscopy. Dietary recommendations are either a low-residue or a full liquid diet until evening the day before the procedure. Patients should receive oral and written patient education instructions for all components of the preparation regimen.

The bowel-cleansing regimen selected should consider the patient's medical history, medications, and bowel preparation adequacy reported in previous colonoscopies. Of the Food and Drug Administration (FDA)-n-approved options, the polyethylene glycol-n-electrolyte lavage solution (PEG-ELS)-n-based cleansing agents in high or low volume formulations provide high-quality results. Other choices include oral sulfate solution, sodium picosulfate, and sodium phosphate. Patients are more likely to be willing to undergo repeat colonoscopy if low-volume agents are used. The FDA has not approved several OTC preparations because their efficacy varies and caution is required for use. Among these are PEG-3350 powder and magnesium citrate. Adjunctive agents are not recommended.

Patient age is an important consideration for bowel-cleansing agent and regimen choice. Care is required when considering patients who are elderly, children, with known or suspected inflammatory bowel disease, with previous bariatric surgery, pregnant women, and those with spinal cord injury or other conditions.

When patients have inadequate preparation, some salvage strategies are possible, but all are supported by poor quality evidence.

Conclusions.—Efficacy of bowel preparation is essential for colonoscopy results. Physicians must choose the approach that will yield the best results for each patient.

▶ Effective colonoscopy is dependent on an adequately prepared colon before the procedure. A multisociety task force recently published this guideline, and important highlights included the following:

1. Procedures in which the preparation is obviously not going to allow adequate evaluation should be terminated early. It is of little use to struggle through a poorly prepared colon when it is clear that an early repeat examination will be needed.
2. Colonoscopies with inadequate preparation should have an early repeat study. The timing of that examination depends on the patients personal and family history.
3. Split dose (part of preparation on the day of examination) preparations are strongly recommended. The final dose should be started 4 to 6 hours and completed at least 2 hours before the procedure.
4. A low-residue or full liquid diet can usually be continued until the day before the procedure.
5. Adequacy of preparation should be noted in reports.
6. At least 85% of examinations should have an adequate preparation.
7. Some low-volume preparations may be similar to a 4-L preparation, especially when given in split doses.
8. Nonpolyethylene glycol preparations may be effective but have increased risk in some populations, particularly older patients and those with kidney disease.

All providers who send their patients for colonoscopy should understand these concepts and do everything possible to maximize the chance of a high-quality examination.

K. R. DeVault, MD

Incidence of Colonic Neoplasia in Patients With Serrated Polyposis Syndrome Who Undergo Annual Endoscopic Surveillance

Hazewinkel Y, Tytgat KMAJ, van Eeden S, et al (Academic Med Ctr, Amsterdam, The Netherlands)

Gastroenterology 147:88-95, 2014

Background & Aims.—Patients with serrated polyposis syndrome (SPS) are advised to undergo endoscopic surveillance for early detection of polyps and prevention of colorectal cancer (CRC). The optimal surveillance and treatment regimen is unknown. We performed a prospective study to evaluate a standardized endoscopic treatment protocol in a large cohort of patients with SPS.

Methods.—We followed a cohort of patients with SPS who received annual endoscopic surveillance at the Academic Medical Centre in Amsterdam, The Netherlands from January 2007 through December 2012. All patients underwent clearing colonoscopy with removal of all polyps ≥3 mm. After clearance, subsequent follow-up colonoscopies were scheduled annually. The primary outcomes measure was the incidence of CRC and polyps. Secondary outcomes were the incidence of complications and the rate of preventive surgery.

Results.—Successful endoscopic clearance of all polyps ≥3 mm was achieved in 41 of 50 (82%) patients. During subsequent annual surveillance, with a median follow-up time of 3.1 years (interquartile range, 1.5–4.3 years), CRC was not detected. The cumulative risks of detecting CRC, advanced adenomas, or large (≥10 mm) serrated polyps after 3 surveillance colonoscopies were 0%, 9%, 34%, respectively. Twelve patients (24%) were referred for preventive surgery; 9 at initial colonoscopy and 3 during surveillance. Perforations or severe bleeding did not occur.

Conclusions.—Annual surveillance with complete removal of all polyps ≥3 mm with timely referral of selected high-risk patients for prophylactic surgery prevents development of CRC in SPS patients without significant morbidity. Considering the substantial risk of polyp recurrence, close endoscopic surveillance in SPS seems warranted. www.trialregister.nl ID NTR2757.

▶ Serrated polyps (SPs) are a somewhat new pathological designation and are frequently diagnosed during screening and surveillance colonoscopy. The diagnosis of serrated polyposis syndrome (SPS) requires one of the following:

- SPs proximal to sigmoid with at least 2 > 10 mm.
- Any SP in a patient with a first-degree relative with SPS.

- > 20 SPs anywhere in the colon.

This disorder is not rare, occurring in somewhere between 1:150 and 1:300 colonoscopies. Some experts have suggested yearly surveillance for patients with SPS.

The data from this study emphasize the challenging nature of these patients. Eighteen percent of SPS patients were diagnosed with cancer at the index colonoscopy, and 11% had so many SPs that they were referred for colectomy before entering the surveillance phase of the study. Yearly colonoscopy in that group prevented the development of cancer, but large numbers of polyps continued to appear and require resection, some of which had advanced pathology. Also more than half of patients had large polyps at either index or follow-up colonoscopy that required endoscopic mucosal resection (EMR), a technique that is not available at all centers. This suggests that patients with SPS should be followed yearly in groups with expertise both in polyp detection and EMR.

K. R. DeVault, MD

Long-Term Colorectal-Cancer Mortality after Adenoma Removal

Løberg M, Kalager M, Holme Ø, et al (Univ of Oslo, Norway; Sørlandet Hosp Kristiansand, Norway; et al)
N Engl J Med 371:799-807, 2014

Background.—Although colonoscopic surveillance of patients after removal of adenomas is widely promoted, little is known about colorectal-cancer mortality among these patients.

Methods.—Using the linkage of the Cancer Registry and the Cause of Death Registry of Norway, we estimated colorectal-cancer mortality among patients who had undergone removal of colorectal adenomas during the period from 1993 through 2007. Patients were followed through 2011. We calculated standardized incidence-based mortality ratios (SMRs) using rates for the Norwegian population at large for comparison. Norwegian guidelines recommended colonoscopy after 10 years for patients with high-risk adenomas (adenomas with high-grade dysplasia, a villous component, or a size ≥10 mm) and after 5 years for patients with three or more adenomas; no surveillance was recommended for patients with low-risk adenomas. Polyp size and exact number were not available in the registry. We defined high-risk adenomas as multiple adenomas and adenomas with a villous component or high-grade dysplasia.

Results.—We identified 40,826 patients who had had colorectal adenomas removed. During a median follow-up of 7.7 years (maximum, 19.0), 1273 patients were given a diagnosis of colorectal cancer. A total of 398 deaths from colorectal cancer were expected and 383 were observed, for an SMR of 0.96 (95% confidence interval [CI], 0.87 to 1.06) among patients who had had adenomas removed. Colorectal-cancer mortality was increased among patients with high-risk adenomas (expected deaths, 209; observed deaths, 242; SMR, 1.16; 95% CI, 1.02 to 1.31), but it was reduced among patients with low-risk adenomas (expected deaths, 189; observed deaths, 141; SMR, 0.75; 95% CI, 0.63 to 0.88).

Conclusions.—After a median of 7.7 years of follow-up, colorectal-cancer mortality was lower among patients who had had low-risk adenomas removed and moderately higher among those who had had high-risk adenomas removed, as compared with the general population.

► Screening colonoscopy with removal of adenomas remains the gold standard method of colon cancer screening. New, less-invasive tests that use stool collections (fecal immunochemical testing or Cologuard) and radiological methods are being suggested as an alternative. Although effective in finding cancer and higher risk adenomas, they are not as effective in finding smaller, low-risk adenomas and do not allow resection of adenomas. This study followed patients for more than 7 years after adenoma removal to help answer questions in this area.

This study provides support for removing even low-risk adenomas as a cancer preventative measure because there was a 25% reduction in colon cancer compared with the population when low-risk adenomas were removed. Interestingly, patients with high-risk adenomas had a 16% increased risk of cancer. Although impossible to prove, this could be related to the long interval between screening and future surveillance colonoscopy in Norway (10 years for patients with high-risk adenoma, 5 years if there are 3 or more adenomas, and not at all if only low-risk adenomas), which is substantially different from the United States. A major weakness of the study is that most patients entered the study when colonoscopy-based screening was not practiced in Norway, so this is really not an asymptomatic, screening population.

This study provides support for the concept of a high-quality colonoscopy with all adenomas removed as an important screening and cancer preventative maneuver. We should not discard colonoscopy in favor of "less invasive" screening at this time. On the other hand, those less-invasive measures may indeed expand screening to those who would not submit to a colonoscopy.

K. R. DeVault, MD

Multitarget Stool DNA Testing for Colorectal-Cancer Screening

Imperiale TF, Ransohoff DF, Itzkowitz SH, et al (Indiana Univ School of Medicine, Indianapolis; Univ of North Carolina at Chapel Hill; Icahn School of Medicine at Mount Sinai, NY; et al)

N Engl J Med 370:1287-1297, 2014

Background.—An accurate, noninvasive test could improve the effectiveness of colorectal-cancer screening.

Methods.—We compared a noninvasive, multitarget stool DNA test with a fecal immunochemical test (FIT) in persons at average risk for colorectal cancer. The DNA test includes quantitative molecular assays for *KRAS* mutations, aberrant *NDRG4* and *BMP3* methylation, and β-actin, plus a hemoglobin immunoassay. Results were generated with the use of a logistic-regression algorithm, with values of 183 or more considered to be positive. FIT values of more than 100 ng of hemoglobin per milliliter of buffer were considered to be positive. Tests were processed independently of colonoscopic findings.

Results.—Of the 9989 participants who could be evaluated, 65 (0.7%) had colorectal cancer and 757 (7.6%) had advanced precancerous lesions (advanced adenomas or sessile serrated polyps measuring ≥1 cm in the greatest dimension) on colonoscopy. The sensitivity for detecting colorectal cancer was 92.3% with DNA testing and 73.8% with FIT ($P = 0.002$). The sensitivity for detecting advanced precancerous lesions was 42.4% with DNA testing and 23.8% with FIT ($P < 0.001$). The rate of detection of polyps with high-grade dysplasia was 69.2% with DNA testing and 46.2% with FIT ($P = 0.004$); the rates of detection of serrated sessile polyps measuring 1 cm or more were 42.4% and 5.1%, respectively ($P < 0.001$). Specificities with DNA testing and FIT were 86.6% and 94.9%, respectively, among participants with nonadvanced or negative findings ($P < 0.001$) and 89.8% and 96.4%, respectively, among those with negative results on colonoscopy ($P < 0.001$). The numbers of persons who would need to be screened to detect one cancer were 154 with colonoscopy, 166 with DNA testing, and 208 with FIT.

Conclusions.—In asymptomatic persons at average risk for colorectal cancer, multitarget stool DNA testing detected significantly more cancers than did FIT but had more false positive results. (Funded by Exact Sciences; ClinicalTrials.gov number, NCT01397747.)

▶ A new test for colon cancer screening (Cologuard) was recently approved and marketed in the United States. That approval was based on studies like the one cited here. The sensitivity for detecting colon cancer with this noninvasive, stool-based test was 92.3% and for detecting polyps with high-grade dysplasia was 69.2%. The false-positive rate was between 10% and 15%. It was more sensitive, yet less specific than an older, albeit much less expensive fecal test (fecal immunochemical test-FIT).

Where should testing of this type fall in our battle against colorectal cancer? It is clear that fecal testing is a viable option for patients who do not wish to have direct screening with colonoscopy. However, the patient should agree that if DNA or FIT testing results are positive, they would then undergo a colonoscopy to find the lesion responsible. DNA testing also is not nearly as effective in finding polyps. Ongoing studies are looking at repeating the test every 3 years over a 9-year period to evaluate its efficacy in preventing cancer despite not finding all or perhaps even most polyps. One major concern facing the gastroenterology community is our response to a patient with a positive DNA test result and a negative colonoscopy finding. DNA testing has a substantial false-positive rate, and colonoscopy has a small but not inconsequential false-negative rate leading many to believe that the numbers in this population will be substantial. Future research will determine whether that patient should have additional DNA tests, early follow-up colonoscopy, or perhaps both. For now, I still consider colonoscopy the gold standard, but DNA testing may well be an option for those who decline colonoscopy, assuming the patient understands the risks and benefits of this approach and is willing to follow-up on a positive test.

K. R. DeVault, MD

54 Pancreas

American Gastroenterological Association Institute Guideline on the Diagnosis and Management of Asymptomatic Neoplastic Pancreatic Cysts

Vege SS, Ziring B, Jain R, et al (Mayo Clinic, Rochester, MN; Thomas Jefferson Univ, Philadelphia, PA; Texas Digestive Disease Consultants, Dallas; et al)
Gastroenterology 148:819-822, 2015

This article has an accompanying continuing medical education activity on page e12.

Learning Objective.—At the conclusion of this exercise, the learner will understand the approach to counseling patients regarding the optimal method and frequency of radiologic imaging, indications for invasive tests like endoscopic ultrasonography (EUS) and surgery, select patients for follow-up after surgery, decide the duration of such follow-up, and decide when to stop surveillance for those with and without surgery.

▶ Asymptomatic pancreatic cysts are a common finding on cross-sectional imaging.[1] These cysts present a management challenge because they are usually benign but can, in some circumstances, be or become malignant. A new guideline has been published addressing this problem. Selected, important recommendations include:

1. Patients must have a clear understanding of the risk and benefits of each approach to a cyst. Patients who are not surgical candidates likely should not enter a surveillance program.
2. Cysts less than 3 cm without a solid component or dilated pancreatic duct should have MRI in 1 year, then if stable, every 2 years for a total of 5 years.
3. Cysts with 2 high-risk features (solid component, increasing size, size > 3 cm) should have endoscopic ultrasound with fine-needle aspiration (FNA). If the FNA is nonconcerning, then the patient can enter an MRI surveillance program
4. Cysts changing in appearance on MRI should have FNA.
5. Surveillance can be discontinued if the cyst is stable for 5 years.
6. Surgery should be considered in patients with a solid component, dilated pancreatic duct, or with a concerning endoscopic ultrasound scan/FNA. Surgery should be limited to experienced centers.
7. If a benign cyst is resected, no radiologic follow-up is needed.

K. R. DeVault, MD

Reference

1. Scheiman JM, Hwang JH, Moayyedi P. American gastroenterological association technical review on the diagnosis and management of asymptomatic neoplastic pancreatic cysts. *Gastroenterology.* 2015;148:824-848.e22.

New Diagnosis of Chronic Pancreatitis: Risk of Missing an Underlying Pancreatic Cancer

Munigala S, Kanwal F, Xian H, et al (Saint Louis Univ School of Medicine, MO; Veterans Affairs St Louis Health Care System, MO)
Am J Gastroenterol 109:1824-1830, 2014

Objectives.—Patients with pancreatic cancer (PaCa) sometimes present with symptoms suggestive of chronic pancreatitis (CP). We evaluated the prevalence of undiagnosed PaCa in patients with new CP diagnosis.

Methods.—This is a retrospective study with data from Veterans Health Administration national medical care data sets from fiscal year 1998–2007. A 3-year washout period was used to identify patients with preexisting PaCa and preexisting CP diagnosis.

Results.—Among 471,992 veterans included, 917 (0.19%) had PaCa, 2,557 (0.54%) had a preexisting CP, and 2,175 (0.46%) had a new diagnosis of CP. PaCa was diagnosed ≤2 years following CP diagnosis in 44 patients, comprising 4.80% of patients with PaCa. Following a new diagnosis of CP, the risk of PaCa diagnosis was most marked in the first year (incidence 18.04 per 1,000 person-years (py), relative risk (RR) 63.43) and became similar to risk in patients with preexisting CP in the third year. The first-year incidence of PaCa was 7.33/1,000 py in the fifth decade and reached 36.91/1,000 py after seventh decade of life. Time to PaCa diagnosis following a CP diagnosis was ≤60 days in 14 patients, 3–12 months in 25 patients, and 13–24 months in 5 patients.

Conclusions.—Approximately 5% of patients with PaCa are initially misdiagnosed as CP, and in two-thirds of these patients the cancer diagnosis is delayed by >2 months. PaCa should reliably be excluded before making a new CP diagnosis in patients who are >40 years old, especially in those without heavy smoking or alcohol history.

▶ Pancreatic cancer (PaCa) is a fairly common malignancy with a very poor prognosis unless diagnosed very early. PaCa often presents with pain and weight loss even when the lesions are small and contained. A problem is that PaCa can coexist with chronic pancreatitis (CP), which might delay the diagnosis. This report used a large Veterans Affairs database to determine how often this happened. They concluded that approximately 5% of patients with PaCa are initially misdiagnosed at the time of CP diagnosis, resulting in a substantial delay in diagnosis. They suggest that this is a particular problem in patients older than 40 years without other risk factors for CP. This risk continued to increase with each decade of life.

How aggressive should one be in searching for PaCa in a patient with CP? It is clear that we should perform advanced imaging in the subgroup without strong risk factors for CP. What is less clear is when that screening should occur, but early is obviously better given the need for early diagnosis and this study's finding of most cancers being diagnosed in the first year after diagnosis of CP. It is possible the PaCa might be missed if the pancreas is inflamed (acute pancreatitis on top of CP), but probably that is a minority of cases. MRI or endoscopic ultrasound scan should then be used in many patients. These modalities not only screen for cancer but also allow a more firm diagnosis of CP in patients with equivocal findings.

K. R. DeVault, MD

55 Liver

Nonalcoholic Steatohepatitis Is the Second Leading Etiology of Liver Disease Among Adults Awaiting Liver Transplantation in the United States

Wong RJ, Aguilar M, Cheung R, et al (Highland Hosp Campus, Oakland, CA; Stanford Univ School of Medicine, CA; et al)

Gastroenterology 148:547-555, 2015

Background & Aims.—Nonalcoholic steatohepatitis (NASH) has been predicted to become the leading indication for liver transplantation (LT) in the United States. However, few studies have evaluated changes in the etiology of liver diseases among patients awaiting LT, and none have focused on the effects of NASH on liver transplant waitlists in the United States.

Methods.—We collected data from the United Network for Organ Sharing and Organ Procurement and Transplantation Network registry from 2004 through 2013, on liver transplant waitlist registrants with hepatitis C virus (HCV) infection, NASH, alcoholic liver disease (ALD), or a combination of HCV infection and ALD. We compared differences in survival within 90 days of registration (90-day survival) and probability of LT among patients with different diseases using Kaplan-Meier and multivariate logistic regression models.

Results.—Between 2004 and 2013, new waitlist registrants with NASH increased by 170% (from 804 to 2174), with ALD increased by 45% (from 1400 to 2024), and with HCV increased by 14% (from 2887 to 3291); registrants with HCV and ALD decreased by 9% (from 880 to 803). In 2013, NASH became the second-leading disease among liver transplant waitlist registrants, after HCV. Patients with ALD had a significantly higher mean Model for End-Stage Liver Disease score at time of waitlist registration than other registrants. However, after multivariate adjustment, patients with ALD were less likely to die within 90 days when compared with patients with NASH (odds ratio [OR] = 0.77; 95% confidence interval [CI]: 0.67—0.89; $P < .001$); patients with HCV infection or HCV and ALD had similar odds for 90-day survival compared with NASH patients. Compared with patients with NASH, patients with HCV (OR = 1.45; 95% CI: 1.35—1.55; $P < .001$), ALD (OR = 1.15; 95% CI: 1.06—1.24; $P < .001$), or HCV and ALD (OR = 1.29; 95% CI: 1.18—1.42; $P < .001$) had higher odds for 90-day survival.

Conclusions.—Based on data from US adult LT databases, since 2004 the number of adults with NASH awaiting LTs has almost tripled. However, patients with NASH are less likely to undergo LT and less likely to survive for 90 days on the waitlist than patients with HCV, ALD, or HCV and ALD.

▶ Common causes of liver disease leading to transplantation include viral infections and alcohol use, among many others. Diseases of the liver caused by fat infiltration have become more common. This article shows that nonalcoholic steatohepatitis (NASH) is now the second leading cause of being placed on a transplant waiting list in the United States (after hepatitis C). The proportion of patients on waiting lists with this indication increased 170% between 2004 and 2013, while there was a modest (14%) increase in patients with hepatitis C and a decrease of 9% in those with alcohol liver disease. Patients with NASH were more likely to die on the waiting list and also had a poorer post-transplant survival.

Obesity and its complications including NASH are major public health concerns leading to vascular disease, increased risk of malignancy, and other problems. Liver disease is an ever-increasing problem in these patients. This article confirms this increase, and many experts believe NASH will become the most common cause of chronic liver disease in the future. It is not clear why these patients were less likely to be transplanted and more likely to do poorly after transplant. One would assume it is related to the multiple organs affected by obesity. It is important to remember that NASH also increases the risk of hepatocellular carcinoma and that patients need to be in appropriate screening programs once they have been diagnosed with fibrosis or cirrhosis. This is a yet another reason that public health measures directed at the control of obesity need to be intensified.

K. R. DeVault, MD

ACG Clinical Guideline: The Diagnosis and Management of Focal Liver Lesions

Marrero JA, on behalf of the Practice Parameters Committee of the American College of Gastroenterology (Univ of Texas at Southwestern, Dallas; et al)

Am J Gastroenterol 109:1328-1347, 2014

Focal liver lesions (FLL) have been a common reason for consultation faced by gastroenterologists and hepatologists. The increasing and widespread use of imaging studies has led to an increase in detection of incidental FLL. It is important to consider not only malignant liver lesions, but also benign solid and cystic liver lesions such as hemangioma, focal nodular hyperplasia, hepatocellular adenoma, and hepatic cysts, in the differential diagnosis. In this ACG practice guideline, the authors provide an evidence-based approach to the diagnosis and management of FLL.

▶ The number of patients with a focal liver image identified is ever expanding with the widespread use of cross-sectional and ultrasound imaging. Some of these patients have gastrointestinal complaints, whereas others will be asymptomatic with the abnormality identified as part of a scan for other issues. I highlight here a few of the concepts and guidelines:

1. When a lesion is noted in a cirrhotic liver, it is a hepatocellular carcinoma (HCC) until proven otherwise. The diagnosis can be confirmed with appropriate MRI or triple-phase CT.
2. MRI or CT can usually diagnose cholangiocarcinoma.
3. Most patients with hepatocellular adenoma can also be diagnosed with imaging. Hormone supplements and steroids should be avoided in patients with adenomas. Large (> 5 cm) or symptomatic lesions should be resected.
4. Hemangiomas, hepatic cysts, and focal nodular hyperplasia should also be diagnosed with imaging and require no specific intervention unless they are producing discomfort.
5. Nodular regenerative hyperplasia is suggested by imaging but should be confirmed with biopsy. Once confirmed, they require no specific intervention unless they are producing discomfort.
6. Bilary cystadenoma and cystadenocarcinoma require careful imaging and, if confirmed, surgical excision by an experienced team.
7. The management of polycystic liver disease is based on cyst burden and can vary from observation to transplantation.
8. Hydatid cysts are best diagnosed with MRI. Surgery or percutaneous approaches are reasonable followed by antihelminthic therapy.

Overall, these guidelines highlight the accuracy of modern imaging, which has decreased the need for biopsy of low-risk lesions in many situations. On the other hand, it supports an aggressive approach for possible and proven HCC.

K. R. DeVault, MD

ABT-450, Ritonavir, Ombitasvir, and Dasabuvir Achieves 97% and 100% Sustained Virologic Response With or Without Ribavirin in Treatment-Experienced Patients With HCV Genotype 1b Infection

Andreone P, Colombo MG, Enejosa JV, et al (Univ of Bologna, Italy; Univ of Milan, Italy; AbbVie, Inc, North Chicago, IL; et al)

Gastroenterology 147:359-365.e1, 2014

Background & Aims.—The interferon-free regimen of ABT- 450 (a protease inhibitor), ritonavir, ombitasvir (an NS5A inhibitor), dasabuvir (a non-nucleoside polymerase inhibitor), and ribavirin has shown efficacy in patients with hepatitis C virus (HCV) genotype 1b infection—the most prevalent subgenotype worldwide. We evaluated whether ribavirin is necessary for ABT-450, ritonavir, ombitasvir, and dasabuvir to produce high rates of sustained virologic response (SVR) in these patients.

Methods.—We performed a multicenter, open-label, phase 3 trial of 179 patients with HCV genotype 1b infection, without cirrhosis, previously treated with peginterferon and ribavirin. Patients were assigned randomly

(1:1) to groups given ABT-450, ritonavir, ombitasvir, and dasabuvir, with ribavirin (group 1) or without (group 2) for 12 weeks. The primary end point was SVR 12 weeks after treatment (SVR12). We assessed the noninferiority of this regimen to the rate of response reported (64%) for a similar population treated with telaprevir, peginterferon, and ribavirin.

Results.—Groups 1 and 2 each had high rates of SVR12, which were noninferior to the reported rate of response to the combination of telaprevir, peginterferon, and ribavirin (group 1: 96.6%; 95% confidence interval, 92.8%–100%; and group 2: 100%; 95% confidence interval, 95.9%–100%). The rate of response in group 2 was noninferior to that of group 1. No virologic failure occurred during the study. Two patients (1.1%) discontinued the study owing to adverse events, both in group 1. The most common adverse events in groups 1 and 2 were fatigue (31.9% vs 15.8%) and headache (24.2% vs 23.2%), respectively. Decreases in hemoglobin level to less than the lower limit of normal were more frequent in group 1 (42.0% vs 5.5% in group 2; $P < .001$), although only 2 patients had hemoglobin levels less than 10 g/dL.

Conclusions.—The interferon-free regimen of ABT-450, ritonavir, ombitasvir, and dasabuvir, with or without ribavirin, produces a high rate of SVR12 in treatment-experienced patients with HCV genotype 1b infection. Both regimens are well tolerated, as shown by the low rate of discontinuations and generally mild adverse events. ClinicalTrials.gov number: NCT01674725.

▶ The advent of new oral antiviral agents has revolutionized the treatment of hepatitis C. Interferon, with its side effects and relatively poor efficacy, is rapidly fading into the history of hepatitis therapy. Many of the current regimens include ribavirin, which has side effects of its own, but newer combinations without ribavirin are under study. This study used a combination of 4 antiviral agents with and without ribavirin and found an outstanding efficacy regardless of the inclusion of ribavirin. Patients in this study had previously failed an interferon treatment and were all genotype 1b.

This and many other studies continue to prove the efficacy of these new agents. These outstanding results in previously treated patients reemphasize the hope of cure in all patients with hepatitis C virus (HCV) including this previously challenging group. There are some differences in efficacy depending on genotype, but all of the common, Western subtypes seem to respond to this type of treatment. The major downside remains cost with many regimens costing well over US $100 000. Any patient with active HCV infection and the ability to afford these agents should be treated. Clearance of HCV may still be cost-effective given the long-term expense of caring for a patient with liver failure, up to and including transplantation.

K. R. DeVault, MD

56 Obesity

Quantitative Gastrointestinal and Psychological Traits Associated With Obesity and Response to Weight-Loss Therapy

Acosta A, Camilleri M, Shin A, et al (Mayo Clinic College of Medicine, Rochester, MN)

Gastroenterology 148:537-546, 2015

Background & Aims.—Weight loss after pharmacotherapy varies greatly. We aimed to examine associations of quantitative gastrointestinal and psychological traits with obesity, and to validate the ability of these traits to predict responses of obese individuals to pharmacotherapy.

Methods.—In a prospective study, we measured gastric emptying of solids and liquids, fasting and postprandial gastric volume, satiation by nutrient drink test (volume to fullness and maximal tolerated volume), satiety after an ad libitum buffet meal, gastrointestinal hormones, and psychological traits in 328 normal-weight, overweight, or obese adults. We also analyzed data from 181 previously studied adults to assess associations betwecen a subset of traits with body mass index and waist circumference. Latent dimensions associated with overweight or obesity were appraised by principal component analyses. We performed a proof of concept, placebo-controlled trial of extended-release phentermine and topiramate in 24 patients to validate associations between quantitative traits and response to weight-loss therapy.

Results.—In the prospective study, obesity was associated with fasting gastric volume ($P = .03$), accelerated gastric emptying ($P < .001$ for solids and $P = .011$ for liquids), lower postprandial levels of peptide tyrosine tyrosine ($P = .003$), and higher postprandial levels of glucagon-like peptide 1 ($P < .001$). In a combined analysis of data from all studies, obesity was associated with higher volume to fullness (n = 509; $P = .038$) and satiety with abnormal waist circumference (n = 271; $P = .016$). Principal component analysis identified latent dimensions that accounted for approximately 81% of the variation among overweight and obese subjects, including satiety or satiation (21%), gastric motility (14%), psychological factors (13%), and gastric sensorimotor factors (11%). The combination of phentermine and topiramate caused significant weight loss, slowed gastric emptying, and decreased calorie intake; weight loss in response to phentermine and topiramate was significantly associated with calorie intake at the prior satiety test.

Conclusions.—Quantitative traits are associated with high body mass index; they can distinguish obesity phenotypes and, in a proof of concept clinical trial, predicted response to pharmacotherapy for obesity. ClinicalTrials.gov Number: NCT01834404.

▶ Obesity is a major public health challenge. The responses of patients to most methods of weight control are disappointing at best. A high-dose, extended-release combination of phentermine and topiramate (ER-PT) was recently found to produce a mean weight loss of almost 10%, but there was a huge variability in the response to that agent. This study attempted to define physiologic and psychological traits that might predict the response to these and perhaps other medications. Some of the findings are predictable but worthy of discussion. For example, it took larger volumes of a standardized nutrition drink to reach satiety in obese patients, which makes sense, but could be used as a marked for future studies. These patients also ate more at a buffet meal prior to satiety. Interestingly, rapid gastric emptying was also more common in obese patients. Finally, the obese patients had increased resting gastric volume. Psychological traits that were increased in obesity included anxiety, depression, and lower body image satisfaction. The response to ER-PT was not reliably predicted by the pretrial trails.

Where does this leave us? First, we have no clear guidance on who might or might not benefit from this medication-based therapy. However, the study clearly shows gastric motor and sensory dysfunction in the obese, which certainly could lead to more targeted therapies. The interplay between psychological and physiologic issues is once again confirmed and is deserving of continued investigation.

K. R. DeVault, MD

57 Miscellaneous

Appropriate and timely antimicrobial therapy in cirrhotic patients with spontaneous bacterial peritonitis-associated septic shock: a retrospective cohort study

Karvellas CJ, For the Cooperative Antimicrobial Therapy of Septic Shock (CATSS) Database Research Group (Univ of Alberta, Edmonton, Canada; et al)

Aliment Pharmacol Ther 41:747-757, 2015

Background.—Spontaneous bacterial peritonitis (SBP)-associated septic shock carries significant mortality in cirrhosis.

Aim.—To determine whether practice-related aspects of antimicrobial therapy contribute to high mortality.

Methods.—Retrospective cohort study of all ($n = 126$) cirrhotics with spontaneous bacterial peritonitis (neutrophil count >250 or positive ascitic culture)-associated septic shock (1996–2011) from an international, multicenter database. Appropriate antimicrobial therapy implied either *in vitro* activity against a subsequently isolated pathogen (culture positive) or empiric management consistent with broadly accepted norms (culture negative).

Results.—Overall hospital mortality was 81.8%. Comparing survivors ($n = 23$) with non-survivors ($n = 103$), survivors had lower Acute Physiology and Chronic Health Evaluation (APACHEII) (mean ± s.d.; 22 ± 7 vs. 32 ± 8) and model for end-stage liver disease (MELD) (24 ± 9 vs. 34 ± 11) scores and serum lactate on admission (4.9 ± 3.1 vs. 8.9 ± 5.3), $P < 0.001$ for all. Survivors were less likely to receive inappropriate initial antimicrobial therapy (0% vs. 25%, $P = 0.013$) and received appropriate antimicrobial therapy earlier [median 1.8 (1.1–5.2) vs. 9.5 (3.9–14.3) h, $P < 0.001$]. After adjusting for covariates, APACHEII [OR, odds ratio 1.45 (1.04–2.02) per 1 unit increment, $P = 0.03$], lactate [OR 2.34 (1.04–5.29) per unit increment, $P = 0.04$] and time delay to appropriate antimicrobials [OR 1.86 (1.10–3.14) per hour increment, $P = 0.02$] were significantly associated with increased mortality.

Conclusions.—Cirrhotic patients with septic shock secondary to spontaneous bacterial peritonitis have high mortality (>80%). Each hour of delay in appropriate antimicrobial therapy was associated with a 1.86 times increased hospital mortality. Admission APACHEII and serum lactate also significantly impacted hospital mortality. Earlier initiation of appropriate antimicrobial therapy could substantially improve outcome.

▶ Spontaneous bacterial peritonitis (SBP) is a common and severe complication of chronic liver disease with a high morbidity and substantial mortality. This study looked at the most severe SBP patients—those presenting with septic shock. Mortality rate was greater than 80%. Importantly, for each hour of delayed antibiotic therapy, there was a 1.86-fold increase in hospital mortality rate.

This important report underscores several points in caring for patients with liver disease. The increased risk of all infections with chronic liver disease should be respected, particularly in those with ascites. Because time delay was an important marker of mortality in this study, one cannot afford to wait for confirmation of infection in patients with significant infection; early antibiotic coverage is the key. Patients should have immediate blood cultures and paracentesis for both cell counts and cultures. Antibiotics should be initiated while those results are pending. The report suggests some common organisms, but the initial empiric coverage may need to vary depending on the location and history of each individual patient, but the bottom line is broader is better!

K. R. DeVault, MD

Proton Pump Inhibitor Usage and the Risk of Myocardial Infarction in the General Population

Shah NH, LePendu P, Bauer-Mehren A, et al (Stanford Univ, CA; et al)

PLoS One 10:e0124653, 2015

Background and Aims.—Proton pump inhibitors (PPIs) have been associated with adverse clinical outcomes amongst clopidogrel users after an acute coronary syndrome. Recent pre-clinical results suggest that this risk might extend to subjects without any prior history of cardiovascular disease. We explore this potential risk in the general population via data-mining approaches.

Methods.—Using a novel approach for mining clinical data for pharmacovigilance, we queried over 16 million clinical documents on 2.9 million individuals to examine whether PPI usage was associated with cardiovascular risk in the general population.

Results.—In multiple data sources, we found gastroesophageal reflux disease (GERD) patients exposed to PPIs to have a 1.16 fold increased association (95% CI 1.09–1.24) with myocardial infarction (MI). Survival analysis in a prospective cohort found a two-fold (HR = 2.00; 95% CI 1.07–3.78; $P = 0.031$) increase in association with cardiovascular mortality. We found that this association exists regardless of clopidogrel use. We also found that H_2 blockers, an alternate treatment for GERD, were not associated with increased cardiovascular risk; had they been in place, such pharmacovigilance algorithms could have flagged this risk as early as the year 2000.

Conclusions.—Consistent with our pre-clinical findings that PPIs may adversely impact vascular function, our data-mining study supports the association of PPI exposure with risk for MI in the general population. These data provide an example of how a combination of experimental studies and data-mining approaches can be applied to prioritize drug safety signals for further investigation.

▶ Proton pump inhibitors (PPIs) are a widely used class of drugs designed to control gastric acid production and treat disorders such as gastroesophageal reflux disease (GERD). They have been felt to be relatively safe, and most are available without prescription. That having been said, reported adverse effects have included an increased risk of gastrointestinal and pulmonary infections as well as interactions with several medications. This large database study suggested an increase in myocardial infarction (MI) independent of the proposed effect on clopidogrel. The methods of the study are important to understand. The authors mined 2 huge databases of more than 3 million patients and then compared these data to yet one-third population. There was little effort to stratify based on other cofactors because the authors feel those should not be significant in this huge data set. Although there was an increased risk of MI (16%), this only translated into a roughly 1:4000 risk.

If the association is true, then why might this be? First, PPIs might actually change something biochemically that leads to MI, and the authors outline a possible explanation, although there are many conflicting data on this issue. Second, the data set of PPI takers could be more ill than the controls or H2-blocker patients, which is not only possible but probable. Finally, taking a PPI might change something else. For example, having less postprandial heartburn might cause patients to eat more or perhaps eat more unhealthy foods that lead to an increased risk of MI. The bottom line is that patients who do not really need a PPI (or any other drug) should not take them. At this point, patients who need PPI can continue to take them but should also pay attention to diet, exercise, and other activities that may alter their risk of vascular disease.

K. R. DeVault, MD

The Risks of Thromboembolism Vs. Recurrent Gastrointestinal Bleeding after Interruption of Systemic Anticoagulation in Hospitalized Inpatients With Gastrointestinal Bleeding: A Prospective Study

Sengupta N, Feuerstein JD, Patwardhan VR, et al (Harvard Med School, Boston, MA)

Am J Gastroenterol 110:328-335, 2015

Objectives.—Anticoagulants carry a significant risk of gastrointestinal bleeding (GIB). Data regarding the safety of anticoagulation continuation/cessation after GIB are limited. We sought to determine the safety and risk of continuation of anticoagulation after GIB.

Methods.—We conducted a prospective observational cohort study on consecutive patients admitted to the hospital who had GIB while on systemic anticoagulation. Patients were classified into two groups at hospital discharge after GIB: those who resumed anticoagulation and those who had anticoagulation discontinued. Patients in both groups were contacted by phone 90 days after discharge to determine the following outcomes: (i) thromboembolic events, (ii) hospital readmissions related to GIB, and (iii) mortality. Univariate and multivariate Cox proportional hazards were used to determine factors associated with thrombotic events, rebleeding, and death.

Results.—We identified 197 patients who developed GIB while on systemic anticoagulation ($n = 145$, 74% on warfarin). Following index GIB, anticoagulation was discontinued in 76 patients (39%) at discharge. In-hospital transfusion requirements, need for intensive care unit care, and etiology of GIB were similar between the two groups. During the follow-up period, 7 (4%) patients suffered a thrombotic event and 27 (14%) patients were readmitted for GIB. Anticoagulation continuation was independently associated on multivariate regression with a lower risk of major thrombotic episodes within 90 days (hazard ratio (HR) = 0.121, 95% confidence interval (CI) = 0.006–0.812, $P = 0.03$). Patients with any malignancy at time of GIB had an increased risk of thromboembolism in follow-up (HR = 6.1, 95% CI = 1.18–28.3, $P = 0.03$). Anticoagulation continuation at discharge was not significantly associated with an increased risk of recurrent GIB at 90 days (HR = 2.17, 95% CI = 0.861–6.67, $P = 0.10$) or death within 90 days (HR = 0.632, 95% CI = 0.216–1.89, $P = 0.40$).

Conclusions.—Restarting anticoagulation at discharge after GIB was associated with fewer thromboembolic events without a significantly increased risk of recurrent GIB at 90 days. The benefits of continuing anticoagulation at discharge may outweigh the risks of recurrent GIB.

▶ Management of anticoagulation medications after an episode of gastrointestinal bleeding is a common and challenging situation. Once the patient is stabilized, the question of when to restart anticoagulation as medication is often unclear. This study provides some important information. The bottom line is that restarting the medications at discharge resulted in fewer thromboembolic events without an increase in rebleeding. The events that occurred include deep venous thrombi, strokes, and a pulmonary embolus. No one died from either a recurrent gastrointestinal (GI) bleed or a thrombotic event. Thrombotic events were particularly common in patients with active malignancy.

In the past, taking patients with GI bleeding off anticoagulants and keeping them off for a period of time has been standard of care. This and other studies have emphasized the risk of that approach. Stroke and other events may produce irreversible morbidity and are likely more risky than a recurrent bleeding event; thus, it is reasonable to recommend an early reinstitution of these medications whenever possible.

K. R. DeVault, MD

PART EIGHT

ENDOCRINOLOGY, DIABETES, AND METABOLISM

DEREK LeROITH, MD, PhD

Introduction

This year has seen significant accomplishments in innovation, clinical trials, and the introduction of new and improved medications. Advances have been particularly notable in the realm of metabolism, i.e., obesity and diabetes.

The bionic pancreas holds promise for Type 1 diabetic patients. In the case of obesity there are now multiple oral tablets for appetite suppression and one injectable.

This compilation of articles and commentaries spans epidemiology, therapeutics, aspects of complications, and some basic science, though most are clinical articles that hopefully will be of value to the practicing health care provider.

Derek LeRoith, MD, PhD

58 Diabetes Mellitus

Preserved β-Cell Function in Type 1 Diabetes by Mesenchymal Stromal Cells

Carlsson P-O, Schwarcz E, Korsgren O, et al (Uppsala Univ, Sweden; Örebro Univ Hosp, Sweden; et al)

Diabetes 64:587-592, 2015

The retention of endogenous insulin secretion in type 1 diabetes is an attractive clinical goal, which opens possibilities for long-term restoration of glucose metabolism. Mesenchymal stromal cells (MSCs) constitute, based on animal studies, a promising interventional strategy for the disease. This prospective clinical study describes the translation of this cellular intervention strategy to patients with recent-onset type 1 diabetes. Twenty adult patients with newly diagnosed type 1 diabetes were enrolled and randomized to MSC treatment or to the control group. Residual β-cell function was analyzed as C-peptide concentrations in blood in response to a mixed-meal tolerance test (MMTT) at 1-year follow-up. In contrast to the patients in the control arm, who showed loss in both C-peptide peak values and C-peptide when calculated as area under the curve during the 1st year, these responses were preserved or even increased in the MSC-treated patients. Importantly, no side effects of MSC treatment were observed. We conclude that autologous MSC treatment in new-onset type 1 diabetes constitutes a safe and promising strategy to intervene in disease progression and preserve β-cell function.

▶ Autologous intravenous administration of mesenchymal stem cells, derived from patients' bone marrow and grown in culture, preserved the beta-cell function in 10 type 1 diabetics compared with type 1 controls patients as measured by a mixed meal tolerance test. In this randomized trial, beta-cell function was measured using C-peptide measurements and demonstrated that as opposed to the deterioration of beta-cell function in the control group of 10 type 1 diabetics, the treated group has preservation of beta-cell function. Mesenchymal stem cell autologous administration has been used successfully in other disorders, and in animal models of type 1 diabetes has been shown to home specifically to the damaged pancreatic islets. Thus, in addition to their important systemic immunomodulatory effects they may have local effects. Interestingly, the 10 treated patients did not demonstrate any noticeable side effects.

D. LeRoith, MD

Assessment of β-Cell Mass and α- and β-Cell Survival and Function by Arginine Stimulation in Human Autologous Islet Recipients

Robertson RP, Bogachus LD, Oseid E, et al (Univ of Washington, Seattle; Pacific Northwest Diabetes Research Inst, Seattle, WA; et al)

Diabetes 64:565-572, 2015

We used intravenous arginine with measurements of insulin, C-peptide, and glucagon to examine β-cell and α-cell survival and function in a group of 10 chronic pancreatitis recipients 1–8 years after total pancreatectomy and autoislet transplantation. Insulin and C-peptide responses correlated robustly with the number of islets transplanted (correlation coefficients range 0.81–0.91; $P < 0.01–0.001$). Since a wide range of islets were transplanted, we normalized the insulin and C-peptide responses to the number of islets transplanted in each recipient for comparison with responses in normal subjects. No significant differences were observed in terms of magnitude and timing of hormone release in the two groups. Three recipients had a portion of the autoislets placed within their peritoneal cavities, which appeared to be functioning normally up to 7 years posttransplant. Glucagon responses to arginine were normally timed and normally suppressed by intravenous glucose infusion. These findings indicate that arginine stimulation testing may be a means of assessing the numbers of native islets available in autologous islet transplant candidates and is a means of following posttransplant α- and β-cell function and survival.

▶ Autologous islet cell transplantation is used to avoid the diabetes that follows total pancreatectomy for chronic, unrelenting pain, and narcotic dependence for patients with chronic pancreatitis. An important question is the status of functional alpha and beta cells years after the procedure. Although blood glucose and HbA_{1c} are useful measures of continued survival of the beta cells, the authors used a more precise test to determine alpha- and beta-cell function. In 10 patients who had autotransplanted islets for up to 8 years, they determined functional capability of the beta and alphas cells by measuring insulin, C-peptide, and glucagon after an intravenous injection of arginine. There was a direct relationship with the responses and the number of transplanted islets as well as with the functionality at various time points after transplantation. Thus, the intravenous arginine test can be useful in following survival and function of islets under these circumstances in patients with autologous islet transplantation.

D. LeRoith, MD

Impact of Islet Autoimmunity on the Progressive β-cell Functional Decline in Type 2 Diabetes

Brooks-Worrell BM, Boyko EJ, Palmer JP, et al (Univ of Washington, Seattle)

Diabetes Care 37:3286-3293, 2014

Objective.—Cross-sectional studies have suggested that islet autoimmunity may be more prevalent in type 2 diabetes (T2D) than previously appreciated and may contribute to the progressive decline in β-cell function. In this study, we longitudinally evaluated the effect of islet autoimmune development on the progressive β-cell dysfunction in T2D patients.

Research Design and Methods.—Twenty-three T2D patients negative for islet autoantibodies (GAD antibody and insulinoma-associated protein 2) and islet-specific T cells were evaluated prospectively for up to 36 months. We investigated the percentage of patients who developed islet autoantibodies (Ab+) and/or islet-reactive T cells (T+) and the effect of the islet autoimmunity on fasting and glucagon-stimulated C-peptide responses. We defined positive islet autoimmunity as Ab+ and/or T+ for at least two study visits.

Results.—Of the 23 patients, 6 (26%) remained negative for islet autoimmunity (Ab−T−), 14 (61%) developed Ab+ and/or T+, and 3 (13%) were unclassifiable because they developed islet autoimmunity at only one study visit. Islet Ab+ was observed to be less stable than islet-specific T-cell responses. Development of islet autoimmunity was significantly associated with a more rapid decline in fasting ($P < 0.0001$) and glucagon-stimulated ($P < 0.05$) C-peptide responses.

Conclusions.—These pilot data suggest that the development of islet autoimmunity in T2D is associated with a significantly more rapid β-cell functional decline.

▶ Islet cell autoimmunity is a sine qua non type 1 diabetes. However, some patients with classic type 2 diabetes may develop these autoantibodies. In this study, 23 patients with established type 2 diabetes and autoantibody negative were followed for up to 36 months. During this time frame, islet autoantibodies and/or islet-reactive T cells became positive in a significant number of patients. Interestingly, the presence of autoimmunity was associated with a more rapid deterioration of beta-cell function as measured by fasting and glucagon-stimulated C-peptide responses. The authors conclude that the presence of the autoimmunity and islet cell decline suggests some degree of islet autoimmune damage.

D. LeRoith, MD

PD-L1—Driven Tolerance Protects Neurogenin3-Induced Islet Neogenesis to Reverse Established Type 1 Diabetes in NOD Mice

Li R, Lee J, Kim M-S, et al (Baylor College of Medicine, Houston, TX; et al)

Diabetes 64:529-540, 2015

A breakdown in self-tolerance underlies autoimmune destruction of β-cells and type 1 diabetes. A cure by restoring β-cell mass is limited by the availability of transplantable β-cells and the need for chronic immunosuppression. Evidence indicates that inhibiting costimulation through the PD-1/PD-L1 pathway is central to immune tolerance. We therefore tested whether induction of islet neogenesis in the liver, protected by PD-L1—driven tolerance, reverses diabetes in NOD mice. We demonstrated a robust induction of neo-islets in the liver of diabetic NOD mice by gene transfer of Neurogenin3, the islet-defining factor, along with betacellulin, an islet growth factor. These neo-islets expressed all the major pancreatic hormones and transcription factors. However, an enduring restoration of glucose-stimulated insulin secretion and euglycemia occurs only when tolerance is also induced by the targeted overexpression of PD-L1 in the neo-islets, which results in inhibition of proliferation and increased apoptosis of infiltrating $CD4^+$ T cells. Further analysis revealed an inhibition of cytokine production from lymphocytes isolated from the liver but not from the spleen of treated mice, indicating that treatment did not result in generalized immunosuppression. This treatment strategy leads to persistence of functional neo-islets that resist autoimmune destruction and consequently an enduring reversal of diabetes in NOD mice.

▶ Type 1 diabetes is characterized by loss of the beta cells, and replacement of sufficient numbers of islets is the Holy Grail of research in this area. To overcome the lack of supply of islets, investigators have studied neo-islet production by the liver using gene transfer of Neurogenin3, the islet-defining factor, along with betacellulin, an islet growth factor. Successful production of neo-islets was achieved as demonstrated by a reduction in blood glucose in diabetic mice; however, prevention of the autoimmune destruction required the overexpression of programmed death-L1 (PD-L1), thereby inducing local immune tolerance without affecting systemic immunity. Thus, these gene transfer experiments may bypass the lack of islets for transplantation in type 1 diabetes to effect a "cure" or significantly reduce the dependence on insulin injections.

D. LeRoith, MD

High Calorie Intake Is Associated With Worsening Insulin Resistance and β-Cell Function in Hispanic Women After Gestational Diabetes Mellitus

Chen Z, Watanabe RM, Stram DO, et al (Univ of Southern California, Los Angeles, CA; et al)

Diabetes Care 37:3294-3300, 2014

Objective.—To assess associations between dietary intake and rates of change in insulin resistance and β-cell function in Hispanic women with prior gestational diabetes mellitus (GDM).

Research Design and Methods.—Sixty-two nondiabetic Hispanic women with pregnancies complicated by GDM completed oral and intravenous glucose tolerance tests and bioelectrical impedance measurements of body fat every 12–15 months postpartum for up to 12 years. Self-reported dietary intake was collected at all visits by structured food frequency questionnaires developed for Hispanics. Mixed-effects models were used to assess the relationship between dietary intake and rates of change in metabolic outcomes during follow-up.

Results.—The median length of follow-up from the first postpartum evaluation was 8.0 years (interquartile range 4.5–10.8 years). At baseline, women were 32 ± 5.7 years old and had a median calorie intake of 2,091 kcal/day. Over the course of follow-up, dietary intake did not change significantly. Higher baseline calorie intake was associated with a faster decline in insulin sensitivity, measured by the insulin sensitivity index (S_I) ($P = 0.029$), and β-cell compensation, measured by the disposition index (DI) ($P = 0.027$), over time. These associations remained after adjustment for baseline characteristics; changes in BMI, calorie intake, levels of physical activity; and additional pregnancies during the follow-up period. The median rates were −0.06 vs. −0.02 units/year for S_I and −810 vs. −692 units/year for DI for women with baseline calorie intake above versus below the cohort median.

Conclusions.—High calorie intake is associated with a faster decline in insulin sensitivity and β-cell compensation in Hispanic women who are at high risk for type 2 diabetes, independent of adiposity.

► The role of obesity in the development of type 2 diabetes is clear-cut. Worldwide the obesity epidemic is driving a parallel increase in type 2 diabetes. However, the precise effects of caloric intake independent of adiposity and body mass index (BMI) were unclear. In 62 Hispanic women with gestational diabetes who were followed for between 4.5 and 10.8 years, the average caloric intake was higher than recommended: approximately 2000 calories per day.

Independent of any variables such as BMI and physical activity, the caloric intake was associated with a faster decline in insulin sensitivity and B-cell compensation as measured by the oral glucose tolerance test and intravenous glucose tolerance test that allowed for the calculation of the insulin sensitivity and disposition indexes. Thus, in predisposed individuals, such as women with gestational diabetes, more emphasis should be placed on caloric intake to slow the progression to type 2 diabetes.

D. LeRoith, MD

Tight Glycemic Control and Use of Hypoglycemic Medications in Older Veterans With Type 2 Diabetes and Comorbid Dementia

Thorpe CT, Gellad WF, Good CB, et al (Veterans Affairs Pittsburgh Healthcare System, PA; et al)

Diabetes Care 38:588-595, 2015

Objective.—Older adults with diabetes and dementia are at increased risk for hypoglycemia and other adverse events associated with tight glycemic control and are unlikely to experience long-term benefits. We examined risk factors for tight glycemic control in this population and use of medications associated with a high risk of hypoglycemia in the subset with tight control.

Research Design and Methods.—This retrospective cohort study of national Veterans Affairs (VA) administrative/clinical data and Medicare claims for fiscal years (FYs) 2008–2009 included 15,880 veterans aged ≥65 years with type 2 diabetes and dementia and prescribed antidiabetic medication. Multivariable regression analyses were used to identify sociodemographic and clinical predictors of hemoglobin A_{1c} (HbA_{1c}) control (tight, moderate, poor, or not monitored) and, in patients with tight control, subsequent use of medication associated with a high risk of hypoglycemia (sulfonylureas, insulin).

Results.—Fifty-two percent of patients had tight glycemic control (HbA_{1c} <7% [53 mmol/mol]). Specific comorbidities, older age, and recent weight loss were associated with greater odds of tight versus moderate control, whereas Hispanic ethnicity and obesity were associated with lower odds of tight control. Among tightly controlled patients, 75% used sulfonylureas and/or insulin, with higher odds in patients who were male, black, or aged ≥75 years; had a hospital or nursing home stay in FY2008; or had congestive heart failure, renal failure, or peripheral vascular disease.

Conclusions.—Many older veterans with diabetes and dementia are at high risk for hypoglycemia associated with intense diabetes treatment and may be candidates for deintensification or alteration of diabetes medications.

► One of the major side effects of the use of oral hypoglycemic agents and insulin is hypoglycemia. Although many of the newly introduced oral agents do not by themselves cause significant hypoglycemia, they are often used in conjunction with sulfonylureas or insulin and therefore enhance the propensity to this complication.

The major ways to avoid this devastating complication is the appropriate use of the medications; monitoring of renal function or other organ dysfunction that may lead to reduced metabolism of the drugs. Another important aspect is education—that is, informing patients regarding early symptoms, maintaining adequate food intake, and techniques to respond to the hypoglycemia.

In this publication, the investigators studied more than 15 000 patients in the Veterans Administration system with diabetes and dementia and used Medicare claims for the study. Interestingly, more than 50% of patients were well controlled with HBA_{1c} levels below 7%. Patients who recently lost weight had better control compared with those with recent weight increase and/or Hispanic background. The use of insulin was significantly common in these older patients and may reflect the cost of newer drugs being introduced recently or the familiarity of the physicians and providers in its use. Thus the investigators conclude that one should avoid tight control in elderly diabetics and those with dementia. In addition, they questioned the widespread use of insulin because it puts these patients at risk for hypoglycemia. An additional reason is that elderly diabetic patients with cardiovascular disease are prone to developing acute cardiovascular events secondary to hypoglycemia.

D. LeRoith, MD

Follow-up of Glycemic Control and Cardiovascular Outcomes in Type 2 Diabetes

Hayward RA, for the VADT Investigators (VA Ann Arbor Healthcare System, MI; et al)

N Engl J Med 372:2197-2206, 2015

Background.—The Veterans Affairs Diabetes Trial previously showed that intensive glucose lowering, as compared with standard therapy, did not significantly reduce the rate of major cardiovascular events among 1791 military veterans (median follow-up, 5.6 years). We report the extended follow-up of the study participants.

Methods.—After the conclusion of the clinical trial, we followed participants, using central databases to identify procedures, hospitalizations, and deaths (complete cohort, with follow-up data for 92.4% of participants). Most participants agreed to additional data collection by means of annual surveys and periodic chart reviews (survey cohort, with 77.7% follow-up). The primary outcome was the time to the first major cardiovascular event (heart attack, stroke, new or worsening congestive heart failure, amputation for ischemic gangrene, or cardiovascular-related death). Secondary outcomes were cardiovascular mortality and all-cause mortality.

Results.—The difference in glycated hemoglobin levels between the intensive-therapy group and the standard-therapy group averaged 1.5 percentage points during the trial (median level, 6.9% vs. 8.4%) and declined to 0.2 to 0.3 percentage points by 3 years after the trial ended. Over a median follow-up of 9.8 years, the intensive-therapy group had a significantly lower risk of the primary outcome than did the standard-therapy group (hazard ratio, 0.83; 95% confidence interval [CI], 0.70 to 0.99; $P = 0.04$), with an absolute reduction in risk of 8.6 major cardiovascular events per 1000 person-years, but did not have reduced cardiovascular mortality (hazard ratio, 0.88; 95% CI, 0.64 to 1.20; $P = 0.42$). No reduction in total mortality was evident (hazard ratio in the intensive-therapy group, 1.05; 95% CI, 0.89 to 1.25; $P = 0.54$; median follow-up, 11.8 years).

Conclusions.—After nearly 10 years of follow-up, patients with type 2 diabetes who had been randomly assigned to intensive glucose control for 5.6 years had 8.6 fewer major cardiovascular events per 1000 person-years than those assigned to standard therapy, but no improvement was seen in the rate of overall survival. (Funded by the VA Cooperative Studies Program and others; VADT ClinicalTrials.gov number, NCT00032487.)

► It has been well established that patients with type 2 diabetes have increased macrovascular and microvascular complications. The causative factors include hyperglycemia, hypertension, and hyperlipidemia. Controlling circulating lipid levels as well as blood pressure has convincingly shown a reduction in complications; however, although tight blood glucose controls delays and prevents microvascular complications, whether there is an effect on macrovascular complications is still not well defined. The most definitive effect of blood glucose control on macrovascular disease was seen with United Kingdom Prospective

Diabetes Study (UKPDS), whereas more recent studies including the Action to Control Cardiovascular Risk in Diabetes, ADVANCE, and Veterans Affairs Diabetes Trial (VADT) studies failed in this respect, although microvascular complications were affected significantly. Two possible explanations are given for these outcomes. First, the UKPDS trial involved new-onset patients who were relatively free of macrovascular disease compared with the older patients in the other trials, which recruited established patients who generally had established disease. Another possible reason was the longer duration of follow-up with the UKPDS trial. Support for this has come from the Diabetes Control and Complications Trial and Epidemiology of Diabetes Interventions and Complications trials in the type 1 diabetic patients. During the first 8 years of the Diabetes Control and Complications Trial, no effect on macrovascular complications was seen, whereas a long-term follow-up (Epidemiology of Diabetes Interventions and Complications) showed a significant reduction in cardiovascular events. In the long-term follow-up of patients in the VADT study, described in the present article, those patients with good control had fewer cardiovascular events compared with those in the standard therapy group. Thus it is clear that early intervention with glucose control is important to reduce vascular complications.

D. LeRoith, MD

Fibroblast growth factor 21 analogue LY2405319 lowers blood glucose in streptozotocin-induced insulin-deficient diabetic mice by restoring brown adipose tissue function

Kim J-H, Bae K-H, Choi Y-K, et al (Kyungpook Natl Univ, Daegu, South Korea; Kyungpook Natl Univ School of Medicine, Daegu, South Korea; et al)
Diabetes Obes Metab 17:161-169, 2015

Aim.—To investigate the effects of LY2405319, an analogue of fibroblast growth factor 21 (FGF21), on glucose homeostasis in streptozotocin (STZ)-induced insulin-deficient mice (STZ mice).

Methods.—Nine-week-old male C57BL/6J mice were administered a single intraperitoneal injection of STZ (150 mg/kg). One week later, after confirmation of hyperglycaemia, saline or LY2405319 (5 mg/kg) was injected subcutaneously daily for 4 weeks. Changes in glucose homeostasis, energy metabolism and brown adipose tissue (BAT) function were assessed.

Results.—The STZ mice had elevated blood glucose and reduced plasma FGF21 levels, impaired glucose uptake in the BAT, and BAT mitochondria with absent or swollen cristae and fewer lipid vacuoles. LY2405319 significantly reduced blood glucose levels and this was associated with increased BAT glucose uptake and changes in gene expression and morphology, indicating improved mitochondrial lipid metabolism in the BAT. Importantly, the ability of LY2405319 to lower blood glucose in STZ mice was compromised after removing interscapular BAT.

Conclusions.—Our results show that LY2405319 reduces blood glucose levels in insulin-deficient diabetes by improving BAT metabolism.

Additional studies investigating the therapeutic potential of FGF21 for the treatment of type 1 diabetes are warranted.

▶ One of the more exciting and potential factors being widely studied in diabetes (especially obesity and type 2 diabetes) is the fibroblast growth factor 21 (FGF21), both as a mediator of metabolism as well as a potential therapeutic agent. FGF21 is a secreted protein that has been shown to regulate glucose, lipid, and energy metabolism. A mechanistic understanding of the pharmacology of FGF21 continues to evolve, but it has been shown that the glucose-lowering properties of FGF21 are partly attributable to increased expression of the insulin-independent glucose transporter 1 (GLUT1), increased production of adiponectin and brown adipose tissue activation. In this article, a variant of FGF21 (LY2405319) was used to examine the effects of LY2405319 on blood glucose levels in streptozotocin (STZ) mice. STZ is used to destroy the beta cells of the pancreas in rodent models and results in an insulinopenic diabetic model that resembles type 1 diabetes in humans. After the injection of STZ the blood glucose levels rose in the mice and following the FGF21 molecule the blood glucose levels were reduced and glycosuria was relieved. In comparison with control mice, STZ mice exhibited a marked decrease in brown adipocyte size and intracellular lipid content, both of which were reversed by LY2405319 administration. These data support the role of insulin in the regulation of intracellular lipid content and show that LY2405319 reverses the delipidation induced by insulin deficiency. The take-home message that can be derived from this study is that FGF21 may be useful in reversing the metabolic abnormalities seen in type 1 and type 2 diabetes and that the role of FGF21 in the adipocyte, especially the metabolically active brown fat cell, is a critical mechanism through which metabolic improvement is mediated.

D. LeRoith, MD

Determinants of Adherence to Diabetes Medications: Findings From a Large Pharmacy Claims Database

Kirkman MS, Rowan-Martin MT, Levin R, et al (Univ of North Carolina School of Medicine, Chapel Hill; American Diabetes Association, Alexandria, VA; Express Scripts, Franklin Lakes, NJ; et al)

Diabetes Care 38:604-609, 2015

Objective.—Adults with diabetes typically take multiple medications for hyperglycemia, diabetes-associated conditions, and other comorbidities. Medication adherence is associated with improved outcomes, including reduced health care costs, hospitalization, and mortality. We conducted a retrospective analysis of a large pharmacy claims database to examine patient, medication, and prescriber factors associated with adherence to antidiabetic medications.

Research Design and Methods.—We extracted data on a cohort of >200,000 patients who were treated for diabetes with noninsulin medications in the second half of 2010 and had continuous prescription benefits eligibility through 2011. Adherence was defined as a medication possession ratio ≥0.8. We used a modified adherence measure that accounted for switching therapies. Logistic regression analysis was performed to determine factors independently associated with adherence.

Results.—Sixty-nine percent of patients were adherent. Adherence was independently associated with older age, male sex, higher education, higher income, use of mail order versus retail pharmacies, primary care versus nonendocrinology specialist prescribers, higher daily total pill burden, and lower out-of-pocket costs. Patients who were new to diabetes therapy were significantly less likely to be adherent.

Conclusions.—Several demographic, clinical, and potentially modifiable system-level factors were associated with adherence to antidiabetic medications. Patients typically perceived to be healthy (those who are younger, new to diabetes, and on few other medications) may be at risk for nonadherence. For all patients, efforts to reduce out-of-pocket costs and encourage use of mail order pharmacies may result in higher adherence.

▶ One of the major problems we face in treating patients with chronic disorders such as type 2 diabetes is compliance (ie, adherence) to medications. Most type 2 diabetic patients require multiple antidiabetic medications. This requirement is often in addition to medications for other conditions that may or may not be associated with the diabetes. For example, many will also be treated with multiple antihypertensive and hyperlipidemic medications. In addition, they maybe suffering and treated for prevention of osteoporosis or arthritis. It has been clearly demonstrated that nonadherence has numerous consequences. However, what has not been well studied are the determinants for medication adherence. This study used a large pharmacy claims database and assessed determinants of adherence to oral antidiabetic medications in more than 200 000 US adults with type 2 diabetes. The results showed that patients new to therapy were 61% less likely to be adherent to their diabetes medication. In addition, younger patients were less likely to adhere. Thus, younger individuals who are otherwise healthy may need more support to help them overcome barriers to adherence, one of which may be accepting the reality of having a chronic illness. Those with higher education and better incomes showed a propensity to adhere to medications. No significant effects were seen when prescribers studied. For example, no difference was found whether primary care or endocrinologists were the prescribers. Thus the result of this study dispels some of our misconceptions and highlights important factors that affect patient adherence. It can therefore be concluded from this study that particular attention should be paid to certain patients to ensure they adhere to medications as prescribed to avoid many of the complications of diabetes.

D. LeRoith, MD

Effects of 60-day head-down bed rest on osteocalcin, glycolipid metabolism and their association with or without resistance training

Yang C, Chen J, Wu F, et al (Haerbin Inst of Technology, Haerbin, China; China Astronaut Res and Training Ctr, Beijing, China)

Clin Endocrinol 81:671-678, 2014

Introduction.—Bone loss and subclinical diabeteslike are developed during long-term spaceflight. Recently, it was demonstrated that bone was able to regulate energy metabolism and testosterone synthesis via osteocalcin. The aim of this study was to determine whether serum osteocalcin level is associated with glycolipid metabolism or testosterone under the influence of microgravity with or without resistive vibration exercise (RVE).

Methods.—A total of 14 healthy adult male volunteers (25–40 years) were randomly assigned to two groups (n = 7 each): control (CON) group and RVE group. Radioimmunoassay kits and ELISA kits were used for measurement of serum indices.

Results.—During 60-day bed rest, serum osteocalcin of both groups increased at day 4 during bed rest. Serum OPG started decreasing and reached its lowest value at day 30 during bed rest. In control group, serum insulin increased at day 4 during bed rest. IGF-I did not change significantly during the entire period of bed rest. The serum glucose decline 10% and 14% in CON and RVE groups at day 4 during bed rest. Relatively, the same results as glucose were found in serum HDL and LDL for both groups. Leptin rose and became highest at day 60 during bed rest in both groups. The level of serum testosterone was declined in control group at day 4 during bed rest. Cortisol kept stable in both group during bed rest. By spearman correlation analysis, serum osteocalcin was significantly associated with serum insulin ($P < 0{\cdot}05$), LDL ($P < 0{\cdot}01$) and Leptin ($P < 0{\cdot}01$).

Conclusion.—Our findings suggested that the mutual regulation may exist between skeletal and energy metabolism under simulated microgravity.

▶ Because space travel is associated with loss of the effects of gravity on bone and the lack of exercise may affect metabolic functions, the authors studied individuals during a 60-day bed-rest experiment. There were changes in circulating levels of osteocalcin and osteoprotegerin, which increased and decreased, respectively. The major change in hormonal status was a decrease in testosterone without any significant change in circulating cortisol levels. There were reciprocal changes in insulin and glucose with changes in low-density lipoprotein and high-density lipoprotein cholesterol levels. The authors conclude that the changes in bone density and the changes in metabolism and other hormonal effects that occur due to prolonged bed rest, and by extrapolation to lack of gravity and exercise, may be interrelated and that osteocalcin may affect metabolism. Thus, there may be a bone-to-islet-cell interaction via certain hormones, as has been suggested by mouse genetic models.

D. LeRoith, MD

Incretin-Based Therapy and Risk of Acute Pancreatitis: A Nationwide Population-Based: Case-Control Study

Thomsen RW, Pedersen L, Møller N, et al (Aarhus Univ Hosp, Denmark; et al)

Diabetes Care 38:1089-1098, 2015

Objective.—To investigate whether the use of incretin-based drugs (GLP-1 receptor agonists and dipeptidyl peptidase 4 [DPP4] inhibitors) is associated with acute pancreatitis.

Research Design and Methods.—The study was a nationwide population-based case-control study using medical databases in Denmark. Participants were 12,868 patients with a first-time hospitalization for acute pancreatitis between 2005 and 2012 and a population of 128,680 matched control subjects. The main outcome measure was the odds ratio (OR) for acute pancreatitis associated with different antihyperglycemic drugs. We adjusted for history of gallstones, alcoholism, obesity, and other pancreatitis-associated comorbidities and medications.

Results.—A total of 89 pancreatitis patients (0.69%) and 684 control subjects (0.53%) were ever users of incretins. The crude OR for acute pancreatitis among incretin users was 1.36 (95% CI 1.08–1.69), while it was 1.44 (95% CI 1.34–1.54) among users of other antihyperglycemic drugs. After confounder adjustment, the risk of acute pancreatitis was not increased among incretin users (OR 0.95 [95% CI 0.75–1.21]), including DPP4 inhibitor users (OR 1.04 [95% CI 0.80–1.37]) or GLP-1 receptor agonist users (OR 0.82 [95% CI 0.54–1.23]), or among nonincretin antihyperglycemic drug users (OR 1.05 [95% CI 0.98–1.13]), compared with nonusers of any antihyperglycemic drugs. Findings were similar in current versus ever drug users and in patients with pancreatitis risk factors. The adjusted OR comparing incretin-based therapy with other antihyperglycemic therapy internally while also adjusting for diabetes duration and complications was 0.97 (95% CI 0.76–1.23).

Conclusions.—Our findings suggest that the use of incretin-based drugs appears not to be associated with an increased risk of acute pancreatitis.

▶ Newly introduced drugs have been evaluated by the US Food and Drug Administration (FDA) and similar regulatory agencies worldwide, following large phase 3 trials to evaluate efficacy of the agent. Outcome from these trials include adverse events to help in the evaluation of the safety of the agent before approval. Although the results give one confidence that the drug is effective and safe, the trials are only a few years in duration, and this is often inadequate to assess the true safety of the drug, similar to the use of the new incretin class of agents. One class is the oral dipeptidyl peptidase (DPP)-IV inhibitors, which have limited side effects, and their mechanism of action is to raise the level of glucagon-like peptide-1 (GLP-1) by inhibiting DPP-IV, which is usually involved in inactivation of GLP-1. The injectable GLP-1 mimetic shows greater reductions in HbA_{1c} and weight loss through appetite suppression. Of concern are the reports that both DPP-IV inhibitors and GLP-1-mimetics may increase the risk and occurrence of acute pancreatitis. This concern has led the FDA and other regulatory bodies to insist on postmarketing surveillance. This article describes a population-based case-control study of 12 868 patients in Denmark, to evaluate the incidence of acute pancreatitis in patients using various antihyperglycemic agents. They adjusted for known causes of pancreatitis, including alcoholism, gallstones, and other comorbidities. The results show that the use of incretin therapy, whether DPP-IV inhibitors or GLP-1-mimetics, were not associated with increased risk for acute pancreatitis, although acute pancreatitis occurs more commonly in type 2 diabetics, perhaps secondary to hypertriglyceridemia and other mechanisms. However, these and other studies do not show any effect of the incretin therapies.

D. LeRoith, MD

Efficacy and Safety of Saxagliptin in Older Participants in the SAVOR-TIMI 53 Trial

Leiter LA, for the SAVOR-TIMI 53 Steering Committee and Investigators (Univ of Toronto, Ontario, Canada; et al)

Diabetes Care 38:1145-1153, 2015

Objective.—To examine the safety and cardiovascular (CV) effects of saxagliptin in the predefined elderly (≥65 years) and very elderly (≥75 years) subpopulations of the Saxagliptin Assessment of Vascular Outcomes Recorded in Patients with Diabetes Mellitus—Thrombolysis in Myocardial Infarction 53 (SAVOR-TIMI 53) trial.

Research Design and Methods.—Individuals ≥40 years ($n = 16{,}492$; elderly, $n = 8{,}561$; very elderly, $n = 2{,}330$) with HbA_{1c} ≥6.5% (47.5 mmol/mol) and ≤12.0% (107.7 mmol/mol) were randomized (1:1) to saxagliptin (5 or 2.5 mg daily) or placebo in a double-blind trial for a median follow-up of 2.1 years.

Results.—The hazard ratio (HR) for the comparison of saxagliptin versus placebo for the primary end point (composite of CV mortality, myocardial infarction, or ischemic stroke) was 0.92 for elderly patients vs. 1.15 for patients <65 years ($P = 0.06$) and 0.95 for very elderly patients. The HRs for the secondary composite end points in the entire cohort, elderly cohort, and very elderly cohort were similar. Although saxagliptin increased the risk of hospitalization for heart failure in the overall saxagliptin population, there was no age-based treatment interaction ($P = 0.76$ for elderly patients vs. those <65 years; $P = 0.34$ for very elderly patients vs. those <75 years). Among saxagliptin-treated individuals with baseline HbA_{1c} ≥7.6% (59.6 mmol/mol), the mean change from baseline HbA_{1c} at 2 years was −0.69%, −0.64%, −0.66%, and −0.66% for those ≥65, <65, ≥75, and <75 years old, respectively. The incidence of overall adverse events (AEs) and serious AEs was similar between saxagliptin and placebo in all cohorts; however, hypoglycemic events were higher for saxagliptin versus placebo regardless of age.

Conclusions.—The SAVOR-TIMI 53 trial supports the overall CV safety of saxagliptin in a robust number of elderly and very elderly participants, although the risk of heart failure hospitalization was increased irrespective of age category. AEs and serious AEs as well as glycemic efficacy of saxagliptin in elderly patients are similar to those found in younger patients.

▶ Treatment of type 2 diabetes involves both oral hypoglycemic agents as well as injectables such as insulin and the GLP-1 mimetics. There are now approximately 12 classes of drugs available to the health care professionals and patients. Generally, providers use medications that are appropriate for patients' characteristics, whether this relates to age, the level of glucose control needed, the predetermined goal, or the cost of medications. When new medications are introduced, it is critical to evaluate their adverse reactions and any effects on long-term outcomes, if any. In the Saxagliptin Assessment of Vascular Outcomes Recorded in Patients with Diabetes Mellitus trial, a subset of elderly patients was evaluated and compared with younger patients in the trial, in which saxagliptin was compared to placebo. Although there were no negative effects on myocardial infarction, ischemic stroke, or cardiovascular mortality rates, they noted an increased hospitalization for heart failure. Thus, the outcome of the trial gives providers confidence in using these intravenous dipeptidyl peptidase (DDP-IV) inhibitors, of which there are a number available. Most DDP-IV inhibitors give a real but modest reduction in HbA_{1c} and are often used as second-line therapy, being added to metformin when HbA_{1c} goals were not met. In general, they are not associated with significant side effects, as opposed to the GLP-1 mimetics that are injected and are often associated with gastrointestinal side effects especially when initially used. The concern with the present trial is the increase in heart failure. It is unclear how this particular DDP-IV inhibitor caused this adverse event and one needs to determine whether it is specific to this agent or class effect. In addition, the mechanism will be quite enlightening, given that DDP-IVs have numerous other effects in multiple tissues.

D. LeRoith, MD

Diabetic Kidney Disease: A Report From an ADA Consensus Conference

Tuttle KR, Bakris GL, Bilous RW, et al (Univ of Washington School of Medicine, Seattle; The Univ of Chicago Medicine, IL; Newcastle Univ, Newcastle upon Tyne, UK; et al)

Diabetes Care 37:2864-2883, 2014

The incidence and prevalence of diabetes mellitus have grown significantly throughout the world, due primarily to the increase in type 2 diabetes. This overall increase in the number of people with diabetes has had a major impact on development of diabetic kidney disease (DKD), one of the most frequent complications of both types of diabetes. DKD is the leading cause of end-stage renal disease (ESRD), accounting for approximately 50% of cases in the developed world. Although incidence rates for ESRD attributable to DKD have recently stabilized, these rates continue to rise in high-risk groups such as middle-aged African Americans, Native Americans, and Hispanics. The costs of care for people with DKD are extraordinarily high. In the Medicare population alone, DKD-related expenditures among this mostly older group were nearly $25 billion in 2011. Due to the high human and societal costs, the Consensus Conference on Chronic Kidney Disease and Diabetes was convened by the American Diabetes Association in collaboration with the American Society of Nephrology and the National Kidney Foundation to appraise issues regarding patient management, highlighting current practices and new directions. Major topic areas in DKD included *1*) identification and monitoring, 2) cardiovascular disease and management of dyslipidemia, *3*) hypertension and use of renin-angiotensin-aldosterone system blockade and mineralocorticoid receptor blockade, *4*) glycemia measurement, hypoglycemia, and drug therapies, *5*) nutrition and general care in advanced-stage chronic kidney disease, *6*) children and adolescents, and *7*) multidisciplinary approaches and medical home models for health care delivery. This current state summary and research recommendations are designed to guide advances in care and the generation of new knowledge that will meaningfully improve life for people with DKD.

▶ A consensus conference was convened on the topic of chronic kidney disease secondary to diabetes. Because there is a growing epidemic of diabetes and it is the major cause of end-stage renal disease, prevention, diagnosis, and treatment of this diabetic complication are entirely worthwhile and important for general education both of patients and health care professionals. Monitoring albuminuria is still an important component of the diagnostic tools in addition to standard blood creatinine level and estimated glomerular filtration rate. Control of dyslipidemia and hypertension are important for prevention and delaying progression in addition to classic glycemic control. Blockade of the renin-angiotensin system with angiotensin-converting enzyme inhibition or angiotensin receptor blockade has been demonstrated to be extremely effective preservation of renal function independent of their efficacy in blood pressure management.

D. LeRoith, MD

Noninvasive In Vivo Imaging of Diabetes-Induced Renal Oxidative Stress and Response to Therapy Using Hyperpolarized ^{13}C Dehydroascorbate Magnetic Resonance

Keshari KR, Wilson DM, Sai V, et al (Memorial Sloan Kettering Cancer Ctr, NY; Univ of California, San Francisco)

Diabetes 64:344-352, 2015

Oxidative stress has been proposed to be a unifying cause for diabetic nephropathy and a target for novel therapies. Here we apply a new endogenous reduction-oxidation (redox) sensor, hyperpolarized (HP) ^{13}C dehydroascorbate (DHA), in conjunction with MRI to noninvasively interrogate the renal redox capacity in a mouse diabetes model. The diabetic mice demonstrate an early decrease in renal redox capacity, as shown by the lower in vivo HP ^{13}C DHA reduction to the antioxidant vitamin C (VitC), prior to histological evidence of nephropathy. This correlates with lower tissue reduced glutathione (GSH) concentration and higher NADPH oxidase 4 (Nox4) expression, consistent with increased superoxide generation and oxidative stress. ACE inhibition restores the HP ^{13}C DHA reduction to VitC with concomitant normalization of GSH concentration and Nox4 expression in diabetic mice. HP ^{13}C DHA enables rapid in vivo assessment of altered redox capacity in diabetic renal injury and after successful treatment.

▶ Diabetic nephropathy is a very common complication of both type 1 and type 2 diabetes and leads to end-stage renal disease in a significant proportion of patients. Chronic hyperglycemia is one of the major factors involved in this deterioration. The exact mechanisms through which hyperglycemia affects the kidney are not well established; however, oxidative stress, which is commonly associated with hyperglycemia, is apparently an important causal factor. Hyperglycemia leads to increased reactive oxygen species and oxidative stress through NAPDH oxidase 4 (Nox4), and Nox4-dependent superoxide generation and oxidative stress have been shown to mediate glomerular hypertrophy and mesangial matrix accumulation, which are key histological features of diabetic nephropathy. Angiotensin-converting enzyme (ACE) inhibitors and angiotensin receptor blockers that are commonly used as antihypertensives protect diabetics from renal injury by inhibition of Nox4. The current study uses a unique technique, namely hyperpolarized (HP) ^{13}C magnetic resonance (MR) spectroscopy that is a molecular imaging technique that allows noninvasive investigation of dynamic metabolic and physiological processes in real time. They demonstrate in diabetic mice that the ACE inhibition effects can be identified as changes in the renal redox state as assessed by this noninvasive technique. Adapting to the clinical situation would be a major step forward in our management of patients with diabetes and renal disease.

D. LeRoith, MD

Insulin Sensitivity Is an Important Determinant of Renal Health in Adolescents With Type 2 Diabetes

Bjornstad P, Maahs DM, Cherney DZ, et al (Univ of Colorado School of Medicine, Aurora; Univ of Toronto, Ontario, Canada; et al)
Diabetes Care 37:3033-3039, 2014

Objective.—Diabetic nephropathy (DN) remains the most common cause of end-stage renal disease and is a major cause of mortality in type 2 diabetes. Insulin sensitivity is an important determinant of renal health in adults with type 2 diabetes, but limited data exist in adolescents. We hypothesized that measured insulin sensitivity (glucose infusion rate [GIR]) would be associated with early markers of DN reflected by estimated glomerular filtration rate (eGFR) and albumin-creatinine ratio (ACR) in adolescents with type 2 diabetes.

Research Design and Methods.—Type 2 diabetic ($n = 46$), obese ($n = 29$), and lean ($n = 19$) adolescents (15.1 ± 2.2 years) had GIR measured by hyperinsulinemic-euglycemic clamps. ACR was measured and GFR was estimated by the Bouvet equation (combined creatinine and cystatin C).

Results.—Adolescents with type 2 diabetes had significantly lower GIR, and higher eGFR and ACR than obese or lean adolescents. Moreover, 34% of type 2 diabetic adolescents had albuminuria (ACR ≥30 mg/g), and 24% had hyperfiltration (≥135 mL/min/1.73 m^2). Stratifying ACR and eGFR into tertiles, adolescents with type 2 diabetes in the highest tertiles of ACR and eGFR had respectively lower GIR than those in the mid and low tertiles, after adjusting for age, sex, Tanner stage, BMI, and HbA_{1c} ($P = 0.02$ and $P = 0.04$). GIR, but not HbA_{1c}, LDL, or systolic blood pressure, was also associated with eGFR after adjusting for sex and Tanner stage (β ± SE: −2.23 ± 0.87; $P = 0.02$).

Conclusions.—A significant proportion of adolescents with type 2 diabetes showed evidence of early DN, and insulin sensitivity, rather than HbA_{1c}, blood pressure, or lipid control, was the strongest determinant of renal health.

▶ Diabetic retinopathy leads to end-stage renal disease and its commonest cause. There are a number of factors that lead to more rapid deterioration in renal function including uncontrolled glucose levels (higher HbA_{1c} levels), hypertension, and hyperlipidemia. Adolescent type 2 diabetes is associated with early renal impairment, and the current study investigated glucose infusion rates as a measure of insulin sensitivity, estimated glomerular filtration rate, and the albumin/creatinine ration as measures of renal insufficiency as well as other implicated factors. The study showed that renal insufficiency was most closely associated with insulin insensitivity. While controlling the known factors that enhance renal deterioration such as blood pressure, lipid, and glucose, the authors strongly advocate the reduction of insulin resistance by reducing body weight using lifestyle changes including diet, exercise, and even metformin therapy.

D. LeRoith, MD

Serum High-Sensitivity C-Reactive Protein Levels Are Associated With High Risk of Development, Not Progression, of Diabetic Nephropathy Among Japanese Type 2 Diabetic Patients: A Prospective Cohort Study (Diabetes Distress and Care Registry at Tenri [DDCRT7])

Hayashino Y, for the Diabetes Distress and Care Registry at Tenri Study Group (Tenri Hosp, Nara, Japan; et al)

Diabetes Care 37:2947-2952, 2014

Objective.—To assess the prospective association between baseline serum hs-CRP concentration and the subsequent risk of development or progression of diabetic nephropathy.

Research Design and Methods.—Longitudinal data were obtained from 2,518 patients with type 2 diabetes registered in a Japanese diabetes registry. To assess the independent correlations between serum baseline hs-CRP and either the development or progression of diabetic nephropathy 1 year later, the Cox proportional hazards model was used and adjusted for potential confounders.

Results.—The mean patient age, BMI, and HbA_{1c} level were 66.1 years, 24.6 kg/m^2, and 7.5% (57.6 mmol/mol), respectively. Baseline serum hs-CRP levels were significantly associated with the urinary albumin-to-creatinine ratio at baseline ($P < 0.001$). Multivariable adjusted hazard ratio for the development from normoalbuminuria to microalbuminuria was 1.31 (95% CI 0.80–2.17; $P = 0.286$), 1.55 (1.16–2.08; $P = 0.003$), and 1.57 (1.22–2.03; $P = 0.001$), respectively, for the second, third, and fourth quartiles of serum hs-CRP levels, showing a statistically significant linear trend across categories ($P < 0.001$). We did not observe a significant association between hs-CRP levels and the subsequent risk of diabetic nephropathy progression (P for trend $= 0.575$).

Conclusions.—Serum hs-CRP levels, independent of possible confounders, were associated with a subsequent risk of developing, not progressing, diabetic nephropathy in type 2 diabetic patients. Serum hs-CRP may be useful for predicting the future risk of developing diabetic nephropathy.

▶ In a study of 2518 Japanese type 2 diabetic patients, serum highly sensitive C-reactive protein (hs-CRP) was associated with the development of diabetic nephropathy, as measured by the albumin/creatinine ratio in a spot urine sample. Although there are a number of concerns with the laboratory measurement used and inherent problems with a cross-sectional study, the large patient sample size strongly suggests that the association is significant. Interestingly, the authors did not find a relationship between the hs-CRP levels and progression of the nephropathy. However, they showed that hs-CRP's prediction was independent of most other variables considered to be relevant, including inflammatory cytokines, HbA1c, and others. As noted by the authors hs-CRP maybe a marker for predicting atherosclerosis, diabetes, and now diabetic nephropathy because a functional role is yet to be determined.

D. LeRoith, MD

Peripheral Neuropathy and Nerve Dysfunction in Individuals at High Risk for Type 2 Diabetes: The PROMISE Cohort

Lee CC, Perkins BA, Kayaniyil S, et al (Univ of Toronto, Ontario, Canada; et al)
Diabetes Care 38:793-800, 2015

Objective.—Emerging evidence suggests that peripheral neuropathy begins in the early stages of diabetes pathogenesis. Our objective was to describe the prevalence of peripheral neuropathy and nerve dysfunction according to glucose tolerance and metabolic syndrome status and examine how these conditions are associated with neurological changes in individuals at risk for type 2 diabetes.

Research Design and Methods.—We studied 467 individuals in the longitudinal PROMISE (Prospective Metabolism and Islet Cell Evaluation) cohort. Peripheral neuropathy was defined by Michigan Neuropathy Screening Instrument (MNSI) scores (>2), and the severity of nerve dysfunction was measured objectively by vibration perception thresholds (VPTs) using a neurothesiometer. Metabolic syndrome was defined using the International Diabetes Federation/American Heart Association harmonized criteria.

Results.—The prevalence of peripheral neuropathy was 29%, 49%, and 50% for normal glycemia, prediabetes, and new-onset diabetes, respectively ($P < 0.001$ for trend). The mean VPT was 6.5 V for normal glycemia, 7.9 V for prediabetes, and 7.6 V for new-onset diabetes ($P = 0.024$ for trend). Prediabetes was associated with higher MNSI scores ($P = 0.01$) and VPTs ($P = 0.004$) versus normal glycemia, independent of known risk factors. Additionally, progression of glucose intolerance over 3 years predicted a higher risk of peripheral neuropathy ($P = 0.007$) and nerve dysfunction ($P = 0.002$). Metabolic syndrome was not independently associated with MNSI scores or VPTs.

Conclusions.—In individuals with multiple risk factors for diabetes, prediabetes was associated with similar risks of peripheral neuropathy and severity of nerve dysfunction as new-onset diabetes. Prediabetes, but not metabolic syndrome, was independently associated with both the presence of peripheral neuropathy and the severity of nerve dysfunction.

▶ Diabetic complications are basically of 2 major groups: microvascular and macrovascular. Whereas microvascular disease affects the retina, kidney, and nerves, macrovascular disease affects the heart and eventuates in ischemic strokes. Type 1 diabetics are usually free of complications at the onset of disease but many develop microvascular complications first and only later may develop macrovascular complications. In the case of type 2 diabetes, many have complications even at the time of presentation, presumably because the disease process began many years before but was either not diagnosed or they had the metabolic syndrome and prediabetes, which also lead to the same complications. The question that these investigators studied was whether there was an increase in peripheral neuropathy and nerve dysfunction in individuals before the development of diabetes. They studied 467 individuals in the Prospective Metabolism and Islet Cell Evaluation and measured neural function using Michigan Neuropathy Screening Instrument scores (> 2), and the severity of nerve dysfunction was measured objectively by vibration perception thresholds using a neurothesiometer. Metabolic syndrome was defined using the International Diabetes Federation/American Heart Association harmonized criteria. Interestingly, they noted that the metabolic syndrome (hypertension, hyperlipidemia, impaired glucose tolerance, and increased waist circumference) was not associated with increased prevalence of nerve dysfunction. In contrast, glucose levels are definitely predictive of nerve dysfunction. The incidence of nerve dysfunction increased with worsening of glucose tolerance. The study therefore proved again that glucose is the major factor involved in neuropathy causation, and not other risk factors involved in diabetes such as blood pressure and lipids. The most important conclusion is that individuals with a risk for developing diabetes need early detection of impaired glucose tolerance and frank diabetes to prevent or delay the neuropathy and probably other complications.

D. LeRoith, MD

Liraglutide and the Preservation of Pancreatic β-Cell Function in Early Type 2 Diabetes: The LIBRA Trial

Retnakaran R, Kramer CK, Choi H, et al (Mount Sinai Hosp, Toronto, Ontario, Canada; et al)

Diabetes Care 37:3270-3278, 2014

Objective.—Clinical studies evaluating the effects of medications on β-cell function in type 2 diabetes (T2DM) are compromised by an inability to determine the actual baseline degree of β-cell dysfunction independent of the reversible dysfunction induced by hyperglycemia (glucotoxicity). Short-term intensive insulin therapy (IIT) is a strategy for eliminating glucotoxicity before randomization. This study determined whether liraglutide can preserve β-cell function over 48 weeks in early T2DM following initial elimination of glucotoxicity with IIT.

Research Design and Methods.—In this double-blind, randomized, placebo-controlled trial, 51 patients with T2DM of 2.6 ± 1.9 years' duration and an A1C of 6.8 ± 0.8% (51 ± 8.7 mmol/mol) completed 4 weeks of IIT before randomization to daily subcutaneous liraglutide or placebo injection, with serial assessment of β-cell function by Insulin Secretion- Sensitivity Index-2 (ISSI-2) on oral glucose tolerance test performed every 12 weeks.

Results.—The primary outcome of baseline-adjusted ISSI-2 at 48 weeks was higher in the liraglutide group than in the placebo group (339.8 ± 27.8 vs. 229.3 ± 28.4, $P = 0.008$). Baseline-adjusted HbA_{1c} at 48 weeks was lower in the liraglutide group (6.2 ± 0.1% vs. 6.6 ± 0.1%, $P = 0.055$) (44 ± 1.1 vs. 49 ± 1.1 mmol/mol). At each quarterly assessment, >50% of participants on liraglutide had an HbA_{1c} ≤6.0% (42 mmol/mol) and glucose tolerance in the nondiabetic range. Despite this level of glycemic control, no difference was found in the incidence of hypoglycemia between the liraglutide and placebo groups ($P = 0.61$). Two weeks after stopping treatment, however, the beneficial effect on ISSI-2 of liraglutide versus placebo was entirely lost (191.9 ± 24.7 vs. 238.1 ± 25.2, $P = 0.20$).

Conclusions.—Liraglutide provides robust enhancement of β-cell function that is sustained over 48 weeks in early T2DM but lost upon cessation of therapy.

▶ A randomized, double-blind trial was undertaken to determine whether the glucagon-like peptide-1 (GLP-1) receptor agonist liraglutide could preserve beta-cell function over a 48-week period. The patients had type 2 diabetes of short duration (2.6 ± 1.9 years) and average HbA_{1c} (6.8 ± 0.8%). The investigators utilized an Insulin Secretion Sensitivity Index (ISSI) and oral glucose tolerance test and determined that during the study period beta-cell function was preserved in the liraglutide-treated patients compared with the placebo group. Immediately after cessation of the liraglutide treatment, the positive effect on ISSI was lost. Of importance was the finding that not only did liraglutide preserve function, but that there was a significant enhancement of beta-cell function on the therapy. Besides its effect on acute beta cell, with release of insulin secretion and inhibition of glycogen secretion, it seems possible that the reduction in glucose levels and removal of significant glucotoxicity effects on the beta cells. Future studies are necessary to identify the mechanisms of preservation on human islet cells, by GLP-1 receptor agonists, such as liraglutide.

D. LeRoith, MD

59 Obesity

Adjusting Glucose-Stimulated Insulin Secretion for Adipose Insulin Resistance: An Index of β-Cell Function in Obese Adults

Malin SK, Kashyap SR, Hammel J, et al (Cleveland Clinic, OH; et al)

Diabetes Care 37:2940-2946, 2014

Objective.—The hyperbolic relationship between insulin secretion and sensitivity has been used to assess in vivo β-cell function (i.e., the disposition index). The disposition index emphasizes the importance of taking into account both skeletal muscle and hepatic insulin resistance to depict insulin secretion. However, we propose that adipose tissue insulin resistance also needs to be accounted for when characterizing glucose-stimulated insulin secretion (GSIS) because elevated plasma free fatty acids (FFAs) impair β-cell function.

Research Design and Methods.—To characterize the adipose disposition index, we used [1-^{14}C] palmitate infusion to determine basal FFA turnover rate/adipose insulin resistance and an oral glucose tolerance test to characterize the first (i.e., 0–30 min) and second phase (i.e., 60–120 min) of GSIS. We validated a simplified version of the tracer infusion calculation as the product of (1/plasma FFA concentration × plasma insulin concentration) × GSIS in 44 obese insulin-resistant subjects.

Results.—The plasma FFA and palmitate tracer infusion calculations of the first- and second-phase disposition index were strongly correlated ($r = 0.86$, $P < 0.000001$ and $r = 0.89$, $P < 0.000001$, respectively). The first- and second-phase adipose disposition index derived from plasma FFA also was tightly associated with fasting hyperglycemia ($r = -0.87$, $P < 0.00001$ and $r = -0.89$, $P < 0.00001$, respectively) and 2-h glucose concentrations ($r = -0.86$, $P < 0.00001$ and $r = -0.90$, $P < 0.00001$).

Conclusions.—Adjusting GSIS for adipose insulin resistance provides an index of β-cell function in obese subjects across the glucose spectrum. Plasma FFA-derived calculations of β-cell function may provide additional insight into the role of adipose tissue in glucose regulation.

► Insulin resistance is commonly seen in obese prediabetic individuals. Once beta-cell dysfunction occurs, type 2 diabetes becomes apparent. Avoiding β-cell dysfunction is therefore critical for the prevention of diabetes and to limit the progression of the disease once it has appeared. This relationship between β-cell insulin secretion and insulin sensitivity has been characterized by the "disposition index," and although it accounts for hepatic and muscle insulin resistance, it does not account for the role of the adipocyte and the circulating free fatty acids (FFA) on β-cell function. These investigators used a isotope labeled palmitate to study basal FFA turnover rate/adipose insulin resistance and an oral glucose tolerance test to characterize the glucose-stimulated insulin release in obese patients. Their results strongly suggest that the adipose tissue plays an important role in affecting insulin secretion, especially in obesity.

D. LeRoith, MD

Anorexia and Impaired Glucose Metabolism in Mice With Hypothalamic Ablation of Glut4 Neurons

Ren H, Lu TY, McGraw TE, et al (Columbia Univ College of Physicians and Surgeons, NY; Weill Cornell Med College, NY)
Diabetes 64:405-417, 2015

The central nervous system (CNS) uses glucose independent of insulin. Nonetheless, insulin receptors and insulin-responsive glucose transporters (Glut4) often colocalize in neurons (Glut4 neurons) in anatomically and functionally distinct areas of the CNS. The apparent heterogeneity of Glut4 neurons has thus far thwarted attempts to understand their function. To answer this question, we used Cre-dependent, diphtheria toxin-mediated cell ablation to selectively remove basal hypothalamic Glut4 neurons and investigate the resulting phenotypes. After Glut4 neuron ablation, mice demonstrate altered hormone and nutrient signaling in the CNS. Accordingly, they exhibit negative energy balance phenotype characterized by reduced food intake and increased energy expenditure, without locomotor deficits or gross neuronal abnormalities. Glut4 neuron ablation affects orexigenic melanin-concentrating hormone neurons but has limited effect on neuropeptide Y/agouti-related protein and proopiomelanocortin neurons. The food intake phenotype can be partially normalized by GABA administration, suggesting that it arises from defective GABAergic transmission. Glut4 neuron-ablated mice show peripheral metabolic defects, including fasting hyperglycemia and glucose intolerance, decreased insulin levels, and elevated hepatic gluconeogenic genes. We conclude that Glut4 neurons integrate hormonal and nutritional cues and mediate CNS actions of insulin on energy balance and peripheral metabolism.

▶ Over the past decade, it has become increasingly clear that the hypothalamus plays a critical role in both satiety and appetite, but additionally, it controls many of the peripheral metabolic programs that we traditionally assigned to hormones such as insulin. Insulin's effect on glucose uptake is dependent on a tissue-specific glucose transporter, GLUT4. Some recent studies demonstrated GLUT4 expression in certain regions of the brain and more specifically in the hypothalamus. In this study, the investigators used a technique to ablate GLUT4-expressing neurons in the hypothalamus—specifically, the orexigenic melanin-concentrating hormone neurons. The resultant reduction in food intake by the mice could be anticipated by ablation of these neurons as well as the increase in energy expenditure. However, there was an additional effect on glucose metabolism—namely, reduced circulating insulin levels and hyperglycemia as a result of increased hepatic gluconeogenesis. Thus, the authors have shown a complicated integration of hypothalamic signals on feeding behavior and peripheral glucose metabolism.

D. LeRoith, MD

Cardiorespiratory Fitness and Incident Diabetes: The FIT (Henry Ford ExercIse Testing) Project

Juraschek SP, Blaha MJ, Blumenthal RS, et al (The Johns Hopkins Ciccarone Ctr for the Prevention of Heart Disease, Baltimore, MD; et al)

Diabetes Care 38:1075-1081, 2015

Objective.—Prior evidence has linked higher cardiorespiratory fitness with a lower risk of diabetes in ambulatory populations. Using a demographically diverse study sample, we examined the association of fitness with incident diabetes in 46,979 patients from The Henry Ford ExercIse Testing (FIT) Project without diabetes at baseline.

Research Design and Methods.—Fitness was measured during a clinician-referred treadmill stress test performed between 1991 and 2009. Incident diabetes was defined as a new diagnosis of diabetes on three separate consecutive encounters derived from electronic medical records or administrative claims files. Analyses were performed with Cox proportional hazards models and were adjusted for diabetes risk factors.

Results.—The mean age was 53 years with 48% women and 27% black patients. Mean metabolic equivalents (METs) achieved was 9.5 (SD 3.0). During a median follow-up period of 5.2 years (interquartile range 2.6–8.3 years), there were 6,851 new diabetes cases (14.6%). After adjustment, patients achieving ≥12 METs had a 54% lower risk of incident diabetes compared with patients achieving <6 METs (hazard ratio 0.46 [95% CI 0.41, 0.51]; *P*-trend < 0.001). This relationship was preserved across strata of age, sex, race, obesity, hypertension, and hyperlipidemia.

Conclusions.—These data demonstrate that higher fitness is associated with a lower risk of incident diabetes regardless of demographic characteristics and baseline risk factors. Future studies should examine the association between change in fitness over time and incident diabetes.

▶ There are studies that suggest that cardiorespiratory fitness may reduce cardiovascular events even in the presence of increased body weight and even in obese individuals. Furthermore, there are a number of studies that have shown that cardiorespiratory fitness results in a reduction in metabolic syndrome, impaired glucose tolerance, and diabetes; the proposed effect is that physical fitness improves insulin sensitivity in muscle and increased glucose disposal. In addition, fitness is often associated with less adiposity and more skeletal muscle; both can play a role in improvements in insulin action. However, it is unclear whether cardiorespiratory fitness will affect incident diabetes in individuals who do not suffer from diabetes. The investigators studied baseline treadmill fitness in more than 45 000 patients in the Henry Ford Exercise Testing Project. The patients were represented by 48% women and 27% blacks. They then followed the individuals for a mean of 5 years and evaluated incident diabetes. Baseline fitness was associated with reductions in incident diabetes. This was shown for all ages, both sexes, and all races. However, investigators demonstrate that this is more obvious in younger individuals, although it was seen in people over age 60 years as well. It was also more obvious in whites than blacks without obvious explanation. The obvious conclusions are that physical fitness is important to reduce the burden of diabetes, although as the investigators pointed out, they measured baseline cardiorespiratory fitness, and studies should be performed on individuals with continual implementation of fitness programs and its effect on incident diabetes.

D. LeRoith, MD

60 Lipoproteins, Atherosclerosis, and Cardiovascular Risk

Preventable Major Cardiovascular Events Associated With Uncontrolled Glucose, Blood Pressure, and Lipids and Active Smoking in Adults With Diabetes With and Without Cardiovascular Disease: A Contemporary Analysis

Vazquez-Benitez G, Desai JR, Xu S, et al (HealthPartners Inst for Education and Res, Minneapolis, MN; Kaiser Permanente Inst for Health Res, Denver, CO; et al)

Diabetes Care 38:905-912, 2015

Objective.—The objective of this study was to assess the incidence of major cardiovascular (CV) hospitalization events and all-cause deaths among adults with diabetes with or without CV disease (CVD) associated with inadequately controlled glycated hemoglobin (A1C), high LDL cholesterol (LDL-C), high blood pressure (BP), and current smoking.

Research Design and Methods.—Study subjects included 859,617 adults with diabetes enrolled for more than 6 months during 2005–2011 in a network of 11 U.S. integrated health care organizations. Inadequate risk factor control was classified as LDL-C ≥100 mg/dL, A1C ≥7% (53 mmol/mol), BP ≥140/90 mm Hg, or smoking. Major CV events were based on primary hospital discharge diagnoses for myocardial infarction (MI) and acute coronary syndrome (ACS), stroke, or heart failure (HF). Five-year incidence rates, rate ratios, and average attributable fractions were estimated using multivariable Poisson regression models.

Results.—Mean (SD) age at baseline was 59 (14) years; 48% of subjects were female, 45% were white, and 31% had CVD. Mean follow-up was 59 months. Event rates per 100 person-years for adults with diabetes and CVD versus those without CVD were 6.0 vs. 1.7 for MI/ACS, 5.3 vs. 1.5 for stroke, 8.4 vs. 1.2 for HF, 18.1 vs. 40 for all CV events, and 23.5 vs. 5.0 for all-cause mortality. The percentages of CV events and deaths associated with inadequate risk factor control were 11% and 3%, respectively, for those with CVD and 34% and 7%, respectively, for those without CVD.

Conclusions.—Additional attention to traditional CV risk factors could yield further substantive reductions in CV events and mortality in adults with diabetes.

▶ As described by the investigators in this study, there are 4 major contributors to cardiovascular disease, namely, coronary artery disease and stroke, in patients with type 2 diabetes. These contributors are elevated blood glucose levels, hypertension, hyperlipidemia, and cigarette smoking. They defined inadequate control as low-density lipoprotein cholesterol level greater than 100 mg/dL and a level of hemoglobin A1C greater than 7% and the systolic blood pressure greater than 140 mm Hg or a diastolic blood pressure (BP) greater than 90 mm Hg and current smoking. They studied more than 850 000 patients that were enrolled in 11 health care organizations and determined the incidence of major cardiovascular events and deaths. Major cardiovascular events were based on primary hospital discharge diagnoses for myocardial infarction and acute coronary syndrome, stroke, or heart failure. Over the 5-year period, the incidence rates varied significantly between those with poorly controlled risk factors. In those patients without obvious cardiovascular disease at baseline, there was an increased risk of myocardial infarction/acute coronary syndrome, stroke, and heart failure, associated with blood glucose and hyperlipidemia, whereas smoking and BP were associated with all-cause mortality. The authors comment on the improvement in control of the general population with regard to BP and lipid management and a significant reduction nationally in cigarette smoking. However, they find that despite these improvements in overall risk factor reduction, there is still room for further improving the reduction of these cardiovascular risk factors in diabetic patients. These improvements will undoubtedly reduce the cardiovascular events that occur at an increased rate in type 2 diabetes. Thus, there will be an improvement in quality of life in our patients and a reduction in the overall burden of health care costs.

D. LeRoith, MD

Metformin Inhibits Monocyte-to-Macrophage Differentiation via AMPK-Mediated Inhibition of STAT3 Activation: Potential Role in Atherosclerosis

Vasamsetti SB, Karnewar S, Kanugula AK, et al (Council of Scientific and Industrial Research (CSIR)—Indian Institute of Chemical Technology, Hyderabad, India; et al)

Diabetes 64:2028-2041, 2015

Monocyte-to-macrophage differentiation is a critical event that accentuates atherosclerosis by promoting an inflammatory environment within the vessel wall. In this study, we investigated the molecular mechanisms responsible for monocyte-to-macrophage differentiation and, subsequently, the effect of metformin in regressing angiotensin II (Ang-II)-mediated atheromatous plaque formation in ApoE$^{-/-}$ mice. AMPK activity was dose and time dependently downregulated during phorbol myristate acetate (PMA)-induced monocyte-to-macrophage differentiation, which was accompanied by an upregulation of proinflammatory cytokine production. Of note, AMPK activators metformin and AICAR significantly attenuated PMA-induced monocyte-to-macrophage differentiation and proinflammatory cytokine production. However, inhibition of AMPK activity alone by compound C was ineffective in promoting monocyte-to-macrophage differentiation in the absence of PMA. On the other hand, inhibition of c-Jun N-terminal kinase activity inhibited PMA-induced inflammation but not differentiation, suggesting that inflammation and differentiation are independent events. In contrast, inhibition of STAT3 activity inhibited both inflammation and monocyte-to-macrophage differentiation. By decreasing STAT3 phosphorylation, metformin and AICAR through increased AMPK activation caused inhibition of monocyte-to-macrophage differentiation. Metformin attenuated Ang-II–induced atheromatous plaque formation and aortic aneurysm in $ApoE^{-/-}$ mice partly by reducing monocyte infiltration. We conclude that the AMPK-STAT3 axis plays a pivotal role in regulating monocyte-to-macrophage differentiation and that by decreasing STAT3 phosphorylation through increased AMPK activity, AMPK activators inhibit monocyte-to-macrophage differentiation.

▶ Metformin is commonly used for the treatment of type 2 diabetes. It is recommended by all diabetes associations, worldwide, as the first oral agent to be used after lifestyle intervention, such as diet and exercise, has not achieved the goal set for blood glucose control. Although metformin has relatively few side effects, and in addition to controlling weight and HbA_{1c} levels quite effectively, its effect on reducing macrovascular disease has only been demonstrated in the UKPDS study. This is probably because other large outcome trials (such as ACCORD, ADVANCE, and VADT) recruited older patients with established cardiovascular disease. Although metformin has been used worldwide for more than 50 years, its mechanism of action has only been studied over the past decade. One of the major effects of metformin is by activating an enzyme AMPkinase, which has many effects at the cellular level. In this article, the investigators studied the effect of metformin on monocyte-to-macrophage differentiation. There is substantial evidence that macrophage infiltration is associated with the atherosclerotic process by secreting inflammatory mediators. apoE knockout developed atherosclerotic plagues, and this can be exaggerated by the use of angiotensin II. The investigators found that metformin by activating AMPkinase reversed many of the effects on monocyte-to-macrophage differentiation. They established that metformin, through AMPkinase, in addition to reducing the macrophage differentiation and infiltration, also reduced the atheromatous plaques and the development of aortic aneurysms in these mice. Thus they have determined the mechanisms through which metformin reduces cardiovascular complications in type II diabetes and should therefore enforce its use in all diabetic patients unless contraindicated.

D. LeRoith, MD

61 Reproductive Endocrinology

Each Degree of Glucose Intolerance in Pregnancy Predicts Distinct Trajectories of β-Cell Function, Insulin Sensitivity, and Glycemia in the First 3 Years Postpartum

Kramer CK, Swaminathan B, Hanley AJ, et al (Mount Sinai Hosp Toronto, Ontario, Canada; et al)

Diabetes Care 37:3262-3269, 2014

Objective.—Glucose intolerance in pregnancy predicts an increased risk of future type 2 diabetes mellitus (T2DM) that is proportional to the severity of antepartum dysglycemia (i.e., highest in women with gestational diabetes mellitus [GDM], followed by those with milder dysglycemia). However, the pathophysiologic changes driving this risk are not known. Thus, we evaluated the longitudinal changes in β-cell function, insulin sensitivity, and glycemia in the first 3 years postpartum after gestational dysglycemia.

Research Design and Methods.—A total of 337 women underwent glucose challenge test (GCT) and oral glucose tolerance test (OGTT) in pregnancy, followed by repeat OGTT at 3 months, 1 year, and 3 years postpartum. The antepartum GCT/OGTT identified four gestational glucose tolerance groups: GDM ($n = 105$); gestational impaired glucose tolerance (GIGT; $n = 60$); abnormal GCT, followed by normal glucose tolerance (NGT) on the OGTT (abnormal GCT NGT; $n = 96$); and normal GCT with NGT ($n = 76$).

Results.—At each of 3 months, 1 year, and 3 years postpartum, the prevalence of glucose intolerance increased from normal GCT NGT to abnormal GCT NGT to GIGT to GDM (all $P < 0.001$), whereas β-cell function, assessed by the Insulin Secretion-Sensitivity Index-2 (ISSI-2), and insulin sensitivity (Matsuda index), progressively decreased across the groups (all $P < 0.002$). Each group predicted distinct trajectories of ISSI-2, Matsuda index, and fasting and 2-h glucose (all $P < 0.001$). Notably, GDM, GIGT, and abnormal GCT NGT predicted varying rates of declining β-cell function and insulin sensitivity, as well as rising glycemia, compared with normal GCT NGT.

Conclusions.—Each degree of gestational glucose intolerance predicts distinct trajectories of β-cell function, insulin sensitivity, and glycemia in the first 3 years postpartum that drive their differential risk of future T2DM.

▶ This study determined glucose tolerance and β-cell function during pregnancy and then 3 months, 1 year, and 3 years postpartum, in 337 women. The results demonstrated that increasing glucose intolerance during gestation predicts a worsening of insulin secretion and insulin sensitivity over the first 3 years postpartum. Of significance is that women with abnormal glucose tolerance during pregnancy have significant β-cell dysfunction that is chronic and therefore predicts future development of type 2 diabetes. Most importantly, the degree of dysglycemia during pregnancy predicts the rate of development of type 2 diabetes: The worse the dysglycemia, the faster the development of type 2 diabetes.

D. LeRoith, MD

Placental Insufficiency Decreases Pancreatic Vascularity and Disrupts Hepatocyte Growth Factor Signaling in the Pancreatic Islet Endothelial Cell in Fetal Sheep

Rozance PJ, Anderson M, Martinez M, et al (Univ of Colorado School of Medicine, Aurora; Univ of Arizona, Tucson)
Diabetes 64:555-564, 2015

Hepatocyte growth factor (HGF) and vascular endothelial growth factor A (VEGFA) are paracrine hormones that mediate communication between pancreatic islet endothelial cells (ECs) and β-cells. Our objective was to determine the impact of intrauterine growth restriction (IUGR) on pancreatic vascularity and paracrine signaling between the EC and β-cell. Vessel density was less in IUGR pancreata than in controls. HGF concentrations were also lower in islet EC-conditioned media (ECCM) from IUGR, and islets incubated with control islet ECCM responded by increasing insulin content, which was absent with IUGR ECCM. The effect of ECCM on islet insulin content was blocked with an inhibitory anti-HGF antibody. The HGF receptor was not different between control and IUGR islets, but VEGFA was lower and the high-affinity VEGF receptor was higher in IUGR islets and ECs, respectively. These findings show that paracrine actions from ECs increase islet insulin content, and in IUGR ECs, secretion of HGF was diminished. Given the potential feed-forward regulation of β-cell VEGFA and islet EC HGF, these two growth factors are highly integrated in normal pancreatic islet development, and this regulation is decreased in IUGR fetuses, resulting in lower pancreatic islet insulin concentrations and insulin secretion.

▶ Fetuses with intrauterine growth retardation (IUGR) have lower plasma glucose and insulin levels and reduced glucose-stimulated insulin secretion during late stages of gestation. In addition, they demonstrate lower pancreatic islet vascularity and a smaller beta-cell population. To study the causes involved, the authors used a model of IUGR in pregnant ewes and isolated islets from

IUGR and control fetuses. Beta cells and endothelial cells (ECs) were cultured, and conditioned media measurements revealed that hepatocyte growth factor (HGF) and vascular endothelial growth factor A (VEGFA) were decreased. HGF is apparently involved in EC cross-talk to islets, and its reduction explains the few beta cells in IUGR, whereas VEGFA is involved in the cross-talk between beta cells and ECs. The reduction in these paracrine factors may therefore play an important role in the reduction in islets in IUGR. Thus, these factors may represent future targets for therapeutic challenges in preventing beta-cell reduction in IUGR fetuses.

D. LeRoith, MD

Article Index

Chapter 1: Osteoarthritis

Chapter 2: Osteoporosis and Other Metabolic Diseases of Bone

Chapter 3: Rheumatoid Arthritis

Chapter 4: Sjogren's Syndrome

Chapter 5: Systemic Lupus Erythematosus

Chapter 6: Drug Toxicity

Chapter 7: Seronegative Spondyloarthropathies

Chapter 8: Myopathies

Chapter 9: Vasculitis

Chapter 10: Miscellaneous Rheumatic Diseases and Therapies

Chapter 11: Gout and Other Crystal Diseases

Chapter 12: Chronic Juvenile Arthritis

Chapter 13: Bacterial Infections

Chapter 14: Vaccines

Chapter 15: Viral Infections

Chapter 16: Tuberculosis

Chapter 17: Clinical Diagnostics

Chapter 18: Health Care Associated Infections

Chapter 19: New Antibiotics

Chapter 20: Miscellaneous

Chapter 21: Supportive Care

Chapter 22: Geriatric Oncology

Chapter 23: Prostate Cancer

Chapter 24: Breast Cancer

Chapter 25: Myeloid Suppressor Cell Tumors

Chapter 26: Cancer Screening

Chapter 31: Diabetes and Kidney Disease

Chapter 32: Acute Kidney Injury

Chapter 33: Selected Topics in Clinical Nephrology

Chapter 34: Issues in Severe CKD and Dialysis

Chapter 35: Asthma, Allergy, and Cystic Fibrosis

Chapter 36: Chronic Obstructive Pulmonary Disease

Chapter 37: Lung Cancer

Chapter 38: Pleural, Interstitial Lung, and Pulmonary Vascular Disease

Chapter 39: Community-Acquired Pneumonia

Chapter 40: Sleep Disorders

Chapter 41: Critical Care Medicine

Chapter 42: Arrhythmias

Chapter 43: Cardiomyopathy

Chapter 44: Chronic Coronary Artery Disease

Chapter 45: Coronary Intervention Procedures

Chapter 46: Non-Invasive Testing

Chapter 47: Risk Factors

Chapter 48: Valvular Heart Disease

Chapter 49: Acute Coronary Syndromes

Chapter 50: Esophagus

Chapter 51: Stomach

Chapter 52: Small Bowel

Chapter 53: Colon

Chapter 58: Diabetes Mellitus

Chapter 59: Obesity

Chapter 60: Lipoproteins, Atherosclerosis, and Cardiovascular Risk

Chapter 61: Reproductive Endocrinology

Author Index

A

B

C

D

E

R

S

T

U

V

W

X

Y

Z

FSC
www.fsc.org
MIX
Papier | Fördert gute Waldnutzung
FSC® C083411

Kolibri 360 GmbH
Ferdinand-Jühlke-Straße 7
99095 Erfurt, Deutschland
produktsicherheit@kolibri360.de